Injury Prevention: An International Perspective

Injury Prevention: An International Perspective
Epidemiology, Surveillance, and Policy

Peter Barss
Gordon S. Smith
Susan P. Baker
Dinesh Mohan

New York   Oxford
Oxford University Press
1998

This work is dedicated to the many young adults
and children everywhere in the world who die prematurely
or are disabled by preventable injuries.

And may we dedicate ourselves to the task of ensuring
that the modifiable risk factors of such injuries are inscribed
in more than the hearts and minds of their loved ones.

Oxford University Press

Oxford New York
Athens Auckland Bangkok Bogota
Bombay Buenos Aires Calcutta Cape Town
Dar es Salaam Delhi Florence Hong Kong
Istanbul Karachi Kuala Lumpur Madras
Madrid Melbourne Mexico City Nairobi
Paris Singapore Taipei Tokyo
Toronto Warsaw

and associated companies in
Berlin Ibadan

Published by Oxford University Press, Inc.
198 Madison Avenue, New York, New York 10016

Oxford is a registered trademark of Oxford University Press

Library of Congress Cataloging-in-Publication Data

Injury prevention : an international perspective epidemiology,
    surveillance and policy / Peter Barss . . . [et al.].
        p.   cm.
    Includes bibliographical references and index.
    ISBN 0-19-511982-7
        1. Wounds and injuries—Epidemiology.   2. health surveys.
    I. Barss, Peter.
RA645.T73I55   1998
362.1'971—dc21   97-45595
                                                        CIP

Cover: A boy crosses a suspension bridge in the highlands of Papua New Guinea, with a rooster under each
arm. While his situation may appear precarious, consider the alternative of fording such rapids. Bridges are
an effective method of drowning prevention for rural
areas of developing countries, although they are usually
installed for transport purposes. [Photo © 1998 Peter
Barss.]

1 2 3 4 5 6 7 8 9

Printed in the United States of America
on acid-free paper

Foreword

William H. Foege

Defining the "unacceptable" is the challenge and burden of public health. The loss of a child to measles has always been a tragedy, but it became unacceptable in the last third of this century as an effective vaccine became available. As public health expanded beyond infectious diseases, the list of unacceptable conditions expanded rapidly. The Surgeon General's report on smoking in 1965 elucidated the natural history of most cases of lung cancer, and lung cancer deaths became unacceptable. As the sum of what is not acceptable continued to grow, so did personal and collective efforts to implement the new findings, with the result that life expectancy for the average American has increased by about 7 hours per day for every day since 1900. The United States has now formalized objectives to reduce the unacceptable in its health goals for the nation, *Healthy People 2000*.

Albert Schweitzer reminded us that pain and suffering constitute a bigger burden than even death itself. Yet death continued to be the conventional way of measuring the impact of a condition because death figures were available and less controversial than morbidity figures. In recent years other approaches have become available to complement our understanding of the burden of disease. Potential Years of Life Lost (PYLL) places emphasis on the problem of early death. Disability Adjusted Life Years (DALYs) attempt to combine suffering and death into a single number. Such approaches make clear that intentional and unintentional injuries are major health problems in both developed and developing areas of the world. The 1993 World Development Report, published by the World Bank, presented DALYs for the entire world for 1990. Five injury categories, vehicle injuries, falls, homicide, suicide and war, when combined, became the second largest health burden in the world, second only to respiratory diseases.

Two challenges emerge. First, the difficulty in convincing people that these are not "accidents." This is not a fatalistic world. There are events that can be described which clarify the cause and effect relationship that is the basis for science. In the words of Stephen Hawking, "Things do not happen in an arbitrary fashion." Second, understanding the causes provides the knowledge for intervention, knowledge that is inadequately utilized. The simplicity of prevention in many cases makes the loss entirely unnecessary and therefore "unacceptable." The great physicist Richard Feynmann once said that it takes very little energy to scramble an egg, but science is totally incapable of reversing that simple process. It takes very little energy to sever a spinal cord, scramble a brain or end a life. Even our very best science is impotent in reversing the process. And yet it is difficult to popularize prevention.

Barss, Smith, Baker, and Mohan have now assembled the expertise of the world for us. It will take action by all of us if the potential power of this book is to be reflected in lives saved and suffering prevented. When Thucydides was asked when justice would come to Athens, the philosopher replied, "Justice will come to Athens when those who are not injured are as indignant as those who are injured." This book is a roadmap to indignation.

The philosophy of public health is to eliminate inequities, to make health knowledge available to all, and to have all people benefit from the skills and knowledge that have accumulated. The motivating principle is social justice. This is a book, therefore, about social justice, assembling what is known about injury prevention so that it is available for use in the entire world. In bringing together the art and science of injury prevention for the benefit of everyone, the book is ambitious, thorough, and helpful. Its publication is a landmark event. Now it must be used.

Preface

The origins of this book lie in the beautiful and intriguing tropical forests and coastal villages of Papua New Guinea, the seemingly endless rolling savannah of Angola, and perhaps even further back, in the coastal villages of eastern Canada. Much as modern traffic crashes might appear exotic to a stone-age villager, injuries from tree falls, grass skirt burns, attacks by needlefish, crocodiles, cassowaries, lions, wasps, snakes, bows and arrows, and suicides of young married women struck me as out of the ordinary and initiated a long process of inquiry.

The writing, research, and practical applications were completed in metropolitan areas of North America, including Montreal, Canada, and Baltimore, USA, but were also influenced by several years of collaboration with injury surveillance in northern indigenous communities. The prime motivation for a task that spans nearly two decades has been the belief that the information in this book would be helpful to various professionals and the public in a range of ecological settings around the world. Special, but by no means exclusive, attention has been given to frequently neglected low-income countries, as well as to isolated and indigenous communities.

Although the origins of the work are modest, our ultimate mission has been to provide a resource for injury prevention and control that will be helpful around the world. Interestingly, when one returns to William Haddon's early publications in America, we find that he too was fascinated by the hazards confronting coastal villagers in Melanesia. Haddon described himself as a medical ecologist, and ecological comparisons of the circumstances of injuries and other health conditions often provide crucial insight into their preventability. An even earlier pioneer (1940) in insisting upon the predictability and preventability of injuries was John Gordon, and it is hardly surprising that his interest in injury control ultimately took him as far afield as villages in the Punjab in India.

While providing surgical care to a province of hundreds of remote villages in Papua New Guinea, I too was struck that the external causes of trauma were quite different from what many of us had come to accept as "normal" back home. What we created in our local environments no longer seemed inevitable, and it was obvious that many hazards should have been subject to societal or individual con-

Ce que nous appelons hasard n'est ne peut être que la cause ignorée d'un effet connu.
—*Voltaire,* **Atomes,** *1770*

trol. While the specific nature of the injuries varied from patient to patient, many of the contributory incidents were almost monotonous in their predictability and preventability.

While many "accidents" among tropical villagers are believed to be wrought by sorcery and malevolence, in industrialized countries our accidents have often been attributed to bad luck, God's will, or even sin. Prevention truly begins when we can accept that most injuries, if not always the incidents, really are avoidable. Carefully collected and analyzed population data on the circumstances of various injuries associated with different activities can do much to dispel fatalism. This is the power of epidemiology and surveillance, as contrasted with anecdotal observation of isolated incidents. Community involvement in planning and conducting injury surveillance and research can rapidly engage people in their own prevention activities.

With good population data in hand, the next steps may be obvious. Nevertheless, the most effective injury control measures often involve sectors other than health, and tend to be multisectoral. For this reason, we have wherever possible suggested some of the policy implications of research and surveillance data. Truly effective long-term interventions, such as national legislation to mandate change in environmental, equipment, or personal risk factors, are often neglected in favor of unproven and uncoordinated educational programs launched by individual organizations or sectors.

It has been a fascinating and often arduous journey from the early field studies that initiated the saga that eventuated in this book. The instruments of discovery evolved along the way, from the surgical knife to paper and pencil, and finally to the modern microcomputer and epidemiologic surveillance and research. The setting and circumstances too evolved, from the acute drama of saving and losing lives and limbs, to reflective consideration of the circumstances of thousands of individual tragedies captured in databases and special questionnaires.

While the reader will find a detailed acknowledgment at the end of this work, I wish to express my warmest thanks to my many dear friends and former patients in the thousands of villages of Milne Bay Province, Papua New Guinea, for welcoming me to work and live with them, and for their patience with my countless questions about how they lived and died. Thanks also to the Canadian government, its various programs, and my employers, colleagues, reviewers, and collaborators, without whose support this work could have been neither initiated nor completed. I am unsure whether I should thank Dr. Richard Feachem of the World Bank for initiating a process that has absorbed so many years of my life, but without his initial encouragement this book would not have been written.

As for my collaborators in the creation of this book, the long-term support, experienced input, and energetic editorial work of Susan Baker and her staff at the Johns Hopkins School of Public Health brought the book to completion. Dr. Gordon Smith's enthusiastic early interest and support initiated the undertaking, and his critical input at various steps along the way was valuable. Dinesh Mohan in India provided a special perspective from his own rich experience and unique cultural sensitivity, such that nothing could be taken for granted.

P. B.

Montreal
March 1998

Contents

Injury Prevention: An International Perspective

chapter 1

Introduction: The Importance of Injuries

In many parts of the world, injuries are the leading cause of death for young adults, adolescents, and children. Injury death rates among the elderly, while overshadowed by deaths from degenerative diseases, are even higher than among the young. The importance of injuries has increased in developing countries and indigenous communities, and will continue to do so as infectious and degenerative diseases are better controlled.

Improved living conditions and urbanization bring about decreases in the rates of certain injuries, including falls from trees, burns from open fires, drownings in rivers, and, perhaps, suicides. However, positive changes can be offset by the uncontrolled introduction of new, high-energy technology such as motor vehicles and machinery, and by greater use of alcohol and other substances that impair brain function. In some populations, rates of death from injuries may even increase as rates of death from other leading causes fall.

Violent or intentional injuries are now leading causes of death in many countries and indigenous communities. Rapid population increases in urban areas, poverty with extreme class disparities, political instability, militarism, and ethnocentrism as reflected in racial or religious intolerance can lead to violence and a rise in homicides and assaults.

Women in isolated communities in some developing countries suffer extremely high rates of suicide that would be regarded as a public health emergency were they to occur in cities of industrialized countries. On the other hand, conditions in isolated indigenous communities in industrialized countries have often led to hopelessness, despair, and unemployment among adolescents and young men, as manifested in solvent and alcohol abuse and frequent incidents of suicide.

The health impact of injuries and their causes is a relatively new study compared to those of other health conditions. The understanding and control of injuries has been delayed because the causes of injuries are often multifactoral, and because prevention can require multisectoral interventions.

The newer concept of prevention, as it developed, was applied almost wholly to disease, to the sick. The injured were largely forgotten...
—John E. Gordon, 1949

The purpose of this book is to help reduce the burden of injuries everywhere. Although there are many examples drawn from industrialized and high income countries, greater emphasis is placed on special needs of developing countries and remote and indigenous populations. This book is for everyone who can help achieve that objective, including the following:

- Public health practitioners who choose, develop, and evaluate surveillance programs to monitor injuries, and assist other sectors who need information to design effective interventions and evaluations;
- Epidemiologists and other researchers who help identify and understand the specifics of injury occurrence;
- Government officials with responsibilities for public safety who work in sectors such as transportation, education, police, and sport;
- Volunteers and staff who work in private organizations such as the Red Cross/Red Crescent, life-saving, and first-aid programs;
- Clinicians, coroners, engineers, economists, and other professionals who wish to make a contribution to injury prevention;
- Policy makers at all levels and people with the power to influence their decisions about priorities, resource allocation, and injury prevention strategies.

In bringing together current knowledge of injury epidemiology and control, the authors have included information relevant to situations in developing countries and remote and indigenous communities in industrialized countries, including injury surveillance and research methods. For areas where routine data sources are limited, examples of injury problems and data from developing areas and industrialized countries often provide an informative contrast. The link between injury surveillance and research and public policy is also essential, and the policy and research options described could be useful starting points for discussion and action in a specific country, region, or community.

This chapter reviews recent changes in mortality from injuries in a few selected countries in different regions of the world. It emphasizes the economic importance of injuries and considers their predictability, causes, and preventability. Before going further, it is important to define what a developing country is and to describe a simple classification system for injuries.

DEVELOPING COUNTRIES, DEVELOPING AREAS, AND REMOTE AND INDIGENOUS COMMUNITIES

The definition of *developing country* is controversial. For example, in spite of significant advances in a number of countries, the present situation in some nations of the third world, and perhaps even in the urban slums of certain industrialized countries, is so grim that they appear to be losing ground in the effort to become more developed. According to a World Bank economist, average income has fallen in nearly one–fourth of the 120 developing countries around the world, leaving their economies worse now than they were in the 1960s (V.

Thomas, 1991). Alternatives to the term *third world* that are sometimes preferred include *less-developed, low-income country,* or *developing area.*

Indigenous populations in some industrialized countries have recently experienced rapid economic development and its many consequences. For example, technological advances have reached the native peoples of northern Canada, the United States, the former Soviet Union, and Greenland, including the Inuit and subarctic Indians. In such settings, the concept of development itself is open to different interpretations depending on the desirability of the changes invoked for the populations exposed to them.

While acknowledging the limitations and contradictions of the term, this book defines a *developing country* by annual per capita gross national product less than $2500 per annum, as listed by the World Bank's annual World Development Report (World Bank, 1989).

The most appropriate and culturally sensitive terminology to describe indigenous peoples varies with the country and time. For our purposes, the terms *indigenous, aboriginal, native peoples,* and *native communities* are used interchangeably. Terms such as *registered Indian, Inuit,* and other names of specific ethnic groups have been used in the context of certain studies. *First Nations* is preferred by many indigenous peoples in Canada but excludes the Inuit.

In an effort to focus attention on the concerns faced by indigenous communities around the world, the General Assembly of the United Nations declared 1993 as the Year of Indigenous People. Intentional and unintentional injuries are now among the major problems of many indigenous peoples in developed countries. While the level of resources in their communities is often substantially greater than it is in rural areas of many developing countries, it is helpful to share information about areas of common interest.

In remote communities, whatever their location, recording, collecting, and interpreting data on the causes and circumstances of injuries is a difficult task. Risks of certain types of injuries are high in many isolated communities, whether they include indigenous or non-indigenous inhabitants: high speed driving on open roads, frequent exposure to hazardous travel over water or ice in small boats and snowmobiles, use of an open flame for cooking and heating, social impacts of isolation, together with limited resources for inspection and enforcement, are prevalent in many rural districts.

INJURY CLASSIFICATION

When discussing injuries, it is helpful to have a framework or classification system that takes into account the cause or mechanism of injury and the intent.

Unintentional injuries occur by a number of mechanisms, including road traffic, water hazards, fire and hot liquids, obstacles leading to falls, and poison. Intentional injuries can occur by some of the same mechanisms, but involve violence and include assault, homicide, and suicide.

Various detailed classifications have been developed for coding and classifying the many types of injuries caused by external mechanisms. This topic is discussed in Chapter 2.

CHANGING PATTERNS OF MORTALITY

Data based on death rates and years of potential life lost from injury are often used to assess the relative importance of injuries as a cause of death as compared to mortality associated with other health conditions. Mortality rates from specific injuries are also used to determine secular (over time) trends in the incidence of different injuries.

In many developing countries there have been recent large decreases in mortality from infectious diseases, something that occurred decades ago in industrialized countries. At the same time, however, the recent spread of AIDS and the resurgence of malaria in developing countries have altered this trend in some countries.

The United States provides an example of changes in causes of mortality in an industrialized country. Between 1910 and 1990 the mortality rate per 100,000 population from gastroenteritis fell from 115 to about 2 and for tuberculosis, from about 155 to similar levels (Baker et al., 1992). Unfortunately, injury rates have not shown such dramatic changes and fell only about 20 percent during the same period. As a result, injuries are now the fourth leading cause of death after the chronic disorders of heart disease, cancer, and stroke.

There have been similar changes in a number of developing countries as their level of development changed (G. S. Smith and Barss, 1991). In Brazil, the proportion of deaths due to infectious diseases fell from 45 percent in 1930 to 11 percent in 1980, while cardiovascular diseases, cancer, and injuries increased (World Bank, 1989). In the 15–30 year age group, injuries accounted for 60 percent of deaths. In Taiwan, unintentional injuries, once the seventh leading cause of death, rose to third between 1960 and 1977 (Selya, 1980). From 1960–80 in Shanghai County, China, the annual death rate from infectious diseases decreased from 78 per 100,000 population to 35, while the death rate from injuries fell from 67 to 49; thus, the injury death rate came to surpass the death rate from infectious diseases, even as injury deaths decreased (Xing-Yuan and Mai-Ling, 1982).

Among indigenous communities in developed countries the impact of injuries as a cause of death among children and adults in their economically productive years is striking. Injuries are more prominent in these communities than in developing countries, because many infectious diseases have been relatively well controlled in indigenous populations in developed countries. Among the regis-

Table 1.1 Injury deaths as a proportion of all deaths among registered Indians in Canada, 1986–1988

Age group	% of all deaths
1–14	64
15–24	87
25–44	64
45–64	22
≥65	4
all ages	31

Source: Muir, 1991.

tered Indian population in Canada, for example, injuries arc the leading cause of death for all age groups from 1 to 64 years (Table 1.1) (Muir, 1991).

As life expectancy in most countries increases, the chronic disorders of later life, cardiovascular diseases and cancer, have become more prominent causes of death. These health problems have received more attention than injuries, at least in part because they affect people whose age and economic status place them in a position to influence policy and because diagnosis and treatment often involve attractive, high-cost modern medical technology.

Due to an increase in the proportion of elderly people in the Chinese population, injuries dropped from second place as a cause of death to fifth, after cancer, degenerative vascular diseases (including cardiovascular diseases and stroke), and respiratory disease. Even so, the death rate from injuries exceeded the death rate from infectious diseases, and injuries are the leading cause of death for both males and females ages 1 through 44 (Li and Baker, 1991; WHO, 1991).

Unlike most deaths from chronic diseases, many injuries affect people long before they approach the end of their projected life span. The birth rates and resulting demographic composition of many developing countries are such that a large proportion of their populations, for at least another generation, will consist of young individuals at relatively high risk for injury. In the older population, the injury death rates are even higher, especially in developing countries (Fig. 1.1), although often they are overshadowed by mortality from diseases.

As already mentioned, in many countries injury death rates have become prominent primarily because of decreases in infectious disease rates; nevertheless, absolute increases in death rates in those countries have sometimes been dramatic (Table 1.2).

The burden of injury mortality is reflected not only in death rates but also in years of potential life lost (YPLL) before a predeter-

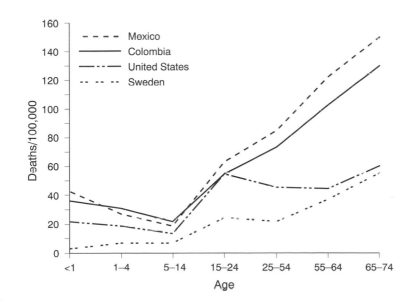

FIGURE 1.1

Male death rates from unintentional injuries, selected contries 1991-93.
Source of data: World Health Organization. *Statistics Annual 1991-93*. Geneva: WHO, 1992, 1993, 1994.

mined age (age 65 is used in most studies). Because injuries affect many children and young adults, they are now the leading cause of lost years of potential life in the United States and many other countries, both industrialized and developing. The YPLL measure can be used not only to establish the relative importance of causes of death but also to examine secular trends. In Taiwan, for example, the age-adjusted YPLL from motor vehicle injuries increased more than fourfold between 1964 and 1988 (T. Baker and MacKinney, 1990).

Specific components of injury mortality have increased markedly in many population groups. Suicide rates rose more than tenfold in recent decades in some North American Inuit communities (Thorslund, 1990), and are extremely high among young Chinese

FIGURE 1.2

Death rates from injuries by country and cause of injury. Source of data: World Health Organization. *Statistics Annual 1994.* Geneva: WHO, 1995.

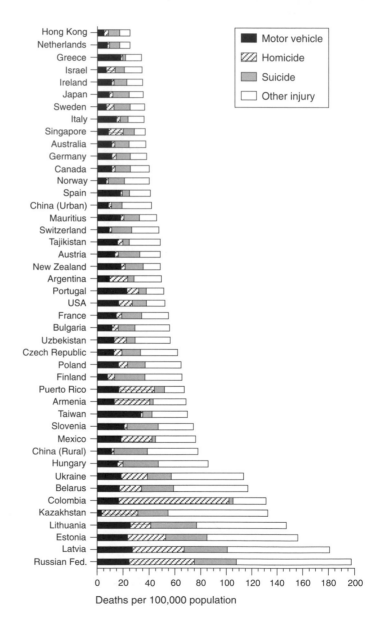

Table 1.2 Examples of changes in injury death rates

Country	Period	Change in death rate/100,000 pop./yr (in thousands)
Taiwan*	1960 to 1977	All unintentional injuries: from 39 to 57
Subarctic Indians, Canada**	1942–44 to 1977–80	All injuries (intentional and unint.): from 140 to 240
São Paulo, Brazil†	1960 to 1984	Homicide: from 4 to 28
Alaska Natives, U.S.A.‡	1960 to 1983–84	Suicide: from 14 to 44
Inuit,‡ Greenland	1962–66 to 1982–86	Suicide: from 9 to 114

Sources: * Selya, 1980; ** Young, 1980; † Jorge, 1988; ‡ Thorslund, 1990.

women who live in rural areas (Li and Baker, 1991). In the highlands of Papua New Guinea during 1971–89, the most significant secular trend in the rural population was a rapid rise in the rate of homicide (Barss, 1991). In Brazil, the homicide rate is rising rapidly; in the city of São Paulo, about half of all deaths among young adults are homicides (World Bank, 1989; Cohen, 1989).

Available data indicate that violent deaths, including homicide, suicide, and other violence, are the major source of exceptionally high injury mortality rates noted in some countries. For example, in Colombia and El Salvador (see Fig. 1.2 and Tables 3.1–3.4), where state terrorism (J. R. White, 1991; Chomsky, 1988) and guerilla warfare have become endemic, violent deaths are commonplace.

The problems associated with violence are not confined to developing countries. In the urban ghettos of the United States, homicide rates have been extremely high among black males for at least 40 years (National Center for Health Statistics, 1990). For U.S. males 15–19 years old, the homicide rate increased threefold between 1984 and 1994.

In developing countries, important factors in the etiology of endemic violence include disruption of traditional life-styles, large and rapidly increasing class disparities, low levels of education and high rates of poverty, problems of individual and community identity and cohesion, lack of local control, stress, and mental illness (Rosenberg and Fenley, 1991). Most of the same factors also contribute to high rates of unintentional injuries.

IMPORTANCE OF ADULT INJURIES

The sudden loss of a productive young adult as a result of death or disability is a serious economic blow to a family and to the community. Not only is that person's potential contribution lost, but also the substantial material and human resources already invested in education and support will not be returned (Barss, 1991).

Injury prevention among young adults in developing countries and aboriginal communities has received relatively little attention (Feachem et al., 1992), despite the fact that the death of a "bread-winner" has far-reaching consequences for dependents, and despite evidence suggesting that many deaths from injury occur so quickly or the damage is so severe that death is unlikely to be prevented by treatment.

The consequences of injuries to the working-age population do not negate the importance of injury morbidity and mortality in the elderly, who throughout the world have the highest injury death rates of any age group (Li and Baker 1991; WHO, 1991). Injuries to children are also important; because they often elicit great concern and may be less apt to involve "blame the victim" attitudes, they can be an opening wedge in injury prevention programs.

IMPORTANCE OF CHILDHOOD INJURIES

In high-income countries, injuries are the leading cause of death for children and youths (Table 1.3). For ages 1–14, injuries account for about one-half of all deaths in both Canada and the United States; for ages 15–19, the proportion increases to about 70 percent in Canada and 80 percent in the United States (Health Canada 1997; S.P. Baker, et al., 1992). In infants, because of high mortality from perinatal and congenital causes, the proportion of deaths due to injury is small, although the rates are high.

Among young children in many low-income countries where high death rates from infectious diseases dwarf the injury rates, injury death rates are substantially higher than in industrialized countries. In illustration, unintentional injury death rates in male children are far higher in Mexico and Colombia than in the United States and Sweden (Fig. 1.1). The lack of uniformity, even among high income countries, is illustrated by Sweden's extremely low rate.

Within any country, there may be great disparity among geographic or economic groups' death rates from childhood injury. In Canada, for example, injury death rates among First Nations aborig-

Table 1.3 Rank of injuries* as a cause of death by age, Canada 1992

| | Rank | | |
Age group (years)	Males	Females	Both sexes
<1	5	4	3
1-4	1	1	1
5-14	1	1	1
15-19	1	1	1
20-44	1	2	1
45-59	3	3	3
60-64	4	5	5
65+	7	8	7
All ages	4	4	4

*Includes all unintentional and intentional injuries.

Source: Canadian Red Cross Society, 1996a.

inal children ages 1–14 are about four times the rates for non-aboriginal children (Health Canada, 1996).

PREDICTABILITY AND PREVENTABILITY OF INJURIES

The most influential factor delaying scientific attention to injury prevention is probably the mistaken notion that injuries are largely unpreventable or can best be prevented by educating people to be more careful. A close look at examples from all over the world reveals that, although injuries are an urgent problem, there are effective measures for preventing them and for lessening their consequences.

Unintentional injuries, and sometimes even intentional ones such as assaults, are often described as "accidents," an imprecise term often applied to the events themselves and to any consequent injuries. Not all accidents result in injuries and, more importantly, the word "accident" for many people suggests an unpredictable and unpreventable random event or "act of God" (Langley, 1988; Doege, 1978; Haddon, 1968). Throughout this book we use the term *unintentional injury* rather than *accident*.

Injuries are not unavoidable events caused by bad luck or fate. While the exact moment of any injury event may not be predictable, injuries generally result from combinations of adverse environmental conditions, equipment, behavior, and personal risk factors, any or all of which can be changed. To illustrate, in some countries about one–half of all motor vehicle fatalities are associated with the use of alcohol but typically involve other factors such as driver inexperience, poor road design, and/or vehicle characteristics. Many injuries from motor vehicle crashes can therefore be prevented by strategies aimed at the risk factors other than alcohol use.

Serious injury often can be avoided by using equipment that provides automatic protection even when education fails to modify the behavior of high-risk individuals. An example is a car fitted with air bags that inflate on impact to protect occupants in a crash, even if they have not attached their safety belts. Similarly, burns resulting from clothing ignition, which is known to be affected by characteristics of fabric, ignition sources, and children's behavior, were greatly reduced in some countries by changing a single factor: flammability standards for children's nightwear.

In many developing countries, successful adaptation to new technologies has yet to be achieved. Nevertheless, the environments in which many people live and work are increasingly artificial ones. Since these environments have been created or modified by people, it should be possible to alter them to provide safer and more user-friendly settings for the activities of daily life and work.

Most injuries are caused by acute exposure to concentrated amounts of various physical agents or energy. A basic principle of injury control is to keep potentially harmful agents from reaching humans in amounts or at rates that exceed the body's ability to withstand trauma (i.e. above the injury threshold) (Haddon, 1980a). Common vectors of agents such as kinetic and thermal energy include equipment, products, and motor vehicles, all of which can be modified to make them safer.

Such alterations need not involve advanced technology. Home-heating systems have been made safer by adding devices that reroute heated air to prevent carbon monoxide poisoning from combustion products. Kerosene poisoning has been avoided by dispensing it in small containers that cannot be confused with soft drink bottles.

ACCIDENT PREVENTION VS. INJURY PREVENTION AND INJURY CONTROL

The term *accident prevention* has largely been abandoned by the injury prevention profession, in part because it ignored many important strategies for reducing the number, severity, and adverse consequences of injuries. It has been replaced by the terms *injury prevention* and *injury control.*

Injury prevention includes, but is not limited to, countermeasures that prevent an injury-causing event. Examples are the construction of special road lanes for pedestrians and bicyclists to separate them from motor vehicles, improved lighting and visibility of cyclists, and the installation of better road signs to prevent confusion and errors by motorists. These measures are termed "pre-event" countermeasures, as further described in Chapter 2, and generally equate with "accident prevention" strategies.

While it is clearly preferable to keep any event that might cause injury from occurring, many injury prevention measures do nothing in this regard but they do reduce the rate of energy transfer and hence the likelihood of injury and its severity. These elements of injury prevention are known as "event phase" measures. For motor vehicles, they include seat belts, air bags, padded dashboards, and safety glass in windshields. Thus, an important conceptual distinction has evolved between accident prevention, which is directed simply at preventing the occurrence of events, many of which do not necessarily result in injury, and injury prevention, in which the focus is on avoiding or reducing injuries.

Injury control includes not only injury prevention but also treatment and rehabilitation to prevent death, progression of damage, or permanent disability from complications such as hypovolemic shock, infection, and scarring or stiffness. For injuries that are not prevented, the adverse impact of nonfatal and some potentially fatal injuries often can be minimized by prompt and efficient first aid and definitive treatment rendered in the "post-event" phase.

In industrialized countries there have been major advances in prevention of traffic injuries by vehicle designs that protect occupants during a crash. In developing countries, however, many injuries involve unprotected road users such as pedestrians, so a greater focus on education may be necessary. This should not obscure the many opportunities for prevention by road designs that emphasize pedestrian safety.

In some countries, great effort and expense have been devoted to treatment and rehabilitation of injuries. In rural areas of developing countries, however, most people with severe injuries never reach hospital. This situation can prevail even in periurban villages near large referral hospitals. For example, in both rural and periurban village populations in Papua New Guinea, over 80 percent of victims of fatal injuries never reached a hospital (Barss, 1991). Similarly, among Native Canadians living near western James Bay in the far north, more than 90 percent of deaths from injuries occurred before involvement of the medical care system (Young, 1983).

The concept of injury control helps to emphasize the importance of developing interventions that are designed to prevent injury–causing events, to reduce or prevent injuries during potentially hazardous events that do occur, and to enhance survival and minimize adverse outcomes when injury does occur.

PASSIVE VS. ACTIVE PROTECTION

Permanent environmental or design changes often provide passive protection against injuries, that is, protection requiring no effort by the individual at risk. Passive protection reduces the need for constant vigilance by individuals to protect themselves or their families and allows for mistakes and momentary lapses of attention due to human error and fatigue, which are inevitable. It also reduces the expense of repeated educational programs for new generations of persons at risk. Examples of passive protection include electrical fuses, flame–retardant clothing, childproof fences around swimming pools, energy–absorbing steering columns, air bags, and rounded corners on furniture.

Because it is more likely to be effective, passive protection is preferred over measures that rely on individual education, behavior change, and repetitive preventive maneuvers (active protection). Either passive or active approaches may be indicated, however, depending upon the specific circumstances.

chapter 2

The Epidemiologic Basis for Prevention

Instead of something set apart from disease and scarcely to be considered within the scope of preventive medicine, injuries are as much a public health problem as measles ... They are amenable to the same epidemiologic approach, and what is least well appreciated, they are preventable and controllable.
—*John E. Gordon, 1949*

*E*pidemiology is the study of the distribution and determinants of health-related events in a defined population and its application to the control of events (Last, 1990). The usefulness of epidemiology is far-reaching and not limited to public health professionals (Gordon, 1940, 1949). The epidemiologic approach is distinguished from the clinical approach in that the focus of epidemiologic investigation and prevention is a group (i.e. a community or population) rather than an individual.

An *injury* is damage to an organism (host) and is defined by the following two factors:

• Damage occurs rapidly and usually is immediately apparent.
• The causative agent is energy or an agent that interferes with energy exchanges in the body.

ETIOLOGY AND NATURE OF INJURIES

Sub-acute exposures to energy over long periods of time cause many chronic diseases and disabilities. It is the acuteness of exposure that differentiates injury from disease. Thus, acute smoke inhalation is generally classified as an injury, while chronic damage from substances such as lead and cigarette smoke are excluded as injuries because toxic effects occur slowly. This distinction is somewhat arbitrary and not rigid, but is conceptually useful for classification, research, and policy purposes.

The establishment of a well-developed theoretical and practical framework for the science of injury prevention has led to replacing the concept of accidents with an etiologic definition of injury events as a health problem (Haddon, 1968; Waller, 1987). Instead of considering injuries as acts of God or unexpected random events without apparent cause, modern epidemiologic concepts of injury control emphasize that injuries result from exposures to specific hazards and affect certain high risk groups more than others.

Therefore, injuries can be analyzed using the same epidemiologic methods as other diseases with attention to host, agent, and environment (Haddon, 1980a) (Table 2.1). In addition, equipment factors and activity at the time of the incident are essential considerations.

Table 2.1 Comparative epidemiology of disease and injury: malaria versus skull injury to motorcyclist

Variable	Health condition	
	Disease	*Injury*
Pathology	Malaria	Brain damage
Incident	Mosquito bite	Crash into tree
Agent	*Plasmodium* parasite	Kinetic energy
Vector/ vehicle	*Anopheles* mosquito	Motorcycle
Activity	Sleeping	Motorcycle travel
Personal/host factors	Low immunity; young child	Alcohol intoxication; youth; male sex; inexperience; fatigue
Equipment factors	Mosquito net, insect screening	Motorcycle helmet, guardrail
Environment factors	Unscreened home near swamp; rain	Unprotected curve near tree; unsafe surface and incline; rain
Time/ visibility factors	Night/darkness	Night/darkness

Methods and Agents

Many of the methods used today to study the epidemiology of injuries originated with the investigation of infectious diseases. For example, to control food-borne outbreaks, it is necessary to identify the nature and source of the agent, such as bacteria from an infected food handler, together with the means of transmission, such as contaminated food. Similarly, to prevent injuries it is necessary to identify the causative agents of injuries and the circumstances in which they occur.

Energy as the etiologic agent for injuries may seem obvious today, but the unifying concept of energy as the causative agent of injuries was not clearly defined until 1961 (Haddon, 1972, 1980a, 1980b). The forms of energy are mechanical (kinetic), chemical, thermal, electrical, and radiant. Tissue damage is caused by rapid transfers of excessive amounts of energy or, in the case of drowning, suffocation, freezing, and certain poisonings, by interference with normal exchange patterns of energy that overwhelms the body's ability to withstand the transfer (Haddon, 1980a). The vector that transfers the agent may be a falling person or falling object, a motor vehicle, a machine, or some other product that transmits energy.

Restricting the definition of injuries to acute damage provides a manageable scope for the field of injury control. Otherwise, injury control would include the unmanageable consideration of many chronic diseases and toxic effects that other disciplines address.

CONCEPTUAL MODELS

If a man will begin with certainties, he shall end in doubts; but if he will be content to begin with doubts he shall end in certainties
　　—*Francis Bacon, The Advancement of Learning, bk 1, v8, 1605.*

Facts which at first seem improbable will, even on scant explanation, drop the cloak which has hidden them and stand forth in naked and simple beauty.
　—*Galileo Galilei, Dialogues Concerning Two New Sciences, Day 1, 1638.*

As for most infectious diseases, agents are now recognized for injuries; however, it is knowing how energy is transmitted that helps develop effective interventions. Just as a mosquito net effectively prevents the vector (mosquito) from transmitting the agent (the malaria parasite, *Plasmodium falciparum*) to the body, a motorcycle helmet can provide a protective barrier in a crash reducing the transfer of energy to the head (Table 2.1). Similarly, a seat belt or air bag absorbs some of the energy from a crash, distributing forces over a large area of the body and increasing the stopping distance needed to decelerate the body. An increase in stopping distance greatly reduces the effect of kinetic energy transmitted to the body by spreading out the transfer over a longer period of time.

When there is an understanding about injury mechanisms or modes of transmission, many interventions become as obvious as the control of food-borne outbreaks through adequate refrigeration.

Injury control includes all preventive measures as well as acute care and rehabilitation. Several models of injury control have been advanced by Haddon and others (Haddon, 1970, 1980a; Waller, 1987). The first involves dividing the factors that determine injury into three phases—pre-event, event, and post-event. Pre-event factors determine if a crash, fall, shooting, fire, or other event will occur. Event factors operate during the incident to reduce or completely prevent injury. Post-event factors determine the outcome once an injury has occurred.

Haddon formed a nine-cell matrix for analyzing injuries by cross classifying these phases of the injury event with factors relating to the injured person, the injury producing vehicle or vector, and the environment (Table 2.2). This matrix has proven to be a successful tool for analyzing injury producing events and recognizing factors important to their prevention (Smith and Falk, 1987; Haddon, 1980a).

For many types of injuries, it is helpful to consider equipment factors rather than, or in addition to, vehicle factors (see Chapter 6). Equipment factors are specific to the type of activity involved and may include the following:

- Hazardous equipment or other products that contribute to an injury;
- Safety equipment that prevents or minimizes the occurrence of an injury or of an incident with potential for injury.

A second model, also developed by Haddon, provides ten basic strategies for the prevention of injuries (Haddon, 1970, 1973, 1980a, 1980c, 1981). Table 2.3 lists the ten strategies with examples of possible applications in developing countries.

As in the case of the Haddon Matrix, the ten strategies stimulate recognition of a variety of factors contributing to the occurrence and

Table 2.2 The Haddon Matrix for injury control: Examples of host, equipment/vehicle, and environmental factors for preventing injuries

Time phase	Personal	Equipment	Environment
MATRIX A: ACTIVITY AND RISK GROUP			
Travel by Motorcycle—Drivers and Passengers			
Pre-event	Avoid alcohol consumption Obey traffic laws	Daytime headlamps Good tires, brakes	One-way streets Special lanes for motorcycles Clear road signs and signals
Event	Put on and strap helmet Physical fitness; exercise bone strength	Good quality, well-fitting helmet Leg guards on cycle Heavy boots and clothing	Energy-absorbing roadside barriers Roadsides clear of fixed obstructions Guardrail along cliff
Post-event	Avoid smoking and lung complications	First-aid kit Emergency radio	Communication network Transportation network Emergency services
MATRIX B: ACTIVITY AND RISK GROUP			
Cooking, Lighting, Warming, Sleeping—Girls and Women; Elderly Persons			
Pre-event	Choose enclosed stoves and lamps; treat epilepsy; supervise young children	Use enclosed stove and lights Electric cooking, heating and lighting	Improve crowded poverty housing, space and enclosure barriers between children and hot liquids, electrification
Event	Choose appropriate clothing design and fabric	Pants of less flammable styles and materials; fabric regulations; fire extinguishers; where feasible, smoke detectors, sprinkler systems	Escape exits in sleeping and cooking quarters
Post-event	Knowledge of first-aid	Bucket of cool water Antibacterial burn creams Intravenous fluids for shock	Communications network Transportation network Emergency services Rehabilitation

Table 2.3 Ten basic strategies for injury control with examples for developing countries

Strategy	Examples
1. Prevent creation of the hazard	Ban production of particularly hazardous substances such as fireworks, certain highly toxic pesticides, or drugs
2. Reduce amount of the hazard	Develop and use shorter varieties of trees (such as hybrid coconut palms) to reduce damage from a fall; enclose open fires to prevent severe burns; restrict the use and availability of toxic chemicals; reduce speed limits
3. Prevent inappropriate release of the hazard	Eliminate sale of kerosene or paraquat in soft drink bottles; childproof caps for all hazardous household drugs and chemicals
4. Modify rate or spatial distribution	Require adequate brakes to slow down vehicles; safety nets to protect construction workers from falls; seat belts, air bags, cushioned dashboards, hydraulic bumpers on vehicles
5. Separate release of the hazard in time or space	Install pedestrian sidewalks and/or bicycle paths along busy roads; reroute high speed through traffic around cities or residential neighborhoods; store poisons in high inaccessible places; spray pesticides at a time of day when people are not around
6. Put a barrier between the hazard and people at risk	Install fences around village ponds; wear helmets to prevent damage from falling coconuts; cover moving machinery belts with protective guards; install guardrail along dangerous sections of roads or between busy sidewalks and roads; enclose cooking fires
7. Change basic nature of the hazard	Modify equipment such as rounding sharp corners or padding the floor; shift to non-leaded, water-based paint to reduce solvent and lead poisonings
8. Increase resistance of people to the hazard	Prevent fractures due to weak bones and osteoporosis by regular exercise or estrogen intake; correct nutritional deficiencies to increase resistance of epithelial surfaces to damage; treat epilepsy to prevent seizure that can result in burns, drownings, and falls
9. Begin to counter damage already done	First-aid, including direct pressure and elevation to control hemorrhage, followed by thorough cleaning and covering of wounds to prevent infection; rapid rescue and resuscitation of trauma victims; induce vomiting for certain ingestions; use antidotes for poisons
10. Stabilization, definitive care, and rehabilitation	Rapid availability of appropriate emergency and long-term treatment, rehabilitation of injured persons; appropriate treatment such as release of burn-scar contractures to correct deformity from injuries

control of injuries. (For more discussion of prevention programs see Baker et al., 1992; National Committee for Injury Prevention and Control, 1989; Smith and Falk, 1987; Waller, 1985; Robertson, 1983, 1992).

Schelp (1988) has proposed a model of community injury prevention for a rural municipality in Sweden that may be applicable to developing countries. It incorporates the following eight steps:

1. Epidemiological mapping
2. Selection of risk groups/environments
3. Formation of intersectoral working and reference groups
4. Joint planning of action programs
5. Implementation of action programs
6. Evaluation of action programs
7. Modification of action programs
8. Transfer of experience to other areas in the district

It is beyond the scope of this book to discuss all of these steps, but it is apparent that the first two steps, by necessity, specify an epidemiologic basis for prevention.

ROLE OF EPIDEMIOLOGY

The initial role of epidemiology includes the following:

- Identifying or establishing data sources appropriate to the surveillance of injuries by external causes; identifying sources of population estimates by age and sex groups;
- Surveillance of intentional and unintentional injuries, including preparation of population-based age- and sex-specific rates of mortality and/or morbidity for major categories of injuries;
- Establishing the relative importance of different specific injuries grouped by external cause, as assessed by mortality, morbidity, lost productive years of life, and service load on the health system;
- Monitoring and investigating significant secular trends in specific injuries for different age and sex subgroups of population(s) under surveillance;
- Determining the circumstances of exposures for specific injuries including the identification of environmental, equipment, and personal risk factors, as well as associated activities.

Clinicians are most interested in the nature of the injury they are about to treat, for example, a fractured tibia, for very practical reasons since their immediate task is to provide therapy appropriate to the injury. On the other hand, epidemiologists are more concerned with the external cause of the injury, for example, a fall or traffic injury. Although the treatment for a fractured tibia is the same whether caused by a fall from a palm tree or from a bicycle collision, the preventive strategies are quite different and involve different organizations and disciplines.

It has been a challenge for injury epidemiologists to identify or develop sources of data on injuries that include not only the nature of the injuries but also the external cause. Minor improvements to existing data sources sometimes turn out to be the most practical solution. In other cases, special injury surveillance systems may need to be established.

Population figures by age and sex are needed to calculate age- and sex-specific rates of different injuries and to monitor secular trends from year to year. While relatively accurate population data are available from national censuses for developed countries and many developing countries, other sources, such as special surveys, may be needed in some developing countries.

Risk factors have the potential to be changed, as in the case of some behaviors, such as binge drinking of alcohol, failure to use safety equipment, and unsafe housing. Others, such as age and, in some societies, socioeconomic status, are largely immutable but are important in identifying high-risk population groups that should be targeted for preventive interventions.

Injury epidemiologists often work cooperatively with professionals in other disciplines. They may collaborate with economists, for example, to establish the direct and indirect costs of injuries; for an illustration of such collaboration in the United States, see Rice and others (1989). The information provided by epidemiologists and/or their collaborators can be used by staff in other disciplines to develop appropriate prevention strategies.

Developing effective prevention measures often requires participation by a variety of different disciplines such as epidemiology, human factors research, psychology, medicine, biomechanics, engineering, law, and economics. To achieve common goals different organizations and sectors must collaborate. Policy makers and politicians are ultimately responsible for the successful implementation, through legislation and regulation, of national and provincial interventions.

In injury studies there is a tendency to identify a single factor as the cause of injury, and this has impeded the development of appropriate prevention strategies (Waller, 1987). Injuries usually involve a complex series of events including environmental factors and the interaction of human performance and the task to be performed.

Intervention is possible at several points in the causal chain once hazardous exposures and circumstances are known. A fall down an embankment at night may involve a number of factors, each of which could form the basis for a prevention strategy. Adequate lighting or the modification of environmental factors, such as provision of a fence, could prevent the fall. Personal factors such as alcohol abuse, untreated epilepsy, night blindness from vitamin A deficiency, or other preexisting medical conditions could all be risk factors for the fall and may or may not be readily modified by interventions.

The reason for an injury producing event can often be traced to policy decisions taken by a society; for example, increases in deaths and disabilities from motorcycle crashes might be attributed to inadequate public transport systems, failure to require that helmets be worn by all riders, or motorcycle licensing, importation, tax, and insurance fees that fail to recover the full costs to society of motorcycle injuries. Haddon emphasized the importance of society's role in collectively reducing the risk of injuries for all citizens rather than placing the blame on individual victims (Haddon, 1980a).

Initially manufacturers of automobiles and other hazardous equipment strongly resisted the public policy approach to injury prevention because it was more expedient and cheaper to blame the victims than to design and build safer products (Nader, 1991). In developed countries, this mode of thinking has changed somewhat in recent years. Expensive lawsuits have been mounted against manufacturers of hazardous products (Teret and Jacobs, 1989), and the public has modified its purchasing patterns as it has become better informed about safety features of products.

One of the challenges for injury epidemiology is not to identify a single cause, which is rarely possible, but to identify those exposures, risk factors, and steps in the causal chain that are most amenable to intervention at reasonable cost.

The cost of any proposed intervention is a constraint to its application, especially in countries with scarce resources. Documentation of the magnitude and economic consequences of the problem is an important aspect of injury studies in developing countries, as it is in industrialized countries. If the costs of injuries are proven to be sufficiently high, they may provide the economic justification needed to divert resources for interventions.

Epidemiologic surveillance of injuries is also an important component in evaluating the effectiveness of prevention programs since outcome indicators of mortality and morbidity are critical measures of success. The incidence of deaths or hospitalizations from various specific injuries can be followed over time to detect significant trends.

Perhaps the greatest challenge to epidemiologists is to recognize the situation in which elaborate study is not necessary. To illustrate, many commuters in Sri Lanka have fallen to their deaths from trains or sustained severe spinal cord injuries because the exterior design of some commuter trains provided footholds and handholds making it easy for people to cling to the outside. Little would be gained from determining the age, sex, or economic groups at highest risk when it is obvious that the solution requires keeping people from riding on the outside of trains.

The epidemiologist's contributions in this situation would be to document the size of the problem, convince decision-makers that educating the riders would not be effective, and contribute to a cost-effectiveness analysis of strategies such as enforcement and redesign of train exteriors. During a time when one could see hundreds of commuters hanging onto the outside of trains in Sri Lanka, one of the authors (SPB) observed that the design of Indonesian trains was such that there were no external protrusions to grasp or stand on and, therefore, no endangered riders.

PROBLEMS OF MEASUREMENT

Definition of Injury

A standardized definition of what should be counted as an injury is important, particularly in surveys of morbidity where there may be uncertainty about including minor injuries. Injuries tend to fall into three major categories—deaths, hospitalizations, and others. Deaths or hospitalizations from injury normally are more easily defined and counted than injuries treated only in outpatient clinics, at home, or not at all.

Criteria such as the presence or duration of temporary or permanent disability, including the inability to work or carry out specified activities of daily living, are sometimes used to define whether an injury is severe enough to be counted for the purposes of a specific survey or for routine epidemiologic surveillance.

Severity scales based upon the nature of the injury(s) sustained have been developed to rate the degree of injury damage in hospitalized patients or fatalities. This makes it possible to group and compare different severities of injury, a classification useful for evaluating the efficacy of tertiary prevention or the case loads of different facilities.

Coding and Classification

Accurate and standard codes for mortality and morbidity from injuries are important to assess the health impact of different injuries and evaluate interventions. Injuries are the only disease group to have two separate coding systems under the World Health Organization's International Classification of Diseases (ICD). The nature of the injury(s) or the body part(s) injured is classified using Nature of Injury codes or N codes from the ICD. These codes describe the type of injury sustained, such as a fractured humerus. There is one principal Nature of Injury code to describe the major injury, while additional Nature of Injury codes describe other injuries. These codes do not describe the external cause, such as a fall or an assault.

At many health care facilities data are often recorded to provide information about only the type of injury, not the cause. While such information can be coded using Nature of Injury codes, it is useful mainly to describe the case loads at clinics or hospitals, and, except for the poisoning codes, is of little use for developing prevention programs.

In response to this deficiency, a separate classification, the Supplementary Classification of External Causes, was developed by the World Health Organization to describe the cause of injury, such as a motor vehicle crash or a fall. Deaths are coded using the Cause of Injury codes, known as E codes in the ninth revision of the ICD and by several letters in the Tenth Revision. Only one External Cause code is assigned to a case, whereas more than one Nature of Injury code can be used.

For nonfatal injuries, data by external cause have only recently become widely available in some industrialized countries, such as the United States (Smith, 1985). In others, such as Canada, external causes of injuries by ICD code have been assigned as a routine by hospital coders for decades, are a routine part of hospital records, and are compiled by provincial and national statistical bodies. Nevertheless, even where external cause codes have been used for years, many are invalid because most health providers fail to include the external cause of injury as part of their diagnoses and hospital summaries (Barss and Masson, 1996).

A national computerized injury surveillance system has been developed in Australia to address the lack of injury data by cause (Vimpani, 1991). This system was adapted for use by a nationwide network of hospitals in Canada to survey injuries presenting in emergency rooms (Pless, 1989).

The Nordic countries found the ninth revision of the ICD,

which was developed mainly for coding injury deaths, inadequate to describe the many important circumstances of hospitalizations from injuries. They collaborated to develop their own Nordic Classification for Accident Monitoring (Nordic Medico-Statistical Committee, 1990), which has been adapted for use in Arctic communities (Frimodt-Møller and Bay-Nielsen, 1992). Improvements in the Tenth Revision, which has gradually been implemented in many countries during the late 1990's, appear to have overcome many of the limitations of the ICD for injury surveillance.

External Cause codes divide injuries into unintentional and intentional; the latter includes homicide, suicide, and war injuries. There is also a category of intent called "undetermined." This is quite large in some developing countries that have many violent deaths, presumably because officials are reluctant to report the deaths as homicides. This category may also be large if there are cultural factors that discourage accurate reporting of suicides.

In some countries, incidents that involve the intentional ingestion of an overdose of medication are often listed by hospital coders as of undetermined intent, rather than as a suicide attempt. This occurs when health professionals do not specify the intentional nature of an overdose as part of their diagnosis.

Homicides and suicides are also sometimes reported as "other violence" (see Table 3.1), a term that may also include war injuries and government executions of criminals or political undesirables.

Underlying and Contributory Causes of Death

Another classification problem that may affect injury rates involves underlying and contributory causes of death. The coding rules are somewhat complex and the correct manner of coding the underlying cause of death may not be obvious if injury occurs in conjunction with a medical disorder, alcohol intoxication, or drug addiction.

Injuries that occur during a seizure of a person with epilepsy should be coded with epilepsy as the underlying cause, whereas injuries that occur in association with most other medical conditions, such as a myocardial infarction, should be coded with the injury as the underlying cause. An exception would be a case in which there was evidence that death from the medical condition occurred before the injury event, such as the victim of a traffic crash who shows evidence of a myocardial infarction but no blood loss from severe injuries. If an injured patient dies of a complication such as pneumonia, the death may be coded erroneously with pneumonia as the underlying cause, particularly if the physician who certifies the cause of death mistakenly lists this on the death certificate as the underlying cause.

Data are scarce on the extent of alcohol involvement in non-vehicular injuries in developing countries. Since alcohol is frequently an important risk factor for many different types of injuries, it is important to ensure that alcohol-related deaths are correctly certified and coded as such by health providers and coders.

For example, among the Inuit of Greenland, 82 percent of all deaths were classified as alcohol-related on the basis of a contributory diagnosis of alcoholism (ICD 303), and only 18 percent on the basis of acute alcohol intoxication (E860 in ICD-8). Of alcohol-related unintentional injuries, 83 percent were classified as such on the basis of a contributory diagnosis (Bjerregaard & Juel, 1990). However, deaths due to ingestion of alcohol by a person other than the victim, such as a drunken driver or parent, were generally not coded as alcohol-related.

The coding of alcohol as a contributory factor is further complicated by the fact that the coding rules for ICD 9 specify that either chronic alcoholism or acute alcohol intoxication be coded, but not both conditions. In many hospitalizations where alcohol intoxication is clearly a contributing factor, it is not consistently included in the codes by hospital coders. These data could be improved if there were a box on the discharge summary sheet for the health professional to specify alcohol as a contributing factor.

Similar coding problems occur when injury deaths are associated with ingestion of drugs such as cocaine and heroin. In ICD-9, deaths from cocaine are coded using the External Cause codes and Nature of Injury codes for poisoning by local anesthetic, since cocaine is classified as a local anesthetic. While there are other more specific codes for contributory diagnoses of cocaine addiction or cocaine use that can be used in addition to the code for poisoning by local anesthetic, these are often omitted.

Physicians and coders need to be trained to consider the sequence of events and important contributory factors that led to death when they certify and code deaths. There is a natural tendency to describe recent events rather than to list the sometimes forgotten or ignored underlying cause and contributory diagnoses. Terminal events, such as cardiorespiratory arrest, often make a dramatic impression upon health care providers, but are of little or no significance to public health and prevention programs. Some jurisdictions have begun to include on death certificates a specific question or data field for important contributory diagnoses such as alcohol abuse or tobacco addiction to ensure that more complete data are obtained on these major determinants of injury and disease.

INFORMATION NEEDS

Truth exists, only falsehood has to be invented.

—Georges Braque (1882–1963), Pensées sur l'Art.

In most developing countries, even the basic descriptive epidemiology is not available to identify the relative importance of injuries, high-risk subgroups in the population, and specific risk factors. Central to the development of basic hazard identification is a need for adequate data on types of injuries and their causes, associated activities, risk factors, and distribution in the community. The types of data needed depend on the level at which activities are conducted.

To determine the magnitude of the injury problem, epidemiologists need population based rates of mortality and morbidity from all injuries and from specific categories (see Chapters 3 and 4). It is important to compare injuries to other leading causes of mortality and morbidity to define the relative importance of injuries.

Indicators of premature mortality, such as years of potential life lost, are also helpful in defining the significance of injuries as a cause of loss of life among the most economically productive age groups. Important measures of morbidity include rates of hospitalization and duration of stay and the incidence and prevalence of permanent disability from various injuries. Because both direct medical costs and indirect costs of lost productivity are important, (see Chapter 5) epidemiologists must collaborate with economists.

Regional and international comparisons provide a broader perspective and may stimulate healthy competition to reduce local injury rates. Large differences in rates of certain injuries among regions can also provide insights into their etiology.

Fatal and severe nonfatal injuries are low-probability events with a serious outcome. To discern the causes and population groups at increased risk for such events, epidemiologists must obtain detailed information about different types of injuries, such as traffic injuries, drownings, falls, burns, poisonings, homicides, and suicides, and define subgroups of the population at highest risk. This requires either that a large population be under surveillance for injury events for a relatively short period, such as a year, or that a smaller population be studied for several years.

In a population with a relatively high overall rate of fatal injury (100 deaths per 100,000 population per year) it is probable that at least 50,000 person-years of observation (a population of 5,000 followed for ten years or a population of 50,000 for one year) are needed to obtain reasonably stable estimates of death rates for specific injuries (Barss, 1991). A substantially greater number of person-years of observation will be necessary to discern high-risk subgroups and hazardous exposures. For less severe injuries that are more frequent, a smaller study population or shorter period of observation may suffice.

INFORMATION NEEDS AT DIFFERENT LEVELS

At global and national levels, epidemiologists need adequate and consistent detail in categorization of unintentional injuries into useful groups, such as drownings, falls, and burns so that they can prioritize specific injuries for more detailed study and action. The major categories of the classification system for external causes of injuries of the ICD provide a basis for standardization and international comparability. Examples can be found in the World Health Statistics Annuals. National and international standardization, comparability of classification, and coding of various data sources should facilitate coordination of data systems within different sectors of a country and allow comparison of improvement or deterioration in health status among regions and countries.

Developing countries may need to work together, preferably in conjunction with WHO, to contribute to injury classification systems suited to their own local conditions, including environment, equipment, and personal factors and activities. During the Tenth Revision of the ICD, a special effort was made to include injuries believed common in developing countries. Some countries may need to develop abridged versions of standard injury coding systems for areas that lack well-trained coders or where coders have heavy workloads and no time to use detailed subcodes. The Tenth Revision of the ICD contains a short list that should accomodate these needs in developing countries.

Abridged classifications should be compatible with major categories in more detailed systems, but could exclude complex and specific levels of detail. Some abridged coding systems for health conditions, including injuries, already exist. Unfortunately, many have not been developed with a view to the special requirements of defining detailed circumstances of injuries and are, therefore, unsuitable for use as a basis for surveillance of specific injuries and development of interventions.

Important causes of injury vary widely from one place to another, and standard systems may have to be adapted to local needs. Detailed data on deaths from specific injuries in rural areas of developing countries are available from studies based upon lay reporting and verbal autopsies (Barss, 1991), which are helpful.

To exemplify the extent of underreporting internationally, the 1988 World Health Statistics Annual, containing data reported to the World Health Organization by member countries included mortality data from only one country in Asia and from no countries on the mainland of Africa. The 1989 and 1990 editions (WHO, 1990, 1991) did, however, include data from large rural and urban surveillance populations in China. International and interprovincial cooperation is needed to establish adequate uniform injury reporting procedures within and among nations.

At a national level, more detail is needed regarding the causes and impacts of specific injuries as important sources of morbidity and mortality. For example, information about hazardous equipment, vehicles, and other products, and information about causes of occupational injuries and the involvement of alcohol in injuries would be useful to develop appropriate regulations, legislation, and training programs for the protection of the general public and the workforce.

Various organizations and sectors of society work independently to compile injury data for their own purposes. Examples include departments of transport, health, labor, and the environment, poison control centers, coroners, hospital insurance commissions, consumer product safety commissions, national safety councils, insurance companies, unions, the Red Cross or Red Crescent, and sports organizations.

To avoid duplication and waste of scarce resources and to standardize coding and optimize the use of different data sources, it is highly desirable to have an effective mechanism or organizing body for intersectoral coordination (Mackay and Petrucelli, 1989; Trinca et al., 1988). The public health sector should be a suitable locus for coordination of injury surveillance if health directors can assemble teams of professionals with appropriate expertise in injury surveillance.

At the local level, a more detailed study of causes of injury, high risk groups, personal risk factors, and hazardous exposures and environments would be useful. It would include tools to detect hazardous areas, such as maps of road traffic deaths or drownings. Where the population is small and events of interest, such as deaths, are relatively rare, the problem of adequate numbers, mentioned above, must be considered. The difficulties of obtaining adequate data in smaller jurisdictions must be balanced against the fact that citizens and decision makers are more motivated to act by local information than by national or international data. However, comparisons of the local injury problem with the situation in larger regional or national populations may provide a useful stimulus for change. For uncommon injuries that require a large population for adequate surveillance, however, it would be unwise to rely upon only local data.

CONCLUSION

Many possible data sources and coding systems are helpful when engaged in routine epidemiologic surveillance or for special studies of the impact of injuries in developing countries. The purposes of collected data and the local resources that are available on a continuing basis should be carefully considered before embarking on ambitious projects.

Data should be collected carefully and consistently in a timely manner using a minimal data set for a few of the most pertinent variables. Complex data sets can bog down data collection (Graitcer, 1992). It is essential to have accurate data on external causes of injuries and to use standard coding systems. Population estimates by age and sex are helpful for the calculation of various injury rates.

Once the requirement has been met for basic surveillance data establishing priority injury groups based on external cause, special surveillance and/or research data must be developed to identify the circumstances of priority injuries. This information guides development and monitoring of effective and efficient policies and interventions.

The measurement of injury mortality, morbidity (including disabilities), and costs are discussed in Chapters 3, 4, and 5. Chapter 6 includes an approach to analysis of specific determinants and circumstances for different types of injuries.

chapter 3

Assessing the Health Impact of Injuries: Mortality

Death is an unambiguous and easily countable outcome of severe injury. Accurate counts of injury deaths and a systematic investigation of the circumstances of each death are a fundamental element of injury surveillance and control. It is therefore surprising, even shocking, to find that official mortality reports are often based upon incomplete counts, biased sources, cursory or no investigations, and erroneous coding. This situation is not unique to developing countries. In remote indigenous communities in developed countries, the circumstances of injury deaths are often documented inadequately.

This chapter describes the process of investigating and reporting injury deaths, the availability of injury mortality data, methods used to measure the health impact of fatal injuries, problems affecting the reliability and validity of data, and community surveys for situations in which official injury data are inadequate. Methods of measuring mortality include crude, age- and sex-specific, and age-adjusted death rates, as well as years of potential life lost. Definition, classification, and coding of injuries were described in Chapter 2. Data available from various regions of the world are discussed to provide insight into patterns and priorities among fatal injuries and to illustrate limitations and biases and the urgent need for improvement.

PROCESS OF MORTALITY REPORTING

In an ideal injury surveillance system with adequate resources and trained personnel, each injury death is considered a unique and essential source of data and is methodically studied to identify hazardous activities and personal, environmental, and equipment risk factors. While the information from a single death can be useful, the power of modern epidemiology to identify causes and determinants of injury is most compellingly revealed only after the compilation and analysis of highly specific data from many deaths of particular types. Population-based analyses are most efficient when there are standards for data collection and computerization of the entire process of death investigation and reporting for provinces, regions, and countries.

One aspect of the investigation of injury mortality that differs from that of disease mortality is that police and medical examiners or coroners are routinely involved in assessing the external cause, circumstances, and intent of each death. The process of investigating an injury death normally begins with a call to police who then investigate and prepare a report. A local coroner reviews the police report and may request a post-mortem examination. In urban areas, this is carried out by a forensic pathologist with specialized training, but in remote areas, the only medical personnel available may be a general medical officer or nurse.

A post-mortem examination may range from a cursory examination of the exterior surface of the body to a detailed autopsy including examination of internal organs and toxicological sampling of blood or other tissues for alcohol, drugs, and other chemical agents. The person carrying out the post-mortem examination and the coroner determine the principal cause of death and associated or secondary causes. In doing so, they use all information available from the history of the circumstances of death and the postmortem. For example, in northern communities it can be difficult to distinguish drowning from hypothermia when a body is retrieved from the water. Since there are no pathognomonic postmortem findings of hypothermia, the immersion time, water and air temperatures, and whether the victim was wearing an adequate personal flotation device should be considered when assigning a primary cause of death.

Formerly, the major emphasis in the investigation of injury deaths was the legal issue of whether the death was a homicide, suicide, or unintentional. Increasingly, coroners have realized that they also have responsibility for public safety and security. Many chief coroners are becoming skillful in defining the circumstances of injury deaths and in reporting to the appropriate agencies having the power to regulate or directly modify the environment, equipment, or personal behavior of individuals. Chief medical examiners and coroners sometimes employ full-time epidemiologists to computerize and analyze data for their annual reports, for special investigations of important topics, and for providing data to public health researchers. However, there are hundreds of individual part-time coroners in any given region whose level of training and expertise varies widely.

In some jurisdictions, all coroners must be physicians or lawyers, but even then their standards of training and interest in investigation of injury deaths vary widely. In other areas, former police officers or other community members are preferred as coroners. Where coroners are elected officials, even illiterate individuals are sometimes chosen.

If an injury victim dies in hospital, a death certificate is completed by a physician and mailed to a national or provincial office for vital statistics. There it is coded and compiled for annual mortality reports. The reported cause of death may change if a coroner's investigation is called and an investigation reveals new findings. However, coroners' investigations sometimes take weeks or months to complete. The final cause(s) of death is supposed to be communicated to the government statistical offices with responsibility for vital statistics, then the cause of death code is corrected using the diagnoses from the coroner's report.

Coding involves the use of External Cause and Nature of Injury codes and this requires well-trained coders. Injury death reports are prepared periodically by province and country, and preferably include population-based death rates for specific injury categories. The denominators for such rates are obtained from census data.

As shown above, the process of investigating and reporting on injury deaths involves several steps. Where resources and trained personnel are scarce, as in many developing countries and remote indigenous communities, the system for investigating and reporting injury deaths may be grossly deficient. Many deaths are never reported, and even if they are, investigations may be inadequate or not done at all. Many injury victims are buried immediately by their families. In such situations, official death reports must be interpreted with great caution and with an awareness of the limitations of each step in the local process. The only way to obtain valid and reliable data is to improve existing data sources or to develop alternative sources.

AVAILABILITY OF OFFICIAL INJURY MORTALITY DATA

Many developing countries have poorly developed health information systems, which means that they do not have reliable data on the local incidence of various health conditions, or even on the leading causes of death (Smith and Barss, 1991). The magnitude of the problem of injuries as a cause of death is inadequately documented in such countries except by special surveys.

The World Health Organization, for example, considered the mortality data for all Southeast Asian countries to be unreliable with the exception of Singapore (Meade, 1980). In the 1988 World Health Statistics Annual, Sri Lanka was the only Asian country that reported mortality data. However, in 1989 and 1990, China did provide data from special rural and urban sampling areas with a total population of 100 million, and in 1990 their reporting was more current than some developed countries, including the United States (WHO, 1990, 1991).

In Africa, there are no recent data from countries on the mainland; only the tiny island nations of Mauritius, the Seychelles, and São Tome and Principe have reported recently on mortality to WHO (WHO, 1990, 1991). In the eastern Mediterranean region, Egypt reported occasionally during the 1980s.

The situation is substantially better in the Americas, including the Caribbean, Central, North, and South America; recent publications from the Pan American Health Organization provide not only mortality rates from several types of injuries, but also some information on years of potential life lost (PAHO, 1986, 1990). However, data concerning specific unintentional injuries such as falls or drownings are not available for many of the countries, and the overall rate for all injuries is not always provided.

The reported rates for different countries often are not comparable because of variability in the completeness of reporting, in classification systems, and even in the definition of what constitutes an injury. Mortality reporting systems were established in a number of countries mainly to serve the needs of colonial administrators, and these systems often have deteriorated because of insufficient supervision and lack of time and resources needed to maintain them.

Sometimes the only deaths recorded are those that occur in hospital and for which a death certificate is completed, while the majority of deaths, which occur at home in villages, go unreported (Barss, 1991). Even the records of deaths that occur in hospital may be relatively useless for public health purposes. Either physicians fail to record the external cause of death or coding may be inadequate.

Thus, for some of the few countries that do report to WHO, there is concern that the available data may seriously underrepresent injury mortality rates since the omission of unrecorded deaths tends to bias the already small numerators, while reasonably accurate census estimates of the total population are used as denominators. Also, data are reported using only a simplified set of codes known as the Basic Tabulations List that gives a limited breakdown of the data into individual injury categories (WHO, 1978a, 1978b, 1986, 1992).

An even greater number of countries have no official mortality reporting system at all or collect data that are heavily biased toward the urban population in proximity to recording centers. In those countries, valid population-based data on mortality or morbidity are unavailable.

Aboriginal communities in developed countries often have different patterns of exposures and risk factors than the general population. It is important that detailed injury mortality data be available to such communities. However, the small size and scattered location of many aboriginal communities often make it difficult to obtain adequate numbers of injury deaths for epidemiological analysis. Long study periods and pooling of data for several similar communities can be helpful. Selection of deaths for analysis is often made by village of residence rather than by location of death in order to delineate aboriginal deaths from those in much larger neighboring nonaboriginal communities.

Because there is a lack of accurate population-based data, it is not possible to evaluate the importance of injuries to society in many countries. This is an important deficiency, since politicians are generally more highly motivated to address a problem on the basis of information about their own country, region, or community than by data from elsewhere. A lack of local or national population-based injury rates also makes international comparisons difficult or impossible.

IMPACT OF INJURIES AS ASSESSED BY MORTALITY RATES

The availability of reliable health statistics is generally a reflection of the level of a country's development. Mortality rates are prepared for populations that have been characterized by a census. Rates are presented using a standard denominator, for example, deaths per 100,000 persons, and for a standard time period, often one year. In small populations, several years of deaths may be pooled as the numerator for the rate and person-years of exposure used as the denominator; such rates are often referred to as incidence density.

Data on injury rates for developing countries with a population

Table 3.1 Unadjusted injury mortality rates by sex per 100,000 population for various developing countries, with other countries for comparison

| | Total all injuries | | Unintentional | | | | Intentional | | | | | | Year |
| | | | Motor vehicle | | Non-motor vehicle | | Suicide | | Homicide | | Other violence | | |
	m	f	m	f	m	f	m	f	m	f	m	f	
AFRICA													
Mauritius	71	21	27	5	22	10	20	4	2	2	0	0	1994
SOUTHEAST ASIA													
China, rural	90	63	20	9	43	55	24	31	3	1	0	0	1994
China, urban	48	31	16	7	22	16	7	7	4	1	0	0	1994
Sri Lanka	116	39	4	1	47	15	47	19	12	2	6	2	1986
Thailand	106	30	21	6	31	11	8	7	47	5	0	0	1981
EASTERN MEDITERRANEAN													
Egypt	50	28	10	3	15	8	0	0	1	0	24	17	1987
AMERICAS													
El Salvador	188	32	20	7	43	11	15	6	66	5	45	3	1984
Colombia	234	32	22	7	36	11	5	1	168	13	4	1	1991
Mexico	106	23	25	7	39	12	5	1	32	3	5	1	1993
Chile	104	28	18	5	21	10	8	1	5	1	51	11	1992

												Year
Guatemala	86	17	2	1	26	7	1	0	5	1	52	7	1984
Uruguay	91	34	18	7	50	21	17	4	7	2	0	0	1990
Panama	80	21	28	6	25	10	6	2	12	2	10	2	1987
Argentina	76	29	14	5	30	15	9	3	7	1	15	4	1991
Costa Rica	62	17	21	5	23	8	7	1	7	2	4	1	1991
Paraguay	61	19	14	5	26	9	3	2	12	2	5	2	1987
Peru	46	15	10	3	27	8	1	0	4	1	5	3	1986
COMPARISON													
Russian Federation	415	102	38	11	191	49	74	13	53	14	59	14	1994
Venezuela	99	23	33	8	27	10	8	2	22	2	9	1	1989
United States	84	31	22	10	25	12	20	5	16	4	2	1	1992
Sweden	67	37	9	4	26	19	22	10	2	1	7	3	1993
Kuwait	45	14	28	6	14	5	1	1	1	0	1	2	1987
Australia	56	22	16	6	19	10	19	5	2	1	1	0	1993

Source: World Health Statistics Annual 1986–1995 (WHO, 1986-1996);

Injury Prevention

Table 3.2 Total deaths from all causes, and numbers and percentages of deaths from all injuries* in the population ≥15 years in various developing countries with other countries for comparison

| | Total deaths | All injuries | | Year |
		Number	Percent	
AFRICA				
Mauritius	6,733	456	7	1994
SOUTHEAST ASIA				
China, rural	308,104	32,973	11	1994
China, urban	349,084	22,173	6	1994
Sri Lanka	82,045	11,421	14	1986
EASTERN MEDITERRANEAN				
Egypt	312,399	12,102	4	1987
AMERICAS				
Guatemala	30,068	3,548	12	1984
El Salvador	20,432	5,428	27	1984
Colombia	140,683	39,612	28	1991
Mexico	344,289	50,107	15	1993
Honduras	11,091	1,823	16	1981
Ecuador	36,642	5,309	14	1988
Panama	7,260	975	13	1987
Surinam	1,819	224	12	1985
Chile	68,336	7,571	11	1992
Cuba	69,085	7,979	12	1990
Costa Rica	10,177	1,081	11	1991
Dominican Republic	17,265	1,705	10	1982
Uruguay	28,587	1,676	6	1990
Argentina	230,066	14,391	6	1991
COMPARISON				
Venezuela	67,156	9,816	15	1989
Russian Federation	2,237,753	347,600	16	1994
United States	2,125,554	136,990	6	1992
Sweden	95,817	4,420	5	1993
Australia	118,418	6,502	5	1993

Source: World Health Statistics Annual 1985–1995 (WHO, 1985-1996)
*Includes all deaths from unintentional injuries, homicide, suicide, and other violence (ICD-9 codes E800-999)

greater than one million that report to WHO are shown in Table 3.1. Higher-income and industrialized countries are included at the bottom of the table for comparison.

It is evident that most of the poorest countries, especially in Africa and Asia, do not report to WHO. Data are usually presented as unadjusted rates. However, the rates available for all injuries, age-adjusted to a standard world population, (WIIO, 1988c, 1992) do not in most cases differ substantially from the crude rates shown. When comparing industrialized and developing countries, however, the younger age distribution of most developing countries should be kept in mind.

While the situation differs from country to country, it is apparent from Table 3.1 that where political or social instability prevails, homicide is a prominent contributor to the overall rate of injury. In general, motor vehicle related deaths are somewhat less prominent as a cause of mortality than the combined effect of the other unintentional injuries in many developing countries. However, the balance is changing in countries where motorization of transport is increasing rapidly. Suicide is an important contributor to overall injury mortality in some countries or regions, but less so in others.

In the Americas, injuries account for 3 to 16 percent of all deaths, depending on the country. However, in the adult population 15-years-old and older (PAHO, 1986), injuries cause up to one-fourth of all deaths (Table 3.2). In several countries in the Americas, unintentional injuries cause more than 40 percent of all deaths of 15 to 24-year-old males (Table 3.3). When suicide and homicide are included, it can be seen that in a number of countries the overwhelming majority of deaths of these prospective "bread-winners" are caused by injuries.

IMPACT OF INJURIES AS ASSESSED BY AGE-SPECIFIC AND AGE-ADJUSTED DEATH RATES

Death rates from unintentional injuries vary considerably by age and sex. Awareness of such differences can be helpful when developing programs for prevention among groups at increased risk. For this reason, it is important to have available age and sex specific mortality rates for specific injuries. However, the calculation of age and sex specific rates requires reasonably accurate information about the composition by age of the population and not just the total number of people at risk. Census data are used to obtain the numbers of individuals in different age and sex groups or strata of the population. Such data may not be available at all or may be available only for selected study populations.

A few examples of high risk groups, as defined by age and sex, are briefly mentioned below to exemplify the practical importance of careful preparation and examination of rates in different age and sex strata. This topic is also considered in Chapter 6 and in some of the discussions of specific injuries in chapters 9–13.

In certain industrialized countries such as the United States, teenagers and young adults are at high risk of injuries, since many have ready access to automobiles, alcohol, and handguns (Smith and Falk, 1987; Waller, 1985; Baker et al., 1992). In developing countries, adult males of working age tend to be at high risk, often because of exposure to environmental (including road traffic) and occupational hazards and, in some countries, to violence. In most countries, the elderly have high mortality rates from non-motor vehicle unintentional injuries (see Table 6.1,) and, in some countries, from sui-

I say "poverty" because they are not able to obtain sufficient good food for their work. It is, therefore, not surprising that for all age groups their mortality rates are higher than in the other classes.

—Louis R Villerme, Tableau de l'etat physique et moral des ouvriers employés dans les manufactures de coton, de laine et de soie, Vol 2, 1840

Table 3.3 Deaths from all causes in 15–24-year-olds and mortality rates per 100,000 population by sex from unintentional injuries* and suicide as a percentage of all causes in various developing countries with other countries for comparison

	Unintentional injuries				Suicide				Deaths from all causes				Year
	Rate		% of all causes		Rate		% of all causes		Number		Rate		
	m	f	m	f	m	f	m	f	m	f	m	f	
AFRICA													
Mauritius	48	10	41	18	25	9	21	16	118	55	119	57	1994
SOUTHEAST ASIA													
Sri Lanka	49	15	24	12	77	48	37	39	3,524	2,072	207	123	1986
China, rural	42	15	44	19	17	33	18	41	5,108	4,128	95	80	1994
China, urban	24	8	45	25	4	6	7	19	2,897	1,622	52	33	1994
EASTERN MEDITERRANEAN													
Egypt	23	13	14	10	0	0	0	0	7,797	5,596	161	127	1987
AMERICAS													
Guatemala	32	9	13	5	1	0	0	0	1,912	1,228	244	162	1984
Mexico	63	11	41	20	6	1	4	2	15,283	5,530	155	57	1993

Country													Year
Chile	27	7	23	15	8	2	6	6	1,472	517	118	42	1992
Colombia	55	11	15	15	8	3	2	4	12,680	2,556	376	77	1991
Panama	55	9	41	16	7	3	5	6	322	129	133	54	1987
Ecuador	66	12	39	12	10	7	6	7	1,794	997	170	97	1988
Uruguay	56	18	54	34	13	3	13	6	258	125	105	52	1990
Argentina	37	11	34	20	7	2	6	4	3,049	1,451	111	54	1991
Costa Rica	37	8	47	21	5	4	6	9	237	115	80	40	1991
COMPARISON													
United States	56	19	39	41	22	4	15	8	26,207	8,341	142	47	1992
Sweden	25	9	42	29	12	7	20	22	347	161	61	30	1993
Russian Federation	127	30	42	34	49	9	16	10	32,271	9,118	304	90	1994
Australia	47	13	49	36	24	4	25	10	1,354	477	97	36	1993

Source: World Health Statistics Annual 1987–1995 (WHO, 1987–1996)

*Injuries include the following ICD-9 codes: unintentional injuries (E800-949 and E980-989) and suicide (E950-959); E980-989 includes injury unknown whether unintentionally or purposefully inflicted.

cide. Young adult females are at high risk of suicide in rural areas of some developing countries, as discussed in Chapter 13 on intentional injuries.

Differences in age distributions between national populations can complicate international comparisons of crude injury rates. This is a problem when comparing an industrialized country, with minimal or no population growth and an aging population, to a developing country with rapid population growth and a larger proportion of children and young adults. However, age and/or sex differences can also complicate comparisons among regions if large migrant populations of young adults are concentrated in certain areas looking for work or other attractions. Such age differences within a country may also complicate the study of trends in injury rates over long periods of time, especially in countries where there have been large demographic shifts in the proportion of young adults in the total population.

Using crude rates, it is possible to adjust for age differences in populations by direct standardization to the World Standard population, which simulates the age distribution of the world's population (WHO, 1988c, 1992). The numbers of injury deaths among different age and sex strata of the standard population are calculated using age- and sex-specific rates separately for each of the different countries compared. A fictitious age-adjusted rate is obtained for each country using the total deaths in all age and sex groups in the standard population; these adjusted rates can then be compared.

The World Standard Population is similar in composition to the population of China, and it has an older age distribution than many of the developing countries, where high birth rates and rapid population growth are typical. For the age adjustment of rates in the Americas, the Pan American Health Organization has used a standard population based upon the estimated age distribution of the entire population of Latin America around 1960 (PAHO, 1986). When comparing two countries an alternative to using one of these special standard populations is to age-adjust the rates of one population to the population structure of the other population. This was done by Li and Baker (1991) for a comparison of injury mortality rates in China and the United States.

Methods of comparing mortality rates among small populations are available in statistical texts. By calculating confidence intervals for adjusted rates or standardized mortality ratios from indirect standardization, there is no undue importance attributed to differences resulting from random variability (Armitage and Berry, 1987).

Age-adjusted data are not available in most WHO publications for all types of injury. However, for the Americas, age-adjusted rates are available for certain unintentional injuries (PAHO, 1986, 1990). Age-adjusted rates have been prepared by the World Health Organization for some countries, and include rates for all injuries, traffic injuries, and suicide (WHO, 1990). Comparisons of injury rates among large countries and between rural and urban areas can provide useful insights to planners and researchers, as in a recent comparison of injury rates between China and the United States and between rural and urban areas of China (Li and Baker, 1991; WHO, 1991).

IMPACT OF INJURIES AS ASSESSED BY PREMATURE MORTALITY

While death rates provide an indication of the relative magnitude of the problem, they may not be the best measure of total health impact. Deaths due to old-age or occurring near the end of life tend to be caused by or attributed to conditions such as stroke, cardiac disease, or cancer. It is, therefore, unwise to rely too heavily on mortality statistics as a basis for policy decisions since this can result in a bias towards geriatric health problems that have relatively little effect on productivity.

The use of premature mortality, years of potential life lost (YPLL, PYLL or YLL) prior to age 65, has been advocated as a better indicator of the impact of injuries on society since it takes into account that injuries have a greater effect on young age groups than most other causes of death (Centers for Disease Control, 1986; Meade, 1980; Romeder and McWhinnie, 1977). In the United States, for example, injuries are by far the greatest cause of premature mortality (Baker et al., 1992; Smith and Falk, 1987). The assessment of YPLL requires the availability of age-specific mortality rates by cause. Such rates are, unfortunately, not available for populations in many of the poorer countries.

The calculation of YPLL involves multiplying the number of deaths within an age group during a period of time, usually one year, by the difference in years between the average age at death within the age group and an endpoint. The endpoint may be fixed or variable.

While a fixed endpoint of age 65 is most commonly used for international comparisons, other endpoints may be more appropriate. Some developed countries with long life expectancies use later ages such as 70 or 75-years-old.

An alternative to a fixed endpoint, such as age 65, is a variable endpoint. If local life tables are available and the life expectancy at different ages is known, the average life expectancy at the age of death for each age interval can be used as the endpoint for that interval. A disadvantage of this approach is that it gives greater weight to diseases of old age (Barss, 1991; Centers for Disease Control, 1986). This is somewhat at odds with the original objectives of the methodology. YPLL was developed to emphasize the economic significance of diseases such as tuberculosis, which, because of their frequency among young adults, have a greater impact than chronic diseases such as cancer (Dempsey, 1947).

As a result of high infant and child mortality rates from nutritional deficiencies and infectious diseases, some developing countries have life expectancies below age 50, and it may at first appear inappropriate to use even age 65 as an endpoint. However, it is important to recognize that low life expectancy at birth is due mainly to high mortality rates in infancy and early childhood. In such countries, life expectancy at age one, age five, or even later is greater than at birth. In a remote population of subsistence villagers in the highlands of Papua New Guinea, remaining life expectancies at different ages were as follows: at birth, 50.5 years; at age one, 53.5; at age five, 52.5; at age 20, 39.0; at age 40, 21.5; at age 60, 9.0; and at age 65, 8.0 (Lehmann, 1984). The effects of different endpoints in priority ranking of leading causes of death were compared to determine the

In order to demonstrate more vividly the seriousness of a disease which may lead to prolonged illness and death in youth or middle age, a computation has been made showing the potential loss in years of life resulting from deaths from heart diseases, cancer, and tuberculosis in 1944.

—Mary Dempsey, Decline in Tuberculosis: The Death Rate Fails to Tell the Entire Story, American Review of Tuberculosis, 1947.

most appropriate endpoint to use in the population (Barss, 1991). A fixed endpoint of 60-years-old gave results that closely approximated those obtained using the variable endpoint of life expectancy at age of death. An endpoint derived by adding five years to the life expectancy at age five, for example, (5 + 52.5) years, also provided results closely approximating those obtained using life expectancy at age of death as an endpoint. However, since the use of age 65 as an endpoint did not substantially affect the relative ranking of different health conditions, this standard endpoint was used in the study to facilitate international comparisons and consistency.

It is inappropriate and potentially misleading to use an early endpoint, such as age 50 or 55, for assessing YPLL from adult mortality. This was done, however, in a study on acquired immunodeficiency syndrome among adults in Africa (DeCock et al., 1990). If analysis of YPLL is restricted to adult age groups, the use of such an early endpoint may exaggerate the importance of certain health conditions and therefore bias the results (Barss, 1991). It is more appropriate to compare age-specific mortality rates for different causes of death.

Another consideration is the inclusion of infant deaths in the calculations. They are sometimes excluded. It may be reasonable to do so, particularly since deaths of infants (and the elderly) tend to be poorly diagnosed and underreported. However, to avoid the possibility of bias, it is best first to present the results of YPLL calculated with all ages from birth to age 64, and then to present alternatives, such as age one to 64.

There are several other possible refinements in the calculation of YPLL. Discounting has been used, particularly by economists (Murray et al., 1992; Murray and Lopez, 1996; Barnum, 1987); however, discounting of health benefits has been challenged and a range of rates should be used, including zero (Lancet editorial, 1992c). Years of life lost have been adjusted for the quality of life, including disability, during different phases of the life span (World Bank, 1993; Loomes and McKenzie, 1989; Robine, 1989). It also is possible to estimate losses of prior economic inputs of deceased persons, measured in years, as well as the losses of potential outputs, also in years. These can be combined to provide estimates of economic years of life lost or YELL (Barss, 1991).

The Pan American Health Organization now includes data on YPLL from various diseases and injuries in its publications of mortality statistics in the Americas (1986, 1988, 1990). YPLL from all causes of unintentional injury, including motor vehicle crashes, are compared to losses from other important health conditions in Table 3.4. Data are available by country for the five leading causes of YPLL in the Americas. One or more injury groups, including homicide, suicide, and unintentional injuries, such as motor vehicle crashes, were the leading cause of YPLL in most countries of the Americas.

In making calculations of YPLL, the Pan American Health Organization chose to group injuries of intent undetermined with unintentional injuries. When interpreting such data, it is important to be aware that state terrorism, the power of the government to terrorize people into submission (White, 1991), is prevalent in some countries. In those countries many homicides or war deaths are recorded as of undetermined intent.

More detailed YPLL data from the early 1980s, provided separately by sex and not restricted to the five leading causes of injuries (PAHO, 1986), show the following:

- In each country of the Americas, injuries as a whole were the leading source of YPLL;
- Unintentional injuries and injuries of undetermined intent were the leading contributors to YPLL for males in the Andean sub-region (Columbia, Ecuador, Peru, Venezuela);
- Unintentional and undetermined intent injuries, followed by homicide, were the first and second sources of YPLL in El Salvador, Guatemala, and Nicaragua;
- YPLL from unintentional and undetermined intent injuries were almost four times the YPLL from the second leading cause (intestinal infections) in Mexico and more than twice the second leading cause (heart diseases) in Brazil.

RELIABILITY AND VALIDITY OF REPORTS ON CAUSE OF DEATH FROM INJURIES

Reports of Injury Deaths

Deaths that occur in hospital tend to be reported; however, in rural areas of some developing countries, the majority of injury deaths occur far from hospital and are never reported (Barss, 1991). This selective underreporting can seriously bias injury mortality data. Common examples include drownings and suicides, since death is often immediate.

Investigation of Injury Deaths

An adequate investigation of the external cause and circumstances of injury deaths that occur in the community involves police, coroners, and pathologists. Poor communications, underreporting of deaths, long delays before reported deaths are investigated, staff shortages, inadequate laboratory tests, and lack of transport to remote areas can all hinder the investigation of injury deaths and reduce the reliability and validity of injury mortality data. A coroner's diagnosis of the underlying cause of death may never be communicated to the vital statistics bureau, and even if it is, the coded cause of death may not be modified in light of this additional information.

Certification and Coding

Some developing countries do have a civil registration system to collect mortality data and other vital statistics. These data are often based mainly upon hospital deaths. Unfortunately, errors are common in the certification of causes of death even for injury victims who die in hospital. Such errors result from incomplete medical certification, inaccurate diagnoses listed on the death certificate, and failure to carefully delineate the sequence of underlying causes of death. Some physicians simply list terminal cardiorespiratory arrest

Table 3.4 Years of potential life lost before age 65 per 100,000 population from leading causes by country* in the Americas

	Injuries			Chronic diseases		Infectious diseases		Total YPLL	Per cap GNP**	Year
	Uninten-tional†	Suicide	Homicide, war, etc.	Heart disease	Malignant neoplasms	Enteritis/ diarrhea	Influenza/ pneumonia			
SOUTH AMERICA										
Colombia	1506		972	524	482	531		7991	1139	1981
Ecuador	1913					1920	1013	12657	1160	1980
Chile	1636			307	659		228	5091	1320	1983
Argentina	1100			932	925		162	5629	2350	1981
Uruguay	753	175		581	945			4314	1900	1984
Peru	920					891	1257	7460	1090	1982
Paraguay	895			383	395	923	525	7400	1000	1984
CENTRAL AMERICA										
Guatemala	2723		3560			4387	2838	23659	930	1981
El Salvador	2341	379	1314	387		626		9922	820	1984
Nicaragua	1280		877	486		1041	346	8513	790	1977

Honduras	1655			443		1252	9010	740	1981
Panama	1192	133		230	389	206	4059	2330	1984
Costa Rica	694	159		276	576		3297	1480	1983
NORTH AMERICA									
United States	993	270	259	672	769		3918	17980	1983
Mexico	2234		532	441	393	639	7594	1973	1982
Canada	894	336		481	745		3210	14120	1984
CARIBBEAN									
Cuba	1622‡			514	596		4077		1983
Dominican Republic	844			464	271	303	5711	710	1981

* Countries with population > one million and 1986 per capita GNP < US$2500; Canada and USA included for comparison; only causes among the top five listed for each country

† All unintentional injuries, including motor vehicle crashes and intent undetermined (in some countries, substantial numbers of homicides and/or suicides may be included in this category)

** Annual per capita gross national product in 1986 U.S. dollars

‡ Includes all injuries, intentional and unintentional

Adapted from *Health Conditions in the Americas 1981–1984* (PAHO, 1986)

as the cause of death. This is useless information since the heart stops in all deaths. Such problems are not unique to developing countries, but are greatly exacerbated by a lack of resources for staff and training.

Even in countries where the majority of injury deaths occur in villages and go uncertified, efforts should be made to ensure that any deaths occurring in health facilities are properly certified and coded, since these deaths often provide the only basis for national statistics on causes of injury. In some cases, improper coding, mixing Nature of Injury codes with External Cause codes, and fragmentation of injury subgroups result in serious misrepresentation and underestimation of the relative importance of injuries as a cause of death (Barss, 1991).

In the Americas, medical certification of the cause of death has ranged from a high of 100 percent of deaths in Uruguay in 1986, to 30 percent in Guatemala in 1981, to a low of 11 percent in Honduras in 1983 (PAHO, 1986). Even with medical certification, the final cause of death may remain uncertain and be classified as "symptoms and ill defined conditions" (ICD 780–799). This "unknown" category varies greatly by country, for example, 9 percent of all deaths were of unknown cause in Costa Rica in 1979, 37 percent in Paraguay in 1980, and 85 percent in Honduras in 1983.

The proportion of YPLL included in the unknown cause category may be a more accurate indicator of the completeness of cause-of-death reporting than the proportion of deaths in this category. Cause-of-death determination is difficult in the elderly, even when competent medical certification is available (Fife, 1987; Fife and Rappaport, 1987), but deaths in old age are excluded in YPLL if a fixed endpoint of 65-years-old is used for the calculations.

In countries that have a well-developed health care and vital registration system, there still can be considerable difficulty in obtaining accurate data on causes of death (Friederici, 1988; Battle et al., 1987; Zemach, 1984; Scottolini and Weinstein, 1983). In the United States and most other developed countries, injury as a cause of death is underreported for the elderly. When injured, the elderly are more likely to die of complications than younger victims. The elderly and others who suffer delayed deaths are more likely to be certified to have died from a complication such as pneumonia, while the initial injury often is not mentioned on the death certificate (Fife, 1987; Fife and Rappaport, 1987). People with epilepsy and other serious diseases are at high risk of drownings, falls, and burns, but such deaths are often coded with epilepsy as the underlying cause. Similar reporting problems are likely to exist in countries with limited health care where complications may be more common.

Even in developed countries, death certificates typically lack details of the circumstances and the contributing factors, such as alcohol consumption. The problem is more severe in remote aboriginal communities where coroners' investigations may not be carried out at all, may be completed by telephone, or may fail to consider risk factors for which data are needed to plan interventions. Special mortality interviews have been developed to supplement the information from official death certification. Examples include the National Mortality Followback Survey in the United States (Seeman et al., 1993; National Center for Health Statistics, 1992; Poe et al., 1991) and surveys of alcohol and other risk factors for injury deaths among Canadian aboriginals (Damestoy and Barss, 1996; Jarvis and Boldt, 1982; Barss et al., 1997).

Misclassification of Intentional Injuries

Suicides are sometimes misclassified as unintentional or intent undetermined, so suicide tends to be underreported in many countries (Sainsbury, 1983; Eastwood, 1980; Jarvis et al., 1991). Underreporting may be more prevalent in countries where there is strong cultural aversion to suicide. The extent of underreporting may vary with the predominant method used, since hanging and firearm suicides are more difficult to conceal than suicide by poisoning or drowning (Monk, 1987).

Because misclassification of suicide among native Americans in Alaska was believed to be serious and suspected to be as high as 80 percent, a special study was carried out in 49 villages during 1979–84 (Marshall and Soule, 1988). Only five suicides had been reported officially by vital statistics, while 38 were recorded in the coroner's files. On the other hand, in Greenland, reports of suicide among the Inuit by the Danish National Board of Health were found to be quite reliable because of a better link between coroners' findings and vital statistics (Thorslund and Misfeldt, 1989).

Where state terrorism is widespread, many homicides and other violent deaths may remain unclassified or be categorized as injuries of unknown intent. In some countries, infanticides may also be misclassified. The rate of infant homicide in rural China was only 1 per 100,000 population during 1989. Hence, the possibility of substantial misclassification of intentional deaths as unintentional may need to be ruled out by more detailed investigation.

In the highlands of Papua New Guinea the situation differs, and overreporting of homicides is frequent (Barss, 1991). In some areas, there is little or no stigma attached to homicide, and death by an enemy warrior confers considerably more prestige and possibility for compensation than does death by disease or old age. As a result, families frequently attribute death by natural causes to old battle wounds sustained years ago. This causes difficulties for mortality interviewers and coders, who must rely almost entirely upon the family's history of the cause of death. Careful enquiry is necessary to avoid classifying deaths from medical illnesses as homicides.

METHODS FOR OBTAINING SUPPLEMENTAL INFORMATION ON CAUSES AND CIRCUMSTANCES OF INJURY DEATHS: COMMUNITY MORTALITY STUDIES

The data presented thus far derive from available statistical reports and do not provide information for the poorest countries. By using special surveys or community-based surveillance and mortality interviews, it is possible to obtain population-based data in countries that lack adequate national systems of vital statistics. Otherwise, where death reporting is poor, relying upon death certificates as the only source of data may cause gross underestimates in the extent of the injury problem.

Table 3.5 Community based studies of injury mortality in developing countries

Place	Investigators	Population	Major findings
North India	Gordon et al., 1962	11 rural villages 12,000 pop.	Burns and injuries from animals were leading causes of fatal injury.
			No deaths from motor vehicles.
			Male mortality 1.6 times that of females.
			Non-fatal injury rate higher in females.
India	Mohan et al., 1989	9 rural villages 25,000 pop.	Deaths and seriously disabling injuries primarily due to mechanized equipment in farming, and transportation.
Bangladesh	Zimicki, 1990; Zimicki et al., 1985	Matlab demographic surveillance area	Drownings were a leading cause of death, especially for young children.
	Fanneau and Blanchet, 1989	Women ages 15–44 in Matlab area	18 percent of all deaths were due to injury.
			Unmarried women at high risk of death from suicide, homicide, and complications of abortion.
Egypt	Grubb et al., 1988	Married women ages 15–49	Injuries the third leading cause of death (14 percent of all deaths), 28/100,000/year.
Nepal	Thapa, 1989	6300 rural villages	Injuries the fourth leading cause of death (10 percent of all deaths), 64/100,000/year (18 month household survey).
Papua New Guinea	Barss, 1991	Rural subsistence hamlets 30,000 pop.	Injuries the fourth leading cause of death, 50 percent intentional.
			Male rate 102/100,000/year; female rate 83/100,000.
			Female homicide and suicide rates exceptionally high.
	Barss, 1991	Periurban villages 6,000 pop.	Injuries the second leading cause of death, 44 percent intentional.
			Male rate 81/100/000/year; female, 110/100,000.
			Female homicide rate especially high.

The results of a few community-based studies are summarized in Table 3.5 to indicate the kinds of information obtained.

Mortality Interviews, Verbal Autopsies, and Psychological Autopsies with Lay Reporting of Mortality

Interviews with relatives or companions of injury victims can be used to determine either or both of the following (Barss, 1991; Damestoy and Barss, 1996; Barss et al., 1997):

- Cause of death, whether injury or medical illness, and if injury, the type of injury by external cause;
- Circumstances of injury deaths, including activity at the time of death as well as personal, environmental, and equipment factors.

In areas where many deaths occur away from a health facility, the causes may never be certified by a health worker. For injury deaths, there may be no systematic investigation by a coroner or autopsy by a pathologist. Even in areas with good reporting of deaths, the circumstances of an injury death often go unrecorded.

Where reporting and certification of deaths are poor, it may be unknown whether a death resulted from an injury or a medical illness. A structured interview of the symptoms prior to death and short history of the events around the time of death can be used by a medical epidemiologist to ascertain the cause(s) of death. Such interviews are a specialized form of mortality interview called *verbal autopsies*.

Verbal autopsies are often used in special study areas together with a system of community demographic surveillance of all vital events. When a community reporter notifies the project epidemiologist of a death, a mortality interviewer comes to the village to conduct a verbal autopsy so that the epidemiologist can code the cause of death (Snow et al., 1992; Gray et al., 1990; Garenne and Fontaine, 1990; Zimicki, 1990; Stephens, 1990; Gray, 1989; Kalter et al., 1989; Zimicki et al., 1985; WHO, 1978a).

Mortality interviews can be designed to determine the circumstances of an injury death. Information about personal, environmental, and equipment factors and about the activity at the time of death can be collected in a systematic manner for analysis. When used to study suicides, mortality interviews are often called *psychological autopsies*. Psychological autopsies can be used to determine if suicides were preceded by chronic psychiatric illness or precipitated by acute problems such as interpersonal conflict or abuse of alcohol and other drugs.

After the causes of death have been established by verbal autopsies, in-depth mortality interviews can be used to follow up and investigate the circumstances of specific types of fatal injuries, such as suicide. Several types of questionnaires may be needed for specific injuries since at least some of the environmental or equipment risk factors for some, such as a drowning or a housefire, may be different from others, such as a suicide or homicide.

A structured questionnaire can be helpful in obtaining details about the circumstances of an injury. For a case reported by verbal autopsy or death certification simply as a road traffic death, it would be helpful, for public health purposes, to have further information, such as the following:

- Whether the victim was a pedestrian, cyclist, motorcyclist, vehicle occupant, or driver;
- Whether the vehicle was a car, bus, motorcycle, bicycle, or open-backed truck;
- Whether the victim was wearing a helmet or seat belt or was ejected from the vehicle;
- The location of the incident, including whether at an intersection or curve;
- Whether collision involved a fixed roadside object;
- Involvement of alcohol.

When verbal autopsies are used to determine the cause of death, structured interviews with relatives are used to establish the conditions, if, for example, diarrhea, skin rash, or cough were associated with the death. Combinations of open-ended and structured questions are used to obtain the basic story of the illness, as well as to establish symptom complexes or syndromes. The open-ended story is generally the most important means of ascertaining the external cause of injuries. However, the structured part of the verbal autopsy interview, including symptoms and their temporal sequence, can be useful to distinguish certain medical causes of death from an alleged injury.

Organized systems of lay reporting and mortality interviews are probably best used to study all causes of death; in this way the relative importance of injuries compared to other diseases can be established (Barss, 1991). In addition, such systems are useful for clinical trials of various treatments, vaccines, and other disease control programs which would otherwise be impossible in rural populations in developing countries (Pacqué-Margolis et al., 1990).

Community-based surveillance of vital events by lay reporting followed by verbal autopsies has been used to determine causes of death in the Matlab area in Bangladesh (Zimicki, 1986; 1990; Zimicki et al., 1985), by the British Medical Research Council in the Gambia, by the French l'Office de la Recherche Scientifique et Technique Outre-Mer in Senegal (Garenne and Fontaine, 1990), by the Papua New Guinea Institute of Medical Research in the Tari Basin (Barss, 1991; Riley et al., 1986; Lehmann, 1984), and by others in Kenya and the Yemen (Snow et al., 1992; Myntti et al., 1991). Demographic surveillance is somewhat costly, requires regular epidemiological supervision, and is feasible mainly on a research basis for selected areas of a country.

Despite the difficulties of underreporting or overreporting intentional injuries, there is reason to believe that, in general, unintentional injury deaths are probably more reliably diagnosed than many other non-injury causes.

Good quality information is, therefore, potentially obtainable, regardless of the level of a country's development (Smith and Barss, 1991). Of all the reported causes of death, the data for unintentional injuries should be the most reliable, and it has even been suggested that cause-of-death reports of injuries could be used as a standard for comparison with reports from other causes (Grubb et al., 1988).

High levels of consistency between two reporting methods in Egyptian and Kenyan studies suggest that it is possible to obtain reliable cause-of-death data on injuries in developing countries, even when the extent of medical certification and the accuracy of diagnosis for other health conditions is low:

- In Egypt, evaluation of the standard vital registration system using detailed interviews of relatives and record reviews for deaths of married women ages 15–49 indicated that 93 percent of injury deaths were correctly registered compared with 53 percent of non-injury deaths. When the cause of injury was reported in both systems there was 74 percent agreement (Grubb et al., 1988);
- In Kenya, verbal autopsy diagnosis for childhood deaths from unintentional injuries had a sensitivity of 78 percent, a specificity of 100 percent, and a positive predictive value of 88 percent when compared to medically confirmed diagnoses (Snow et al., 1992).

A household epidemiological study was conducted in nine villages in India with the help of village youths. For policy purposes, the importance of injuries was established with respect to other health priorities (Mohan et al., 1989). The study showed that a large number of rural injuries are never reported in official statistics, and that public perceptions of the relative importance of various agents may be inaccurate. This is not surprising, given the rarity of death from any particular injury in a single village. These misperceptions emphasize the importance of surveillance of an adequate population base for an appropriate duration to establish the impact of injuries and their patterns in the community.

Problems of underreporting and misclassification using lay surveillance and structured mortality interviews are of potential concern (Chandramohan et al., 1994), but concerns are minor in many developing countries given the extensive underreporting of village deaths in non-surveillance areas and inadequate medical certification and coding of injury deaths in hospitals (Barss, 1991).

Other Mortality Surveys

For injuries that are rapidly fatal, simple community surveys of representative villages, perhaps as part of other surveys or a census, may help to determine whether a serious public health problem exists in a district. This may be particularly important for certain fatal injuries where victims seldom survive to reach a hospital, such as drowning and suicide.

Short retrospective questionnaire surveys of staff who work in rural health center networks are often useful, since permanent employees in a rural area with a stable population are often able to recall many of the injury deaths in their locality for the previous several years. Recall is better for deaths, particularly of adults, than for minor illnesses (Gray et al., 1990). This approach was useful in Papua New Guinea (Barss et al., 1984). A hospital study had shown that falls from trees were a serious source of morbidity in a rural province; a subsequent survey of key informants at rural health centers showed that such falls were also a significant source of unreported mortality.

Key informants from small aboriginal communities may be able to describe causes and preventable factors for most injury deaths in their communities for a recall period of at least ten years. Barss, meeting with rural aboriginals from northern Québec for 1 hour using this approach, obtained information that matched or exceeded data that had been collected routinely by rural health facilities for 10 years. Community representatives were able to provide information about circumstances of injuries not recorded in official data sources. These included personal factors such as alcohol intoxication for traffic injuries, and, for drownings, environmental factors such as wind, wave, and ice conditions and equipment factors such as whether a boat or snowmobile was involved.

INJURY MORTALITY DATA SOURCES IN OTHER SECTORS

The creative investigator or policymaker will seek out or gradually learn about potential data sources in other sectors. Even in jurisdictions where coroners investigate and prepare reports on many injury deaths, these valuable data are often relatively neglected and may never be communicated to vital statistics databases or otherwise published. These data include homicides, and suicides, and unintentional injuries such as drownings and traffic deaths.

Two weeks spent abstracting data from records in the Instituto Medico-Legal in Rio de Janeiro, Brazil, allowed Baker (1977) to determine the circumstances and population-based rates of pedestrian deaths in the city by identifying cases listed in the log book as either pedestrian, MVA (motor vehicle accident), or simply "accident", and then reviewing the death certificates and medical examiner records for those cases.

Police reports are also a potential source of information about road traffic deaths and intentional injuries. At community levels, police data can be obtained directly from local files of crash reports. At regional or national levels, summary reports may be available. Simple computer programs are being introduced into developing countries for entry and analysis of police crash reports and should simplify and speed up research on traffic injuries (Transport and Road Research Laboratory, 1991).

While police records are often useful for obtaining information about motor vehicle injuries, considerable underreporting occurs even in developed countries (Hutchinson, 1987; Barancik and Fife, 1985; Sande and Thorson, 1975). More often, injuries of pedestrians and cyclists are underreported than those involving two motor vehicles, since victims may be taken to hospital before the police become involved. In Rio de Janeiro, Baker found that police counts of traffic deaths failed to include any later deaths in hospital resulting in an underestimation of traffic fatalities by 75 percent.

Other sources can be even more misleading. For example, the Railway Board of India reported 213 railway deaths in 1975–76, while the Ministry of Planning's statistical report listed 10,393 (Mohan, 1984). The Indian Railways apparently did not include in their mortality statistics people who fell from or were struck by trains. Their definition of "accident" excluded at least 98 percent of the deaths.

Records of occupational injuries are sometimes available from sources such as departments of labor, unions, or occupational hygienists in industry. The availability and validity of such sources vary greatly by country, depending on their purpose and the skills and resources of staff who oversee and maintain them. Insurance companies are another potential source of mortality data, since actuaries need reliable information about the probability of death at various ages to establish their rates.

Political agreements that provide compensation to aboriginal residents for environmental damage, loss of land, or other reasons can validate the completeness of other sources of information on deaths. One example is the death list of the Beneficiaries of the James Bay Agreement in Québec, Canada (Damestoy, 1994).

Particularly valuable sources of information are local newspaper accounts of deaths and hospitalizations from injuries. They often contain information about the age and sex of the victim as well as the cause and agent of injuries and poisonings. For certain types of unintentional injuries, such as drownings and fires, these stories can be relatively complete and contain more useful details about preventable factors for injury deaths than do coroners' reports (Rainey and Runyan, 1992). The Canadian Red Cross Society uses volunteer retirees to collect files of newspaper clippings on drownings. Commercial services provide clippings, and articles in major newspapers are referenced in special computer databases. On the other hand, while newspaper reports often provide detailed information about specific intentional injuries, they seriously underreport the numbers of such events and are unreliable for surveillance of suicides and assaults (Jones et al., 1992).

chapter 4

Assessing the Health Impact of Injuries: Morbidity

A nonfatal injury is more ambiguous than a death. Questions of severity and duration of injury are largely irrelevant in the surveillance of injury deaths, but they are important considerations in epidemiologic studies of morbidity. In the study of injury morbidity, it is necessary to consider the following:

- External causes and circumstances of injuries;
- Nature and severity of different types of injuries;
- Nature and duration of disability.

The definition of an injury varies and determines the scope of injury morbidity. Surveillance or research on nonfatal injuries includes injuries managed in hospitals and emergency rooms, at outpatient clinics or doctors' offices, and at home. The complexity and cost of treatment offer a guide to the severity of an injury; however when access to care is limited, severe injuries may be treated at either a simple health facility or not at all.

Specific severity scales quantify the severity of an injury based on the nature of the injuries sustained (Committee on Injury Scaling, 1990; Robertson, 1992; Osler et al., 1997) rather than by the type of treatment facility; however, such data are seldom available for routine surveillance of injury morbidity in developing countries. The duration of hospitalization and/or disability from injury is another index of severity and becomes an issue when it is necessary to quantify the incidence or prevalence of long-term disability from various types of injury.

In the absence of specific injury severity scores, severity may be crudely estimated by considering the following variables:

- Outcome (death/survival);
- Nature of the treatment facility;
- Numbers and types of injuries;
- Duration of hospitalization;
- Duration and nature of disability.

Estimates tend to be most valid when there is reasonable access by the population to all levels of the health system, including primary, secondary, and tertiary care facilities.

This chapter considers existing processes of surveillance and reporting of injury morbidity, availability of official injury morbidity data, quantification of injuries by level of care, reliability and validity of injury morbidity data, classification of impairment, disability, and handicap, data sources in other health sectors, and a few practical examples of community oriented injury research from a district hospital.

PROCESS OF REPORTING MORBIDITY

While most countries have at least a token system for investigating and reporting on fatal injuries, reporting of nonfatal injuries is often unregulated and less standardized. Although a spinal fracture with paralysis or a head injury with permanent loss of intellectual function may cause a lifetime of disability for the victim and be far more costly for the family and community than a death, few countries have an established system of mandatory reporting and investigation into the circumstances of nonfatal injuries. While relatively minor infections such as food-borne diarrheal outbreaks often command mandatory reporting and costly investigations, there are no formal procedures for reporting or investigating severe traffic injuries, falls, burns, or suicide attempts.

Ambiguity may explain why investigations of nonfatal injuries are so sporadic. The definition of an injury that should be counted for clinical or research study or legal action is arbitrary, whereas death is unequivocal.

Relatively minor infectious diseases often trigger definitive responses from the public health system because a culture-positive infection is generally considered to be clear-cut and easy to count. This is actually not always the case, since positive cultures often occur without clinical disease. This suggests that as injury definitions improve and the surveillance of morbidity from injuries improves and becomes more systematized, the public health response for injuries may become more definitive and immediate.

Data from health facilities are most useful and provide a representative portrait of injuries when there is a relatively well-defined population with good access to the health facilities in its area. A defined service population, together with census data, allows for calculating hospitalization or clinic visits as rates per unit of population per year by age and sex; this allows comparisons of incidences of specific injuries among different regions. Population-based injury analysis is relatively simple on a small island with only one facility and no roads, but extremely complex in a metropolitan area where many clinics, health centers, and hospitals serve the same population.

Problems of Definition

Cultural and other factors often determine what constitutes an injury. The United States National Health Interview Survey definition requires that, to be counted, an injury must have caused the person to seek medical attention or have resulted in more than one day of restricted activity (National Center for Health Statistics, 1985).

Because of limited access to medical care in many countries, it is difficult to compare injury morbidity rates between countries, even if the same coding is used for the type, cause, and severity of injury. In addition, other conditions, such as back pain, may or may not be reported as injuries, depending upon whether they are recognized to be the result of a specific episode of trauma.

While injuries are important as a cause of premature death, they are also a significant cause of disability days, which are days lost from normal activities such as subsistence farming or paid employment. Although temporary disabilities are obviously most frequent, injuries are also the source of many long-term or permanent disabilities. Even seemingly minor injuries often result in various disabilities that may be relatively prolonged, lasting a month or longer (Yates et al., 1991).

Assessing the Nature and Severity of Injuries

While injuries can be classified on the basis of duration of disability or severity of injury, for routine epidemiologic surveillance and public health policy it is most practical to simply analyze the number of hospitalizations and their duration for different types of injuries, and the numbers of emergency room and clinic visits. However, when clinicians compare treatment results for severe injuries between hospitals, a scale of severity ensures comparability of cases.

If patterns of hospitalization and availability of beds are known, the average duration of stay and the range in days provides a rough estimate of the severity (and cost) of different types of injuries. Brief hospitalizations of one day or less often involve simple observation of minor injuries and acute poisonings or are used to arrange referrals for victims of suicide attempts or domestic assaults to more appropriate care. Hospitalizations of one day are also used for observation of possible head injuries or to monitor the circulation of a fractured limb that has been immobilized in a plaster cast and might become too tight from swelling. If the principal Nature of Injury code specifies a minor injury such as a bruise, there were probably no serious injuries.

Separate tabulation of the number of cases hospitalized for only one day allows the number of more severe cases to be quantified, although in isolated facilities with poor transport or with many vacant beds, prolonged hospitalizations may occur for social rather than for medical reasons. The duration of hospitalization also provides a crude estimate of the direct costs of treatment, and average durations for different types of injuries and diseases can be compared.

Purpose of Recordkeeping at Health Facilities

Hospitalization data are the most ubiquitous sources of information about injury morbidity, since most hospitals keep patient records for treatment, administrative, and financial purposes. Nevertheless, there are many hospitals in developing countries where the quality of records is poor, and there may be no system for storage or retrieval. Records in emergency rooms and clinics tend to be worse and, if they exist at all, often consist of only a few words scribbled on a single line of the form used to record the number of treatments provided each day.

Injury Morbidity in the Community

Injuries that receive no formal treatment remain totally unrecorded except in the rare instances of special interview surveys in the community. Confidential population surveys are needed to obtain data on unreported injuries such as acute poisonings and suicide attempts. Data on the prevalence of chronic impairment, disability, and handicap from injuries is generally available only if a special disability survey has been conducted in a population, and surveys of the incidence of disability are even rarer.

The process of obtaining injury data from hospitalizations and clinic visits will be discussed first since these record systems and procedures are common, albeit imperfect.

PROCESS OF REPORTING INJURY MORBIDITY DATA FROM HEALTH FACILITIES

Inpatient Wards

Physicians or other health providers record the nature of injuries in treatment records. Depending upon their interest in prevention, they may record the external cause and circumstances of the injuries; this is the exception rather than the rule even in high-income countries. An admission diagnosis may be recorded by a ward clerk or nurse in a summary record book of all admissions.

When the patient is discharged from hospital, the health provider is often required to provide a discharge diagnosis for the patient's chart. If the hospital is fortunate enough to have a medical records clerk, these discharge diagnoses are compiled and sent to a provincial or national registry for centralized coding and tabulation. In some countries, there are trained coders at every hospital; in such facilities, WHO ICD codes are assigned to each case at the hospital. One External Cause code and any number of Nature of Injury codes are assigned, but there is one principal Nature of Injury code. Unless coders are very knowledgeable about the relative severity of injuries, a minor injury may be coded as the principal injury if it was listed first by the physician.

Data from patients admitted to hospitals can be useful sources of information, but only if attention is given to maintaining basic recordkeeping and ensuring that physicians record the external causes of injuries in patient histories and discharge diagnoses. It is easier to avoid double counting of injuries if records distinguish new admissions from readmissions for the same health conditions, if transfers to or from other health facilities are recorded, and if chronic sequelae of injuries are properly coded as such.

Emergency Departments

Few hospitals have computerized emergency department records, even in developed countries. In developing countries, sometimes only the nature of the injury and treatment are recorded on a common daily treatment record for all patients seen.

Special surveys can assess external causes and nature of the injuries that present to emergency rooms; however, facilities must be carefully selected to ensure that they represent the situation for a defined population, and survey forms should include a space for the external cause of injury. If regular staff who collect data are responsible for clinical services, data collection may be abandoned when they are overworked or occupied with resuscitation and treatment of a severe case. For this reason severe injuries are sometimes omitted from recording data and these omissions can introduce bias.

Emergency room surveillance cannot be sustained in all hospitals, but surveillance in a few selected hospitals helps estimations of injury patterns in a community. In illustration, preventive medicine residents spent two months abstracting emergency room data on Hopi Indians treated in the two United States Indian Health Service hospitals, where virtually all Hopis are treated. The residents were able to describe the circumstances of all emergency room-treated injuries that occurred during a two-year period in a defined Native American population, and to determine that almost half of all injuries occurred in the 15–29-year age group. This group had especially high rates of self-inflicted injury, motor vehicle crashes, and assaults (Simpson et al., 1983).

A permanent emergency room injury surveillance system developed in Australia and used at a sample of emergency rooms throughout Canada has been adapted for continuous injury surveillance in all hospitals and clinics serving aboriginals and other inhabitants of the Northwest Territories.

Outpatient Clinics, Health Centers, and Aid Posts

In some areas, nurses and other health providers may have to see dozens, even hundreds, of patients each day. Detailed record keeping may be completely impractical in undeveloped countries. Nevertheless, most staff do keep a one line record of each patient to note the problem and treatment. The most that can be extracted from such records are summaries of the numbers of lacerations, burns, sores, etc. that were seen. A space on the forms for external causes would improve the utility of such data for injury surveillance.

AVAILABILITY OF POPULATION-BASED INJURY MORBIDITY DATA FROM HEALTH FACILITIES

While hospital case reports and case series about injuries are common, few come from hospitals with a well-defined catchment population with good access to the facility. Nor do they include figures for the population at risk, used as denominators for calculation of injury rates. Exceptions include studies from Papua New Guinea of falls from trees and other tree-associated injuries (Barss et al., 1984), clothing burns associated with grass skirts, and untreated epilepsy (Barss and Wallace, 1983). The approaches used are described as practical case studies at the end of this chapter.

IMPACT OF INJURY MORBIDITY AS ASSESSED BY SPECIFIC INJURIES AND BY AGE AND SEX

In a defined population, hospitalization rates for different injuries can be compared by age and sex. Even when this is not possible, the proportion or percent of hospitalizations or bed days from various injuries and diseases can be compared by age and sex. Hospitalization data for specific external causes of injury by age and sex are useful in identifying high risk groups, as discussed below in the section about case reports of tree-related falls and burns from open fires in Papua New Guinea.

The rates or proportions of clinic visits at different levels of the health system (primary and secondary care facilities) provide a complementary view of the burden of less severe injuries.

The burden of morbidity from specific types of injuries suggests different or additional priorities than those using only mortality data. In many developing countries and aboriginal populations, falls are among the leading two or three causes of hospitalization for injury, but are an uncommon cause of death. In populations with a large proportion of elderly persons or with extensive tree agriculture, falls are an important cause of mortality. Traffic injuries are often a common cause of both mortality and morbidity. In contrast, drownings are a common cause of death but a rare cause of hospitalization in many developing countries. In industrialized countries with large numbers of home swimming pools, near drowning may be more common than fatal drownings.

RELIABILITY AND VALIDITY OF INJURY MORBIDITY DATA FROM HEALTH FACILITIES

Assessing the Limitations of Injury Data from Health Facilities

Injury data from health facilities should be reviewed with the awareness that serious biases can result from potential problems at all steps in the recording, reporting, coding, and tabulation of data. The facility's accessibility to the population and the public's confidence in the staff must also be considered.

Clinical and Epidemiological Diagnoses in Health Facilities

Clinicians are most interested in the nature of an injury(s) since this determines the type of treatment and operation required. Hospital administrators are interested in the nature of injuries and the ensuing surgical procedures since these determine budgets, facilities, and personnel needed for treatment. Epidemiologists, on the other hand, are more interested in whether a fall was from a motorcycle or a tree than in the precise details of the injuries and treatment. Fortunately, it is relatively simple to modify hospital records and coding to provide the information needed for injury control.

Coding of Hospital Injury Data

As a consequence of inadequate population or community based data, much of the information about injury morbidity is derived from hospital records. These records tend to emphasize more severe nonfatal injuries. Since hospital data are based upon clinical records, only nature of injury data may be available (Barss and Masson, 1996).

Even when data are coded by external cause, there can be a lack of important details if codes are not used at an appropriate level of detail. For example, in Taiwan, the failure of coders to use the fourth digit codes for traffic injuries made it impossible to distinguish between injuries from motorcycles and those caused by other motor vehicles (Wu and Malison, 1990). This was a serious omission, since motorcycles comprised 83 percent of registered vehicles in Taiwan.

For the study of morbidity, hospital and health center data would be more useful if external cause coding for all injury cases in hospital discharge and clinic records were used (see Chapter 2 for a discussion of injury coding). This would require, first, that physicians or other health providers briefly record the external cause of injury in the patient's record, and second, that the record later be coded correctly by staff in the hospital medical records department or, at a provincial or national level, by using the coding manuals of the International Classification of Diseases (ICD) (WHO, 1978b, 1992) or an adaptation of another system such as the Nordic injury classification for hospitals discussed in Chapter 2.

A brief supplementary version of the external cause codes is available in the ICD manuals. This version is relatively simple to use and can be reduced to fit onto a few pages; it contains the major headings for different injury groups (WHO, 1992). However, where patient loads are heavy and record keeping is poor, extra resources may need to be available to maintain even minimal records.

Impact of Access and Trust on Validity of Injury Data from Health Facilities

The validity and utility of hospital data as a reflection of disease patterns in the community depend upon a number of factors. If most patients who die from a particular injury do so before reaching a hospital, it may be assumed mistakenly that the injury is not a serious public health problem in the community. Drowning and suicide are examples of injuries with such a high immediate fatality rate that victims seldom reach hospitals, especially in remote areas.

Similarly, hospital statistics are misleading as a record of the overall patterns of serious nonfatal injury in the community if the general public does not have access to facilities, if public confidence in the health system is low, or if the primary care and referral system for transferring injured patients to hospitals is poor.

The capability of referral is affected by the confidence of rural health workers in a hospital and its staff, the availability and efficiency of communication, and the suitability and speed of transportation networks for patient transfers. Referrals from remote areas are unlikely if rural peasants are made to bear all transportation costs from their own limited resources. Referral patterns to hospital may differ for different age and sex groups. For example, male children may be taken long distances to health facilities for serious illness more often than females (Chen et al., 1981).

In spite of the limitations of information from hospitals, such data are usually readily available and can be useful as a guide to the more severe non-fatal injuries in an area. Hospitals in isolated areas with a defined catchment population may be more useful for sampling purposes than hospitals in areas where patients have other choices.

Rural health centers are another potential source of injury data, but limitations similar to those for hospitals may apply. Patients sometimes bypass health centers to seek care at a hospital.

Simple Estimates of Validity of Health Facility Data

A review of sample records can provide estimates of the number of patients from outlying areas. Such estimates help ascertain if the population of patients in the hospital represents more severe cases in the catchment region. This is obviously not the case if most patients reside in villages or neighborhoods close to the hospital.

If there is a well-developed primary care and referral network, the hospital population may reasonably represent rural as well as urban areas. If so, it may be possible to use hospital data to estimate lower limits for true incidence in the population of nonfatal severe injuries of various types, such as spinal cord injuries. When comparing injury hospitalization rates between urban populations and rural populations, it is important to consider that people from rural communities often must be admitted to their district hospital for diagnostic X-rays and other simple treatments that are outpatient services for city residents who live near a hospital. In countries where there are many private health providers, injured persons are often seen in private clinics instead of hospitals.

In fact, most of the available literature about injuries in developing countries consists of hospital reports, particularly the information about specific types of injuries. Injuries most likely to reach hospital include falls, burns, poisonings, traffic injuries, wounds from cutting tools, and penetrating wounds. Some victims of animal bites may reach hospital, although it is believed that in certain countries, a majority of snake bite victims do not seek medical care because of traditional beliefs and the remoteness of villages (Warrell, 1990).

INJURY MORBIDITY DATA FROM COMMUNITY SURVEYS

The lack of community-based injury morbidity data may be rectified because of recent interest in using special surveys to obtain population-based data on the incidence of various diseases, including injuries (Kroeger, 1983). Morbidity is often studied in conjunction with mortality (Gray, 1989) during special surveys or by community surveillance with lay reporting.

In general, smaller samples or shorter study periods are adequate for morbidity surveys, since for any given cause of injury, nonfatal injuries are usually many times more frequent than deaths. There are occasional exceptions, as in the case of drownings.

In contrast to other diseases, identifying and coding information about injuries rely on external cause coding instead of a complicated medical diagnosis. Information necessary for coding can often be obtained in surveys by simple histories from lay observers without a need for more detailed histories of symptom complexes and/or medical investigations required to diagnose medical illnesses. Many health and demographic surveys are conducted in developing countries; the inclusion of simple questions about injuries in these surveys could provide invaluable and reasonably reliable information upon which to base prevention programs.

A potential problem with community surveys of morbidity from injuries is that people often forget nonfatal events. Only the most severe or most recent injuries are reported during an interview unless a short recall period or frequent reinterviews are used; this greatly increases the cost of surveys.

The results of an international collaborative study of the incidence of nonfatal injuries in children and adolescents under 20 years of age in Brazil, Chile, Cuba, and Venezuela showed that falls were the leading cause of unintentional injury in all four countries (Bangdiwala et al., 1990a). The survey used both household interviews and institutional data from hospitals.

Table 4.1 summarizes three surveys in Nepal that illustrate urban-rural differences in causes of nonfatal injuries, and the different results from a population-based community survey and a tertiary health facility.

IMPACT OF INJURY MORBIDITY ON IMPAIRMENT, DISABILITY, AND HANDICAP

Long-term and permanent disabilities from injuries are a serious burden for affected individuals and their families. The study and classification of disabilities in developing countries is still at a rudimentary stage with little published literature (WHO, 1991; Colodey and Griew, 1982). Recognition of the importance of disabilities is reflected in the concept of disability-adjusted life years lost (DALYS), a combination of years of life lost and years lived with a disability; by 2020, major depression and motor vehicle injuries are projected to

Table 4.1 Injury morbidity: community and hospital-based studies of nonfatal injury in Nepal

Place	Year	Population and method	Most common nonfatal injuries
Rural Nepal	1985-86	Periodic household interviews of 6300 rural villagers	Injuries as frequent as the most common illness (diarrhea)
			Cutting/piercing, 64%
			Burns/scalds, 13%
			Falls, 8%
Urban Kathmandu	1987	Survey of casualty department attendees in tertiary hospital	Falls, 40%
			Traffic-related, 20%
			Burns/scalds, 3%
			In children <15 yr., falls, 62%
		Survey of admissions to tertiary hospital	Traffic-related, 46%
			Burns/scalds, 25%
			Poisoning, 12%

Source: Thapa, 1989.

become respectively the second and third leading causes of DALYS (Murray and Lopez, 1996).

The United Nations (UN) has compiled disability statistics from national household surveys, population censuses, and population-based administrative record systems from 55 countries, including several developing countries (WHO, 1991). This information is contained in the United Nations Disability Statistics Data Base (DISTAT) (United Nations, 1988). From this source, the UN Statistical Office has published a Disability Statistics Compendium (United Nations, 1990). To assist in establishing an international standard for classification of disabilities, the World Health Organization developed the International Classification of Impairments, Disabilities, and Handicaps (WHO, 1980).

Impairment, disability, and handicap are important technical terms used in surveys for disabilities from injuries and other conditions (Yates et al., 1991; Colodey and Griew, 1982; Mitchell, 1981). Inconsistent use of these terms to define affected individuals in different surveys has complicated the international comparison of results.

An *impairment* is a loss or abnormality of psychological, physiological, or anatomical structure or function. Examples include blindness, deafness, paralysis or amputation of a limb.

A *disability* is a restriction or lack of ability to perform an activity within the range considered normal for humans. This includes a functional limitation or restriction of activity resulting from an impairment. Examples include difficulty in seeing, talking, hearing, walking, moving about the house, going to market, gardening, feeding oneself, cooking, and lighting a fire.

A *handicap* is a limitation resulting from an impairment or disability that prevents or inhibits the affected individual from fulfilling a normal role. The term also describes the social and economic roles of impaired or disabled persons that place them at a disadvantage compared to others in a specific environment or culture. Examples include inability to work, underemployment, being bedridden, confinement to home, social isolation, and inability to use public transport.

Prevention or control strategies differ for impairments, disabilities, and handicaps. Primary or secondary prevention is focused on preventing impairment; tertiary prevention is focused on preventing or reducing disability, and on equalizing opportunities within society for people with handicaps.

A classification list for causes of impairment has been prepared based on the International Classification of Diseases by the United Nations Expert Group (United Nations, 1984). Several of the listed causes include injury—motor vehicle accidents [*sic*], other transport accidents, accidental poisoning, falls, fire, operations of war, and other external causes, including natural and environmental factors. The list is broad and general, and WHO states that further evaluation and refinement are needed. They suggest using the classification in conjunction with the International Labor Organization's Classification of Industrial Accidents According to Agency.

The UN Expert Group on disability statistics recommended that disabilities from injury should be classified by External Cause codes, such as for a fall, rather than by the Nature of Injury, such as a fracture. Most countries are not using this classification, and, as a result, there is still marked variation in reporting injury data by cause. The

Expert Group recommended preparation of a standardized short list of causes based upon the ICD for use in surveys and censuses.

Estimates of the percent of the population disabled are affected by which set of questions, impairment or disability, is used to designate the disabled, and by what is perceived as an impairment or disability within a specific country. Impairment questions, such as those used in the presence of blindness or paralysis, generally give lower estimates than disability questions, such as those used when the subject has difficulty seeing, moving, or reaching (United Nations, 1990; Chamie, 1989).

Many disability surveys are difficult to compare because in some the results are expressed as a population-based rate, while in others, no denominator is provided and a simple percentage distribution of different causes is given. When a rate is provided, it may be unclear if this is an incidence rate of new disabilities during a defined time period, such as one year, or the prevalence of all disabilities found to be present at one time during the survey. It is sometimes unclear whether the term "accident" is being used to describe only unintentional injuries or includes intentional injuries.

Various detailed classifications for measuring the severity of temporary and permanent disabilities after injury are currently being developed and tested (Yates et al., 1991). Such systems may be useful for developing countries, although they must be simplified and adapted to suit local conditions (Colodey and Griew, 1982; Griew and Colodey, 1982).

With respect to specific disabilities, injuries are important causes of physical disabilities, less so for disabilities of hearing/speaking, vision, reduced mental capacity, and psychological disabilities. However, if consideration is limited to currently preventable causes, excluding categories such as old age, unknown, congenital, etc., injuries would be relatively more important.

Injuries are a prominent cause of disability in developing countries. In illustration, in a survey in rural Nepal, Thapa (1989) found that 2.6 percent of villagers were totally disabled, and that 25 percent of these disabilities had resulted from injuries. Of all disabilities from injuries, 19 percent were attributed to falls and 17 percent to burns.

The contribution of injuries to impairment and disability in several countries is described in Table 4.2. Population-based prevalence rates are presented in Table 4.3.

The incidence and prevalence of disability from injury is high in very remote rural communities where wounds and fractures are neglected for prolonged periods and become complicated by infection, deformity, and stiffness. For example, an open wound of a joint or tendon may lead to septic arthritis or to scarring in a tendon sheath with permanent loss of function. This is supported by reports of disabilities from rural Nepal and India (Thapa, 1989; Gordon et al., 1962), and by reports from rural Haryana, India, of prolonged recoveries from agricultural injuries as a result of inadequate first aid and treatment (Varghese and Mohan, 1990a). In most surveys, little information is obtained about the causes of disabling injuries, including environmental hazards, equipment, and personal factors. It would be useful to develop a supplementary section of questions about external causes for inclusion in questionnaires. Examples of information that could be helpful for injury control include:

Table 4.2 Injury morbidity: injuries as a proportion of all impairments or disabilities

Country	Date	Survey results
Zimbabwe	1981	Impairments: 32% due to unintentional injury; 13% to war
		Age range of majority (61%) of injury-impaired people: 15–59 years
		War-related impairments: most victims (77%–93%) were civilians
		Mental handicaps: 33% from unintentional injury; 13% from war
		Ocular impairments: 29% from unintentional injury (43% of near-total bilateral losses and 67% of monocular impairments from injuries at home); 7% from war
		Upper limb impairments, excluding paralysis: 52% from unintentional injury; 19% from war
Kenya	1981	Impairments: 12% due to injury
		Paraplegia from unint. injury: 45% from home injuries; 26% from traffic injuries
China	1987	All causes of physical disability: 31% due to injury; injury leading cause
		Preventable causes of physical disability: 31% due to injury
		Preventable causes of hearing/speaking disability: 22% due to injury (includes noise-induced hearing loss)
		Preventable reduced mental capacity: 13% due to injury
		Preventable disability of vision: 2% due to injury
Nepal	1980	Disabilities: 18% due to injury
		In the hills: 27% of male and 17% of female disabilities due to injury
		In lowlands: 12% of male and 8% of female disabilities due to injury
India	1981	In urban areas: 28% of amputations, 42% of dysfunctional joints, and 22% of limb deformities due to injury
		In rural areas: 22% of amputations, 42% of dysfunctional joints, and 27% of limb deformities due to injury

Source: World Health Statistics Annual 1990 (WHO, 1991).

- If disabilities from spinal and head injuries were caused by falls from trees or roofs, or crashes of bicycles, motorcycles, open trucks, or cars;
- If blindness had a preventable cause, such as poisoning by abuse of chemical agents such as methyl alcohol. For monocular blindness, penetrating injuries from industrial grinding and home tasks such as chopping are preventable.
- If severe scars with contractures are from burns caused by open fires, kerosene lanterns and stoves, or loose flammable clothing;

Table 4.3 Injury morbidity: prevalence of impairment from injury per
100,000 population

Country	Date	Impairments from injury
Egypt	1979–1981	Urban areas: 229/100,000 population
		Rural areas: 104/100,000
		Age 50–59: 448/100,000 in urban areas; 326/100,000 in rural areas
		Age >60: 1243/100,000 in urban areas; 485/100,000 in rural areas
Philippines	1980	Paraplegia: 21/100,000 population
		Quadriplegia: 12/100,000
		Single limb paralysis: 120/100,000
Sir Lanka	1981	Paraplegia: 9/100,000 population in males; 3/100,000 in females
		Total visual impairment of both eyes: 8/100,000 in males; 4/100,000 in females
		Loss of hand or leg: 50% more common in rural males than in urban males
		Loss of hand: 10 times more common in rural males than in females

Source: World Health Statistics Annual 1990 (WHO, 1991).

- If hands or extremities are impaired by previous wounds, what type of tool use led to the injury, and if there were problems in obtaining appropriate treatment;
- In all injury cases, if common personal risk factors affected the level of consciousness, such as alcohol abuse or untreated epilepsy.

　　Disabilities from injuries have an important impact on young adults, and the prevalence of such disabilities increases with age. The economic and social consequences of physical disabilities, such as spinal cord injuries with paralysis or mental disability from a head injury, are severe and long lasting, unless the person dies during the acute episode. Such disabilities not only prevent many victims from playing useful economic roles in the community, but frequently tie up other family members who must provide care and cannot be otherwise employed.

　　Unfortunately, in many countries, data on disabilities from injuries have not been well integrated into the range of health indicators used to guide policy development for injury control (Robine, 1989). Standards used to define disabilities, better classification by external cause, and the use of population-based incidence and prevalence rates should improve the utility of disability surveys. It would also be helpful if surveys placed greater emphasis on defining the causes of preventable disabilities, such as injuries.

　　In some countries, the prevalence of disabilities is so high that even a cursory observational survey can serve to document or confirm reports of a major public health problem. In Angola, newspapers reported that 40 percent of the population are amputees from land mines because there are nine million mines scattered about in the country and a population of 10.6 million (Vincent, 1993); other reports provide estimates of 4 percent. With such a high prevalence, a small sample size would be adequate to verify or adjust these shocking figures.

INJURY MORBIDITY DATA IN OTHER SECTORS

In some developing countries, police reports are the only source of data for motor vehicle and intentional injuries, particularly for nonfatal cases. However, if data are based upon police reports, there is serious underregistration for incidents in which there is a disincentive to involve police.

A study from New Delhi showed that as a result of underreporting of serious injuries in police data, the problem has been underestimated by a factor of ten (Mishra et al., 1984). Research in the United States and Holland indicates that police underreporting of traffic injuries is most severe for bicyclists, pedestrians, and occupants in single vehicle crashes (Harris, 1990).

Records on occupational injuries are sometimes maintained by government departments of labor and industry. Departments of agriculture may maintain information on exposures to chemicals such as pesticides (Maddy et al., 1990).

In certain countries, poison control centers are a potential source of information on acute poisonings among the general public and in industry (Blanc et al., 1990; Bresnitz, 1990a, 1990b; Litovitz et al., 1990). However, unless a poison center separates its cases by the degree of morbidity, most of the data may describe relatively minor exposures or calls for information. Poison control centers are not a useful source of data on fatalities.

CASE STUDIES USING SIMPLE EPIDEMIOLOGIC DATA FOR PLANNING INJURY PREVENTION IN PAPUA NEW GUINEA

To initiate appropriate injury control programs, it is essential to obtain local data about which types of injuries are the main sources of morbidity and mortality, and to define their causes and the population groups at highest risk. Research can be time consuming and expensive; however, it is possible to carry out useful research at a relatively low cost even in countries where organized data collection is rudimentary. This can be done by making modest improvements to existing record-keeping systems at health facilities, and by simple questionnaire surveys of rural health centers.

Examples from Barss's experiences during an appointment as a medical superintendent at a rural provincial hospital in Papua New Guinea, which served a population of 130,000 subsistence cultivators, are presented here. This research was completed with neither grants nor epidemiological/statistical expertise; however, essential assistance was provided by several medical students who helped to summarize and analyze data from hospital records, by the hospital records clerk who filed and retrieved the records, and by rural health center staff who made local inquiries and completed questionnaires.

An interest in the research developed when it became apparent over time that many injuries filling a substantial proportion of the hospital's beds had resulted from only a few important causes. Another factor that facilitated injury research was a well-established primary care network of 190 aid posts and 30 health centers that referred patients to the provincial hospital. The local government's willingness to provide support for emergency transfers of patients to hospital by boat or light aircraft improved rural patients' access to hospital care.

Studies of morbidity from two types of injuries, falls and burns, are presented as examples of low cost research; however, other injuries may be of greater interest in a different environment. These two examples are presented here because they show how population risk groups and causes can be quite different for specific injuries. This illustrates the need to collect basic descriptive and etiologic data prior to embarking on prevention programs.

While routine data from health facilities can be helpful in identifying important sources of morbidity from injuries, more costly community surveys are often used to study causes of mortality. However, as will be seen, inexpensive questionnaire surveys can also provide information on mortality to supplement data from health facilities.

Case Study 1: Falls and Tree Agriculture

Hospital Morbidity Survey

It became apparent that a substantial proportion of the injuries requiring hospitalization resulted from falls from trees. Accordingly, when patients were admitted, brief notes were made in their records about the external causes of their injuries.

Basic demographic information was recorded as a hospital routine, including the age and sex of the patients, although the age of some adults had to be described simply as "adult". Files of injured patients could be retrieved by reviewing hospital admission and discharge books, which contained simple one-line descriptions of all admissions and discharges. Information was also obtained by reference to operating theater records of surgery for trauma.

It was found that during the four-year period from 1978–82, 37 percent of trauma admissions had resulted either from falls from trees or other tree-associated injuries (Table 4.4) (Barss et al., 1984; Barss, 1984a). Tree-associated injuries included various injuries from falling trees or branches, head injuries from falling coconuts, and fractures and penetrating wounds from tripping over and falling off of logs. The majority of head and spinal cord injuries in the province had resulted from falls from trees.

A simple analysis of the age and sex of the victims then revealed that 75 percent were ages 3–16 and 84 percent were males.

To obtain further information about the cause of these falls, the types of trees involved in the fall injuries were analyzed (Table 4.5).

Although some records were incomplete, there was still enough information to suggest that many of the most serious injuries resulted from falls from trees that are widely used in tree agriculture. Information was then obtained from horticulturalists about the height of several locally important tropical trees (Table 4.6). A fall from the taller trees would appear to be at least equivalent to falling from a ten-story building.

Table 4.4 Trauma admissions, Provincial Hospital, Milne Bay Province, Papua New Guinea 1978–82

Cause	No.	Percent
Fall from tree	97	27
Tree-associated	35	10
Other trauma	223	63
All trauma	355	100

The hospital records showed that the average duration of hospitalization from tree fall injuries was 40 days, while other injuries were hospitalized an average of 27 days; the long durations were partly a result of difficulty in obtaining transport back to remote islands and mountainous villages. The longest hospitalization from a tree fall injury was 355 days.

Health Center Mortality Survey
All of the above data provided useful information about the causes and population groups at highest risk of tree fall injuries. However, it was still unknown whether such injuries were a significant source of mortality.

Although it might have been possible to obtain such information by a large community survey, it would have been prohibitively expensive. Accordingly, a simple one-page questionnaire was prepared and sent to all 30 rural health centers in the province. The staff were requested to talk to long-term residents and older members of the community who would be aware of such deaths in the surrounding area.

With a response rate of 80 percent (24/30), it was learned that at least 28 villagers had died by falls from trees during 1978–82; many had died instantly in the village, while a few had survived long enough to reach the nearest health center. There were five deaths due to falls from coconut trees, five from breadfruit trees, four from betel palms, four from bush trees, and ten from unspecified trees. As a result of this information, it became possible to calculate a mortality rate, providing an estimate of the lower limit of mortality from such falls for the population.

Table 4.5 Trees implicated in fall injuries, Milne Bay Province, Papua New Guinea, 1978–82

Type of tree	No.	Percent
Coconut	18	20
Mango	14	16
Betel palm	10	11
Other	11	13
Unspecified	35	40
Total	88	100

Table 4.6 Maximum height of some trees important in tropical agriculture

Tree	Maximum height (m)
Mango (*Mangifera indica*)	40
Coconut (*Cocos nucifera*, var. *typica*)	35
Betel palm (*Areca catechu*)	30
Breadfruit (*Artocarpus altilis*)	20

Summary of Findings for Case Study on Falls

As a result of the simple analyses above, it was learned that falls from trees and related injuries were an important cause of both morbidity and mortality in the population. The types of trees implicated in the most serious falls and the population groups at greatest risk were also identified.

This information and various suggestions for prevention were disseminated to the people by radio broadcasts and in village talks by health educators. Over time, safer harvesting methods and new varieties of trees may also help to reduce the impact of falls on the community.

Case Study 2: Burns, Grass Skirts, and Epilepsy

During the period when the analysis of falls was ongoing, it was noted that many patients who presented to hospital with major burns severe enough to need treatment for shock and extensive skin grafts were young girls. An analysis of the 21 burns severe enough to require admission showed that 48 percent had resulted from grass skirts catching fire and 24 percent from seizures of uncontrolled epilepsy (Barss and Wallace, 1983).

Whereas most victims of grass skirt burns were young girls, the majority of burns from other causes, including falls into open fires during seizures and burns from kerosene stoves and lamps, had involved adult males. This simple study thus helped to establish the two most important causes of burns in the community and to identify population groups at high risk for each cause.

It was learned that many of the girls who were burned had been left alone near an open cooking fire by their parents; when their clothes ignited they panicked and ran. The burn victims with epilepsy had not been taking anticonvulsant medications and had been left alone near open cooking fires; some required amputation for extensive damage to limbs. In this study, no community or health center survey was done to ascertain the unreported mortality related to fires. If such a survey had been done, it might have revealed a significant number of deaths due to housefires as a result of the use of open fires in houses constructed of highly flammable local materials; however, with no data, the true burden of burn mortality remains unknown.

The above information was widely publicized to the population by radio and by village health education talks. Over the next few years significantly fewer severe burns from grass skirts and epilepsy were seen.

Conclusions from Case Studies

The two examples that have been presented should serve to emphasize the feasibility of using simple epidemiologic data collection and analysis to identify the leading causes of locally important injuries and the population groups at highest risk.

With such information, it becomes possible to provide accurate information to the public, to health workers, and to policy makers. However, when using morbidity data from health facilities, it is essential not to overlook important causes of mortality, such as drowning, suicide, and homicide, where victims may not survive long enough to reach a health facility.

It is, therefore, important to supplement health facility data with simple surveys whenever possible, so as to avoid overlooking an important public health problem in the community. This is especially important in countries where most deaths occur at home and are, therefore, never reported by a death certificate. To ensure a good response, questionnaires that are sent to busy primary health care workers must be short and focus on a single problem.

Another example of research on a neglected injury problem is a survey to identify and quantify various chronic disabilities from injuries, and to identify causes and population groups at greatest risk. A community survey of drownings could provide useful information, particularly in areas where people are exposed to rivers, the ocean, or other open bodies of water such as lakes and reservoirs created by dams. Surveys of suicides and homicides might be useful in areas where violent deaths are believed to be common.

Studies to determine rates of morbidity and mortality from injuries in different age and sex groups, together with rates of other significant health problems in the community, can help to establish the relative importance of injuries as a source of morbidity and mortality, including disability. Such data might convince policy makers and educators of the importance of taking the necessary steps to prevent injuries in their community.

chapter 5

Assessing the Community Impact of Injuries: Costs

While measures of morbidity and mortality are most familiar to the public health community, economic indicators are often of greater interest for politicians, policymakers, and business leaders. Although the focus of this book is on the use of epidemiology and policy in the study and control of injuries, a brief overview of certain economic aspects is included here, since no one who is seriously interested in injury control can afford to ignore the costs of injuries or economic strategies for prevention. Cost estimates show the impact of injuries on the following:

- Health expenditures;
- Productivity and assets of individuals, families, communities, and countries.

They also serve to highlight the importance of the following:

- All injuries in relation to other health and social problems;
- Specific types of injuries, such as traffic injuries;
- The economic burden of specific determinants of injury, such as alcohol abuse;
- Economic policy and legislation to reduce the demand for hazardous products.

Data on the health costs and economic impact of injuries that can be provided are often crude estimates that may range widely, depending upon the methods and assumptions used for the calculations. Nevertheless, such information is needed to persuade policymakers and politicians that expenditure on injury control is an appropriate and worthwhile investment, compared to other demands competing for scarce resources.

Comparative cost analyses of different interventions can be useful as one component of feasibility analyses (Robertson, 1992). The feasibility of controlling specific types of injuries depends not only upon the availability of appropriate interventions, but also upon their costs and public acceptability.

LINK BETWEEN EPIDEMIOLOGIC SURVEILLANCE OF INJURIES AND COST ESTIMATES

The reliability and validity of estimated costs of various injuries is greatly affected by the completeness and detail of epidemiologic surveillance of injuries. Accurate reporting of rates of death, hospitalization, and disability from specific injuries by age and sex provides a foundation for construction of estimates of their economic impact. If one does not know how many injury events occurred and their outcome, it surely will be difficult to calculate their costs.

DIRECT AND INDIRECT COSTS OF INJURY

Immediate health costs and material losses are somewhat simpler to estimate for specific categories of injuries than are losses of productivity. Nevertheless, it is essential to estimate the costs of lost productivity from deaths and permanent disability, since such costs are high when the victims are young adults, as is true for many injuries.

Direct health costs include expenditures on hospitalization, plus other medical and rehabilitative costs. Indirect costs include loss of production in the workplace and in the household, including loss of production by family members who forego paid employment to care for people with acute injuries or long-term disabilities. Direct health costs provide estimates of the immediate economic impact of mortality and/or morbidity from different health conditions, while indirect costs provide a measure of the longer-term implications of lost productivity.

The slow death of an elderly person in hospital may result in high direct costs from hospital bills but little or no indirect cost. On the other hand, the sudden traffic death of a young adult might incur minimal or no direct costs, but be associated with large indirect costs in the form of lost economic output of lifetime earnings, together with the sudden loss of all of the resources previously invested in the victim by family and community. Morbidity costs, based upon rates and durations of hospitalizations, emergency visits, and temporary or permanent disability, are also important, particularly since the number of nonfatal injuries greatly exceeds fatalities, but also because of the large costs of many disabilities.

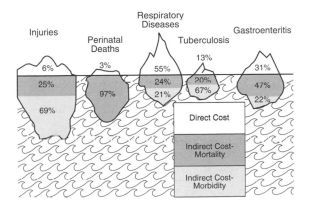

FIGURE 5.1

Proportional contributions of direct and indirect costs of illness by disease groups, Itabuna, Brazil, 1977.
Source: DeCodes J. *Measuring the Economic Impact of Illness in Brazil* (Dissertaion). Baltimore MD: Johns Hopkins School of Hygiene and Public Health, 1979, Reproduced with permission.

In Brazil, it was estimated that 69 percent of the total cost of injury resulted from disability-related losses of productivity, 25 percent from losses of productivity due to fatalities, and six percent from direct costs (DeCodes et al., 1988). Injuries accounted for only 12 percent of direct costs for all diseases and injuries; however, because injuries caused the disability and death of many young adults from injuries, they accounted for 28 percent of indirect and 26 percent of total costs (Fig. 5.1).

Many injuries also involve immediate material losses, such as destruction of a truck or bus or sinking of a vessel. Material losses may be relatively unimportant in a developed country compared to medical costs, but this is not necessarily the case in countries where the cost of a vehicle or small boat represents several lifetimes of pooled earnings. The destruction of such assets could have a substantial long-term impact on the wealth, productivity, and well-being of a community.

Pain and suffering are another cost of injury. It is difficult to put a monetary value on these, but this is often done in legal settlements for injury.

METHODS FOR ESTIMATING INDIRECT ECONOMIC COSTS OF INJURIES

Two alternative methods may be used to estimate loss of production. The human-capital approach places a value on human life by estimating future productivity on the basis of the earning capacity of the individual according to the person's age and sex. A cost is also assigned for loss of domestic work (Rice et al., 1989).

The willingness-to-pay approach, on the other hand, values human life based upon estimates of the amount that an individual would be willing to pay for a change to reduce the probability of death; both direct and indirect costs are included in the estimates. The change could include the introduction of enclosed stoves to prevent burns from open fires or some other intervention. Estimates obtained using a willingness-to-pay approach are highly subjective and would be culture-specific.

Miller et al. (1989) claimed that rational investment levels for increased safety can be estimated by summing the amount that individuals pay for small increases in their safety together with the total costs to society for a death or injury. Society's costs included transfer payments from welfare, unemployment insurance, and workers' compensation.

Most people place a higher positive value on immediate benefits than those far in the future and a higher negative value on immediate losses. Thus, discounting of future productivity losses and direct costs is often part of economic analyses. Six percent per year has been used in some injury studies (Rice et al. 1989), but the results can be expressed using more than one discount rate to provide a range of estimates under different assumptions.

The choice of an incidence or prevalence approach is another methodological consideration in economic analysis; however, most analyses are made using the prevalence approach because it is simpler. Prevalence analyses estimate the total costs of all past and present injuries, including disabilities, during one year. Incidence analyses estimate the total lifetime costs of all injuries that occur during a defined period of time, usually one year; this is more complex and discounting is used for future costs.

Readers who are interested in economic analyses may find it helpful to review the methodology used in the major cost of injury study that was done in the United States by a team of economists and epidemiologists, Cost of Injury in the United States, A Report to Congress 1989 (Rice et al., 1989). This is available from the Centers for Disease Control, Injury Control Division, 1600 Clifton Road, Atlanta, GA, 30333, USA.

The economists on the team prepared cost estimates with the collaboration of epidemiologists, who developed incidence categories and provided incidence rates for different types and severities of injuries. Epidemiologists also helped to estimate the potential savings from various injury interventions.

Because it is important for economists to determine the cost of road injuries, the Transport and Road Research Laboratory in the United Kingdom has prepared a manual that describes how to carry out such analyses in developing countries. Costing Road Accidents in Developing Countries (1994) is available from their Overseas Unit in Crowthorne, Berkshire, U.K., RG11 6AU.

VALIDITY OF COST ESTIMATES

Validity relates directly to the quality of the epidemiologic surveillance data used for calculations. For certain aspects of cost estimates based on data of uncertain quality or upon subjective assumptions, a range of possible costs can be used to show the sensitivity of results to different assumptions. Direct costs to society will be seriously underestimated unless the true total costs, and not just the costs to individual patients, are included for injuries treated at government or government-subsidized health facilities.

A limitation of many cost studies based upon losses of potential years of life is that large economic inputs to the victim prior to injury by family and community are often ignored (Barss, 1991). A much greater investment has been made in a young adult than in an infant, and the economic impact of the loss of a newly productive provider is much more serious for the family and the community than the loss of an infant, as discussed in Chapter 3. Recent health analyses have begun to adjust for this factor, with maximum losses estimated at an average age of 25 years when calculations are made using disability-adjusted life years (World Bank, 1993; Murray and Lopez, 1996). The loss of a provider is accentuated by the high birth rates and large dependency ratios in many developing countries and indigenous populations.

COSTS OF INJURY AS A PROPORTION OF GNP

Total costs for all injuries are not known even for most developed countries. However, a number of cost studies have been carried out for road traffic injuries. These have shown average costs of 1 percent of the gross national product (GNP) for traffic injuries in many developing countries (Transport and Road Research Laboratory, 1991), including some countries with as few as 1.5 motor vehicles per 1000 persons. Some studies have reported higher costs for traffic injuries, ranging between 1 and 3 percent of GNP (Mackay and Petrucelli, 1990; WHO, 1987; Ayati, 1990; Gekonge, 1990).

Estimates are needed for the total costs of all unintentional and intentional injuries as a percent of GNP. The total cost of injury could be of sufficient magnitude to neutralize or exceed any gains in GNP from economic development and growth.

COSTS OF SPECIFIC INJURIES: TRAFFIC INJURIES AND PER-CAPITA GNP

The results of a rough comparison of the US and Indian estimates of the costs of road fatalities were surprisingly similar after appropriate adjustment for the differences in per capita gross national product between the countries (Table 5.1). In 1988, the per capita GNP in the United States was $17,980, and in India was $290 (World Bank, 1988), a ratio of 62:1. Dividing the cost per road fatality in the United States in 1985, $352,000, by the cost per fatality in India, $5,000 in 1978, gives a ratio of 70:1. If adjustment for inflation were made to the Indian currency values to bring them to their 1985 equivalent, these ratios would probably be even closer.

If this comparison is valid, it suggests that it may be possible to obtain rough estimates of the costs of deaths from injuries in developing countries using estimates from the United States or other countries, if adjustment is made for differences in per capita GNP between the countries. This should, however, be verified by other similar comparisons.

COSTS OF DISABILITIES

Estimates of the direct and long-term indirect costs of disabilities should be included in the costs to society of projects with high rates of severe and fatal injury, such as logging and mining. In countries where it is rare to own an automobile and where most labor is manual, loss or damage to a single limb by injury may render a person permanently unfit for work.

Cost estimates should include the lost production of family and

Table 5.1 Estimates of costs of traffic-related injuries

Country	Year	Cost per injury case ($U.S.)	Per-capita GNP	Cost per fatality/ per-capita GNP
India*	1978	Fatality: $5,000	$290	17:1
U.S.A.**	1985	Fatality: $352,000	$17,980	20:1
		Hospitalized: $43,000		
		Non-hospitalized: $1,600		
Kuwait†	1990	Fatality: $500,000	$13,890	36:1

Sources: *Central Road Research Institute, 1982, **Rice et al, 1989, †Jadaan, 1990

community members involved in caring for the disabled victim. Economic analyses of the lifetime impact of preventable disabilities on rural and urban families and communities, including estimates of direct and indirect costs for the entire family unit and the community, would be useful.

More estimates are needed of the costs of disabilities from injuries in developing countries, since disabilities can be far more expensive than fatalities. In the United States, the average cost in 1986 dollars of complete quadriplegia was estimated to be over $700,000 and of paraplegia $500,000 (Miller et al., 1989); current estimates are substantially higher. About half of the costs were attributable to direct care and the other half to lost productivity. The costs for a totally disabling head injury were about $1.2 million. The average costs of lost productivity and hospitalization for a fatal injury were $317,000.

A national sample survey of disabled persons carried out in India in 1981 revealed that there were about 12 million physically disabled persons in India, representing about 1.8 percent of the population (Mohan, 1986a). The impairments included 424,000 amputations, of which at least one-fourth had resulted from injuries. It is believed that the actual number due to injury was substantially higher, since the cause of 60 percent of amputations was unspecified.

Although we have not attempted to estimate the costs of these disabilities, many of the amputees were teenagers or young adults. Therefore, the lifetime costs of lost human capital would be very high, particularly in countries with little or no capability for rehabilitation, such as the fitting of artificial limbs.

Modern warfare often leads to even greater numbers of civilian disabilities (Aboutanos and Baker, 1997). These would be expected to have a major negative impact on productivity, particularly in countries dependent mainly on manual and subsistence labor. The indirect costs of disability from traumatic injury must be staggeringly high in the 62 countries of the world where 100 million land mines lie scattered about, since up to 4 percent of some populations are reported to have suffered traumatic amputations from these explosives (International Committee of the Red Cross, 1992, 1993; Vincent, 1993).

The costs of rehabilitation and artificial limbs, which must be renewed or repaired periodically, could easily reach several percent of GNP and absorb the entire health budget for a nation. Economic estimates of the total costs of the hundreds of thousands or millions of amputations and deaths, together with the costs of loss of use for agriculture of as much as one-quarter of a country's arable land, are compelling reasons for a United Nations ban on such horrible devices and for class action suits by governments and victims to recover from manufacturers the costs of treatment and lost income (Ashtakala and Barss, 1996).

INJURIES AND ELASTICITY OF DEMAND WITH PRICE

Economic evaluations are important in assessing the contribution of pricing policies on certain products in the etiology or prevention of both overall injuries and specific injuries. Elasticity of demand with respect to price is an important concept in assessing the impact on consumption of certain products' price changes and the resulting increase or decrease in injuries.

If demand for a dangerous product is highly elastic with respect to price, demand can be decreased by increasing taxation on the product. An important example is alcohol, since alcohol abuse is associated with many types of injuries. Price is the most powerful variable that can be modulated to regulate alcohol consumption.

In developed countries, consumption of spirits and wine has been observed to decrease rapidly as prices rise. Consumption of beer, however, is less elastic, with one important exception. Young adults, an injury-prone group, tend to have lower incomes than older individuals and therefore reduce consumption more rapidly as prices rise (Adrian et al., 1986, 1993, 1994; Rankin and Ashley, 1992). Similar considerations may apply for other products associated with injuries, such as motorcycles and cigarettes. Children may initially be attracted to expensive brands of cigarettes with appealing images; once addicted, they switch to cheaper brands (Cavin and Pierce, 1996).

The reverse effect may be desirable with products that protect against injuries. Special programs have been developed to provide products such as bicycle helmets at low cost in order to increase demand. On the other hand, high insurance costs for dangerous vehicles and other products can help to discourage their purchase and use and shift consumption to safer products.

OPPORTUNITY COST AND INJURY INTERVENTIONS

All resources are finite, and their use for one purpose means that there is less available for another. An opportunity taken means that another must be sacrificed. *Opportunity cost* is the economic term for this concept. In planning alternative programs and interventions for injuries, it is useful to keep this concept in mind, since, even if you do not, most policy analysts and politicians will.

COST ESTIMATES AS A JUSTIFICATION FOR INJURY SURVEILLANCE AND RESEARCH

When the total costs of a single death or permanent disability from injury are compared to the costs of injury surveillance and research, it is often found that the costs of one injury exceed the annual operating costs of an efficient surveillance system or research survey for injuries. If injury surveillance and research can be shown to prevent even one death or disability from injury per year, they should quickly pay their own way. Cost estimates for deaths, hospitalizations, and disabilities from different types of injuries that are common in local communities can therefore be helpful in obtaining adequate funding for injury prevention programs.

chapter 6

Determinants of Injuries

Analysis of specific determinants for different types of injuries is an essential element of injury control. Before this analysis, priority injuries must be identified on the basis of mortality, morbidity, and cost.

The most important groups of injuries are then subjected to more detailed studies of their circumstances. When the circumstances of injuries are known, it is easier to identify determinants susceptible to modification and develop appropriate interventions.

The probability of an injury for an individual is affected by the following circumstances:

- Hazardous activities;
- Personal factors;
- Equipment factors;
- Environmental factors, including physical and psychosocial;
- Temporal factors, such as time of day, day of the week, and season.

In assessing the circumstances of different types of injuries, the above list can be used as a framework for systematic consideration of each of the major categories of determinants.

It is circumstance and proper timing that give an action its character and make it either good or bad.
—Agesilaus, 444–400 B.C.E., in Plutarch, Lives.

IDENTIFICATION OF RISK FACTORS AND INJURY DETERMINANTS

High Risk Versus Population Approaches

Specific types of injuries tend to occur most frequently in certain subgroups of a population. It is often helpful to identify these high-risk groups by personal or other factors so that they can be targeted for appropriate interventions. However, it is also important to consider interventions for the general population at lower risk, especially if most injuries occur among low-risk individuals.

Fixed and Modifiable Risk Factors

Certain personal risk factors, such as age and sex, are fixed while others, such as alcohol consumption, untreated epilepsy, level of education, interpersonal skills, and self-esteem, are potentially modifiable. Since equipment is man-made, equipment factors are often highly modifiable. Physical and psychosocial environmental factors are also potentially modifiable. The physical environment includes both man-made and natural components. Modification of the man-made environment to prevent injuries is most feasible during design and construction phases. The psychosocial environment is complex, but is potentially modifiable at household, community, societal or even global levels.

Interaction of Injury Determinants

The synergistic interaction of certain combinations of personal, environmental, and equipment factors associated with various activities greatly increases the probability of an injury-causing event. The exact moment when such an event will occur is not predictable, since it depends upon the complex interaction of multiple variables. Nevertheless, the modification of even a single determinant can be enough to substantially reduce the probability of injury. This effect may be mediated either by preventing an injury-causing incident from occurring or by minimizing the resulting damage.

It is, therefore, essential to define the likeliest risk factors and other circumstances for the most common types of serious injuries in a community, region, and country.

Indirect or Underlying Determinants of Injury

These are sometimes referred to as "causes of causes". What initially seems a straightforward cause for an injury may, after careful consideration, turn out to be merely the effect of another more pervasive and insidious underlying cause. For example, many unintentional and intentional injuries are associated with abusive consumption of alcohol, low levels of education, and unemployment, which are in turn associated with poverty, which may in turn be associated with a repressive political system. In the causal sequence, indirect or underlying determinants are closest to the source while proximate determinants more immediately precede the effect.

Thus, social, economic, educational, and employment status, rural/urban residence, and the individual's household environment are often predictors of injury risk (Millar and Adams, 1988). Personal factors, such as occupation and employment status, may be attributable to pervasive socio-environmental characteristics. Level and pace of development may also be important determinants of certain injuries. These factors are important underlying causes, not only of injuries, but also of many diseases.

While it is useful to identify factors amenable to immediate and direct intervention wherever possible, it is important to discern more general underlying patterns of causality so that fundamental and long-lasting multisectoral interventions can be developed and implemented. Such interventions would target underlying problems at a community or societal level, rather than focus on individuals affected by injury.

HAZARDOUS EXPOSURES

Participation in or exposure to various activities obviously affects the risk of injuries. Many activities are related to personal factors such as occupation, age, and sex. The risk of injury associated with various activities can be substantially reduced by appropriate modifications of personal, equipment, and environmental factors.

It is important to distinguish between the concepts of risk and exposure. While subgroups of a population may appear to be at increased risk of injury by virtue of their personal characteristics, their increased risk may be a result of frequent exposure to hazardous environments, equipment, or activities.

There is often a tendency to place the burden of protection on the individual by focusing on personal factors while ignoring hazardous equipment or environments. Fortunately, this "victim blaming" has begun to diminish as professionals and politicians recognize and assume their responsibilities for protecting the public from hazards.

An example may help to clarify the importance of distinguishing between personal risk factors and environmental exposures. In certain areas of the highlands of Papua New Guinea, adult males had an unusually high drowning rate (Barss, 1991). Because of clan hostilities and fighting, many adult males moved about the countryside on foot. Since there were few bridges, they had to ford many cold and fast-flowing rivers. The high rate of drowning observed in this subgroup of the population had more to do with the frequency of hazardous exposures than with the intrinsic characteristics of the victims, such as their age and sex.

By clearly assigning the important contribution of exposure to the high death rate among adult males, it becomes possible to reduce such exposures with permanent environmental modifications. For example, one solution might be to construct sturdy footbridges at a few key crossing points where risks are high. Constructing roads and bridges for motor vehicles as part of the general development process could have an unanticipated beneficial impact.

In the delta of Bangladesh, on the other hand, young children had the highest drowning rates (Zimicki, 1990; Zimicki et al., 1985). This resulted from both personal risk factors and hazardous exposures. Many homes are surrounded by water, and children live in constant proximity to unprotected open bodies of water. However, the extraordinarily high drowning rates among young children in this environment also reflected the fact that toddlers are somewhat unstable, curious, and relatively unaware of hazards. During a momentary lapse of attention by parents or siblings, toddlers often wander to a nearby body of water and tumble in, and are incapable of rescuing themselves.

In communities where drowning hazards are ubiquitous, the best preventive measure may be education at the household level with attention to both personal and environmental factors. This educational approach would provide a less permanent solution than the preceding example of environmental intervention, since long-term prevention of drownings would require sustained vigilance and the need for repeated educational campaigns.

International Travel Risks

Developing countries are an increasingly popular travel destination for business or pleasure. Travelers share some of the same environments as the local population and are at risk for similar preventable injuries. Yet few travelers are aware of the excess risks to which they are exposed in many countries.

For young adult travelers and certain destinations, such as Mexico, injury is the number one cause of travel-related death, primarily from motor vehicle crashes and drownings (Hargarten and Baker, 1985; Guptill et al., 1991). Serious nonfatal injuries, including falls and motor vehicle crashes, account for a significant proportion of evacuations of tourists from developing countries (Hargarten and Bouc, 1993). Every year about 1200 United States citizens die while traveling abroad (Hargarten et al., 1991). Data from other countries suggest that the number of overseas travel-related deaths worldwide is at least several thousand (Steffen and Lobel, 1994; Paixao et al., 1991). Approximately one-fourth of all travel-related deaths are due to injuries.

Injury prevention strategies for the international traveler include education not only for travelers, but also for their health advisors, about hazards likely to be encountered. Pre-travel advice about injury prevention has the same importance as immunization and chemoprophylaxis (Hargarten, 1994; Steffen and Lobel, 1994).

Travelers' opportunities to reduce their exposure to environmental risks include selecting airbag and seat belt-equipped cars when renting automobiles (Hargarten, 1992), traveling in large buses instead of small open-backed vehicles, wearing helmets at all times when riding motorcycles and bicycles (when safer modes of travel are not available), using flotation devices such as life jackets in boats, and abstaining from alcohol during driving, swimming, and boating (Lowenfels and Wynn, 1992).

FIGURE 6.1

Commercial jet airplane crashes with hull losses per million movements (landings or takeoffs) during 1984-93. Source of data: Enders J. and Dodd R. S. Airport Safety: A Survey of Accidents and Available Approach and Landing Aids. Flight Safety Foundation. *Flight Safety Digest*, March, 1996, p9.

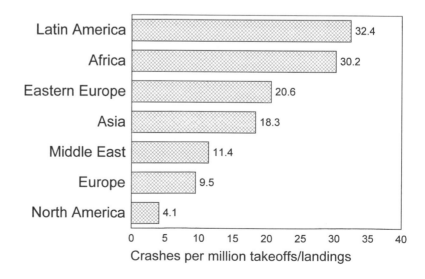

Travel by commercial air carriers often involves greater risks in developing countries than on major carriers in developed countries, due to inadequacies in pilot training, air traffic control, and aircraft equipment. Difficulties in communication between pilots and air traffic controllers has led to some crashes. Many airports in developing countries lack sophisticated weather forecasting and landing guidance systems. Travel on unscheduled flights and on small aircraft may involve exceptionally high risk, especially when bad weather is likely, and should be undertaken only when absolutely necessary. A survey of crashes involving substantial damage to commercial jet aircraft at airports revealed that rates in Latin America and Africa were seven times the rate for North America (Fig. 6.1) (Enders and Dodd, 1996). Differences among individual countries are even greater.

PERSONAL RISK FACTORS

Personal factors are associated with the etiology of many injuries. Nevertheless, it is important to consider personal factors, such as abusive alcohol consumption, objectively and avoid unproductive victim blaming, since adverse personal factors often reflect poverty, a risk prone occupation, or other unfavorable environmental conditions.

Certain risk factors can be modified by immediate changes while others can be modified by long-term solutions. In societies where there is stratification by income and occupation, personal factors such as level of education, employment status, occupation, and income level can be important and should be considered in formulating policy and research. Alcohol, epilepsy, and a number of other physical and medical conditions alter the risk of injury because of their effects on the function of the central nervous system.

Being aware of the importance of modifiable personal risk factors help to develop preventive interventions. For example, regular treatment of epilepsy with anticonvulsant medications may prevent or reduce the frequency of seizures and help to prevent drownings, burns, and falls. Policies to decrease the use of alcohol, or at least to limit its use in hazardous environments, such as at the wheel of a motor vehicle or during the operation of machinery, will modify drinking and help to prevent injury.

Age and sex are often important predictors of risk of injury. Most analyses of risk factors consider the demographic variables of age and sex. This includes calculations for rates of specific types of injuries in different age groups for males and females.

It is fortunate that age and sex are recorded routinely for many administrative purposes. Nevertheless, reliable information about age is frequently difficult to obtain in developing countries, particularly for adults. Other personal attributes of individuals, such as education and alcohol consumption, may also be important determinants of injury; however, information about such variables is seldom available without recourse to special studies.

Obviously, an individual's age and sex are fixed and not susceptible to change in the interests of better injury control. Nevertheless, awareness of an increased probability of specific injuries associated with certain age and sex groups facilitates targeting prevention to specific subgroups of the population at greatest risk. It may also facilitate identification and detailed analysis of other modifiable risk factors and exposures that affect high-risk subgroups.

Although age and sex of individuals are fixed at birth, the age and sex composition of populations are sometimes affected by government policies. Labor, migration, and rural development policies, for example, may affect the ratio of males to females, and of young adults to the rest of the population in certain areas, thereby altering the proportion of the population at greatest risk of certain injuries.

Age

Injury rates vary dramatically with age, reflecting differences among age groups in their activities, behavior, and injury thresholds (Tables 6.1 and 6.2; see Chapters 7–11). In many developed countries, the lowest injury mortality rates are during infancy and between the ages of 5 and 14 years; toddlers (1–4 years old), teenagers, young adults and the elderly are at greatest risk. However, the situation differs in many developing countries such as China, where injury death rates in infancy are high (see Table 6.1). It is important to examine death rates for infants separate from those for toddlers since the two age groups have different experiences for many injuries because of differences in mobility.

Often, injury deaths of infants are not included under the more common categories of drownings, falls, burns, etc., but are listed under the rubric of "other injuries." Some of these deaths could represent infanticides misclassified as unintentional injuries. Infanticide is not a problem confined to developing countries. In the United States, homicide was the leading cause of injury death among infants in many states during 1980–85, and also in the nation's capital, the District of Columbia, where 42 percent of injury deaths in infants were due to homicide (Baker et al, 1996).

In children under 5 years of age, falls are generally the leading cause of nonfatal injuries, but most deaths result from traffic injuries, drownings, and fires. The prevalence of specific injuries is affected by the local environment. For example, in rural areas of many developing countries, drownings are an important cause of death, while in urban areas, traffic injuries of young pedestrians predominate.

In the 15–24 year age group, almost one-half of all deaths in many countries result from unintentional injuries. This age group has especially high mortality rates from traffic injuries and suicide, and in certain countries, from firearm homicides and political violence.

For adults up to the age of 45 years, traffic injuries are the single largest cause of injury death in most countries. However, violent deaths have often been more prevalent in certain countries, such as El Salvador, where state terrorism, guerrilla warfare, and low-intensity conflict were endemic. Violent deaths have also increased rapidly in other countries with large socioeconomic disparities, such as Brazil, where homicides accounted for more loss of life than motor vehicle crashes (World Bank, 1989). Domestic violence is an important problem in many developed and developing countries. Occupational injuries are also important in the adult age group for workers in high-risk industries.

Mortality rates for all unintentional injuries combined are highest among the elderly in developed countries, because of their reduced threshold for fractures and other tissue damage and their susceptibility to complications following injury. Review of available age-specific mortality rates published annually by the World Health Organization (WHO) for all non-motor vehicle unintentional injuries shows that rates are very high for age groups over 55 years in developing countries (Table 6.1). Falls are of particular concern in the elderly, as a cause of both morbidity and mortality, and are likely to assume increasing importance as that proportion of the elderly population rises. In developing countries that report to WHO, such as rural China, falls are an important contributor to high injury mortality rates among the elderly. Nevertheless, in many developing countries where motor vehicles are scarce the elderly remain physically active ameliorating the impact of such demographic trends, because of the positive effects of exercise on bone strength (Barss, 1985a; Ford, 1989; Wickham et al., 1989; O'Brien and Vertinsky, 1991).

The incidence of other injuries, especially burns, is also high among the elderly (Feck et al., 1977), probably due in large part to decreased sensory perceptions and slower reaction times, and possibly to the high prevalence of central nervous system disorders, such as dementia. Housefires are an important cause of death among the rural elderly in a number of developing countries. The problem is accentuated by the use of open flames for cooking, lighting, and warmth in highly flammable huts, some of which have only a single small exit (Barss, 1991). Suicide rates are frequently high among the elderly in both developed and developing countries.

Sex

Overall injury mortality rates for males are two to seven times the rates for females in developing countries that report to the World Health Organization (see Table 3.1). In some developing countries, these sex ratios are substantially larger than in developed countries. This is probably because in many developing countries, greater gender differentiation persists in attitudes, social status, education, occupations, daily household activities, and recreation.

Sex ratios for injury rates can change dramatically over time. For example, in Greenland, mortality rates from unintentional injuries among the Inuit were estimated to be 700 per 100,000 person-years for males and 50 for females during 1861–1900, 540 and 70 during 1901–39 (Bertelsen, 1935), 270 and 80 during 1957–60 (P. Smith, 1961), and 202 and 72 during 1968–85 (Bjerregaard, 1990a). Thus, over the course of a century, the male-to-female ratio of death rates changed from almost 8:1 to less than 3:1 as the rate for males decreased by 70 percent and the rate for females increased by almost 50 percent. Such dramatic shifts may be a reflection of changes because of development in occupational and recreational exposures of males and females, as discussed below under occupation.

The male-to-female ratio of injury mortality rates also varies significantly with different types of injuries and with the local culture.

Table 6.1 Age- and sex-specific mortality rates per 100,000 population per year for non-motor vehicle, unintentional injuries for various developing countries, with other countries for comparison

	Sex	<1	1–4	5–14	15–24	25–54	55–64	65–74	75+	All ages	Year
AFRICA											
Mauritius	M	9	16	13	21	22	38	45	29	22	1994
	F	10	10	4	6	10	9	12	81	10	
SOUTHEAST ASIA											
China, rural	M	173	79	36	27	36	44	67	167	43	1994
	F	196	59	20	43	49	64	117	235	55	
China, urban	M	40	20	14	15	18	19	46	223	22	1994
	F	32	13	6	4	6	12	36	285	16	
Sri Lanka	M	26	17	18	45	63	80	110	133	47	1986
	F	28	16	11	14	15	20	33	48	15	
EASTERN MEDITERRANEAN											
Egypt	M	18	10	11	16	17	16	32	30	15	1987
	F	8	7	6	11	8	8	13	25	8	
SOUTH AMERICA											
Colombia	M	36	23	12	34	42	62	82	157	36	1991
	F	25	15	6	6	7	18	26	103	11	
Costa Rica	M	17	8	4	21	23	55	58	269	23	1991
	F	13	4	3	4	3	5	19	252	8	

Ecuador	M	61	27	16	37	55	96	144	24	44	1988
	F	45	17	8	6	10	22	33	156	13	
Mexico	M	40	20	11	35	49	75	95	243	39	1993
	F	32	13	5	6	7	15	28	185	12	
Uruguay	M	174	16	14	39	47	56	86	217	50	1990
	F	134	15	5	8	9	20	35	132	21	
COMPARISON											
Sweden	M	3	5	5	9	14	30	43	182	26	1993
	F	9	2	1	3	3	5	17	152	19	
United States	M	18	14	6	16	24	27	39	129	25	1992
	F	15	9	3	3	5	9	18	95	12	
Russian	M	85	39	26	82	273	334	194	148	191	1994
Federation	F	61	29	11	17	55	87	61	84	49	

Sources: World Health Statistics Annual 1990–1995 (WHO, 1991-1996)

The male mortality rates for non-motor vehicle unintentional injuries tend to be about two to four times the female rates in most age groups (Table 6.1). Adult males are often at higher risk of drowning and occupational injuries. Adult females and children, on the other hand, are frequently exposed to the hazards of open fires and are at high risk for burns. Increased risk reflects the interaction of personal risk factors and environmental hazards, such as age, sex, occupation, clothing styles and fabrics, and types of cooking fires or stoves.

Throughout the world, motor vehicle injury mortality rates for males tend to be several times those of females (Table 6.2). In developed countries, the gender difference is decreasing as more females join the work force, travel to work, and consume alcohol, thereby gaining exposure to many of the same hazards as males (Popkin, 1992).

The male-to-female ratio of traffic injury rates varies according to road use and is usually much higher for motorcyclists and bicyclists. In Delhi, India, the male-to-female ratio of traffic injury rates ranged from 3:1 for pedestrians to 20:1 for bicyclists (Mohan and Bawa, 1985). The latter ratio reflects high levels of exposure of males to the hazard of bicycling in heavy traffic.

Suicide rates tend to be about 2 to 4 times higher among males. High suicide rates are common among young males in Micronesia and in aboriginal communities in North America and Greenland (Young et al., 1992; Rodgers, 1991; Middaugh, 1992; Thorslund, 1990; May, 1987). In some societies, however, including certain rural areas of Bangladesh, Papua New Guinea, and China, the situation differs, and rates among young females exceed those for males by several times (Smith, 1981; Fauveau and Blanchet, 1989; Barss, 1991; Li and Baker, 1991; WHO, 1991). The sex ratio for suicide attempts is sometimes the reverse of that for completed suicides. In North American aboriginal communities, suicide attempts are more common among females, and completed suicides among males (May, 1987).

Death rates from homicide and war range from 2 to 16 times as high for males as for females in many developing countries. However, in many villages of the highlands of Papua New Guinea, rates of female homicide nearly equal, and sometimes exceed, those for males (Barss, 1991).

In the few available studies of nonfatal injuries, overall rates for males are usually only slightly higher than for females. However, in a study of injuries from rural areas of India, it was found that, for the population above 15 years of age, the male-to-female injury ratio was 4:1 (Mohan and Qadeer, 1988). For some nonfatal injuries, such as falls from trees, male rates are often several times female rates (Barss et al., 1984), while other injuries such as clothing burns occur almost exclusively in females (Barss and Wallace, 1983). Other burns, such as scalds, are also more common among females, probably as a result of frequent exposure to domestic activities (Thapa, 1989).

Alcohol

Ethyl alcohol is classified by toxicologists as an aliphatic organic solvent. It has profound acute and chronic effects on the central nervous system. During ingestion, there are acute effects on neuronal membranes, on the conduction of electrical impulses along nerves, and on neuroreceptors. Chronic alcoholism results in structural brain damage and permanent cognitive deficits. There are also a number of neuropsychiatric syndromes of dependency and abuse that can be attributed to the addictive properties of alcohol.

It is hardly surprising that alcohol is a major risk factor for all types of injuries in many developed countries, especially for severe and fatal injuries (Secretary of Health and Human Services, 1987). Alcohol is an important risk factor for many types of injuries in aboriginal communities in developed countries (May, 1992; Bjerregaard, 1992; Young et al., 1992). Although data are scarce from developing countries concerning the importance of alcohol as an etiological factor for injuries, alcohol abuse is widespread and its use is often underestimated (Edwards, 1979; Weddell, 1981; Wyatt, 1980).

As data on alcohol accumulate, it becomes evident that using alcohol involves a continuum of risk (Rankin and Ashley, 1992) affected by personal, environmental, and equipment factors and activities. For some individuals and situations, the only safe level of alcohol is zero.

Validity of Data on Alcohol and Injuries

The reported degree of association between alcohol and injuries depends upon the data source used. Significant differences abound in completeness and accuracy of reports from police, hospital staff, and coroners. Such differences can arise from biases in estimates of intoxication based upon observations of behavior as compared with more objective tests for alcohol concentration in the blood or breath. The most reliable evidence associating alcohol with various types of injuries is obtained using blood samples from fatalities and hospitalized victims. Blood samples for alcohol must be taken as soon as possible after the injury and, whenever feasible, before treatment with intravenous fluids (Östrom et al., 1992; Wintemute et al., 1990).

Police and coroner records may underestimate the extent to which alcohol involvement in traffic injuries because persons considered unlikely to have been drinking are not tested. In illustration, one of the authors (SPB) found that among traffic fatalities in Rio de Janeiro, Brazil, women were rarely tested for alcohol, and males age 60 or older were tested less commonly than young adult males. In Australia, it has been found that actual blood alcohol concentration tends to be about twice that estimated by the police, who are generally conservative in their estimates (Ryan, 1990).

Blood alcohol is routinely measured in only a few countries in the Americas, and many countries have never established fixed levels above which a person is considered to be legally intoxicated (PAHO, 1990). In some countries, such as Taiwan and Papua New Guinea, legislation to permit alcohol testing by police has been requested by the police departments but not passed by politicians (Wu and Melison, 1990; Ryan, 1989b).

The importance of alcohol as a risk factor for injuries is underestimated not only because injured persons are not tested, but also because symptoms of intoxication or blood alcohol levels are rarely reported for uninjured persons, even though they may have been re-

Table 6.2 Age- and sex-specific mortality rates per 100,000 population per year for motor vehicle injuries for various developing countries, with other countries for comparison

	Sex	<1	1–4	5–14	15–24	25–54	55–64	65–74	75+	All ages	Year
AFRICA											
Mauritius	M	9	2	3	27	36	62	40	86	27	1994
	F	19	0	0	4	5	9	12	40	5	
SOUTHEAST ASIA											
China, rural	M	4	6	6	15	27	26	37	45	20	1994
	F	5	6	5	6	9	14	16	18	9	
China, urban	M	1	4	5	9	19	24	32	41	16	1994
	F	1	3	3	4	7	11	13	20	7	
Sri Lanka	M	0	0	1	4	6	11	11	20	4	1986
	F	0	1	1	1	1	2	4	5	1	
Taiwan	M	9	10	9	69	48	86	117	130	51	1995
	F	7	9	6	20	14	36	48	53	18	
EASTERN MEDITERRANEAN											
Egypt	M	2	4	7	7	18	11	16	8	10	1987
	F	1	2	4	2	3	3	5	5	3	

SOUTH AMERICA

Colombia	M	2	7	9	20	31	41	48	73	22	1991
	F	1	4	4	5	7	15	22	24	7	
Costa Rica	M	2	5	5	16	33	43	54	79	21	1991
	F	0	5	2	4	6	13	13	12	5	
Ecuador	M	6	12	12	30	48	63	72	125	31	1988
	F	5	6	7	5	9	17	29	64	9	
Mexico	M	3	7	8	28	36	46	52	88	25	1993
	F	2	5	4	6	7	12	19	32	7	
Uruguay	M	7	2	5	18	20	25	30	48	18	1990
	F	0	12	1	10	6	8	9	17	7	
COMPARISON											
Sweden	M	0	2	2	17	8	8	12	22	9	1993
	F	0	2	2	6	4	5	5	8	4	
United States	M	4	5	6	40	23	18	23	42	22	1992
	F	3	4	4	16	9	9	13	19	10	
Russian Federation	M	3	7	10	45	51	39	33	39	38	1994
	F	2	5	6	14	10	12	14	19	11	
Australia	M	2	5	4	33	16	10	13	32	16	1993
	F	2	3	3	10	5	6	10	12	6	

Source: World Health Statistics Annual 1990–1995 (WHO, 1991-1996) and *Health and Vital Statistics Republic of China 1995* (Department of Health, The Executive Yuan, 1996)

sponsible for the deaths or injuries. Thus, if a drunken adult causes the deaths of others, the association between alcohol and the deaths is not recorded (Bjerregaard, 1992). This type of underreporting causes underestimation of alcohol's role in housefires and boat-related drownings in aboriginal communities, and in traffic injuries caused by drunken drivers.

Drinking Patterns

The frequency and quantity of alcohol ingestion is important. Occasional use of alcohol in moderate amounts in appropriate circumstances need not be a risk factor for injuries. However, serious problems often arise when there is rapid ingestion of large quantities of alcohol, and when consumption occurs prior to high-risk activities or during periods of depression or other psychologic and interpersonal crises. High-risk activities after ingestion of alcohol include not only driving a motor vehicle but also many other activities, such as cycling, walking, boating, and swimming.

Binge drinking is the rapid consumption of several drinks. It is often defined as the ingestion of five or more drinks on a single occasion. Binge drinking is of particular concern with respect to both unintentional injuries and violence. In the Americas, adolescents tend to consume alcohol intensely and sporadically, away from home with peers rather than on a daily basis (WHO, 1989c). Pathological patterns of alcohol use often develop during adolescence.

In many aboriginal communities in North America, the overall prevalence of drinking may be less than in non-aboriginal communities (May, 1992). The prevalence of binge drinking among disturbed individuals or families, however, may be extremely high. Among subarctic Indians, alcohol consumption has been reported as mainly binge drinking. This pattern of intermittent consumption of large quantities of alcohol resulted in sudden deaths from unintentional injuries and violence rather than prolonged illness from liver cirrhosis and other medical complications of chronic alcoholism (Young, 1988). However, cirrhosis and alcoholism have been important public health and social problems in some Canadian aboriginal communities (Jarvis and Boldt, 1982).

In the Americas, including Argentina, Brazil, Chile, Colombia, Costa Rica, Ecuador, Mexico, Peru, and Puerto Rico, the median prevalence of alcohol dependence syndrome among men was reported to be 10 percent, with a range of 4–24 percent (Levav et al., 1989). In Argentina, Brazil, Chile, Colombia, Costa Rica, Mexico, and Puerto Rico, the median prevalence of alcohol abuse was 17 percent, with a range of 7–28 percent.

Drinking patterns vary with gender and education as well as over time. In Brazil the prevalence of alcoholism was estimated to range from 6 percent to 13 percent in males, and was about 1 percent in females, figures similar to those in the United States (Cardim et al., 1989). A study in Porto Alegre found that 18 percent of men and 2 percent of women drank alcohol every day, and that uneducated men were three times as likely to do so as men with post-secondary education (Achutti et al., 1989). In Taiwan, the per capita consumption of alcoholic beverages increased 300 percent between 1961 and 1986 (Baker and MacKinney, 1990), although part of the increase may have been attributable to demographic changes in the age composition of the population.

Alcohol and Traffic Injuries
Studies of the involvement of alcohol in motor vehicle injuries have been conducted in only a few developing countries; those studies which include reports of blood alcohol concentrations have generally revealed that a substantial proportion of victims had high alcohol levels. Several reviews have also documented that alcohol is a serious problem in motor vehicle crashes in developing countries and among aboriginal populations (Patel, 1977; Jacobs and Sayer, 1983; May, 1992).

Unfortunately, most studies in developing countries did not measure the concentration of alcohol in blood or breath, but used police estimates, which usually underestimate the role of alcohol, to determine the extent of alcohol involvement. In a study in Papua New Guinea, police estimated that alcohol was involved in 27 percent of drivers admitted to hospital after crashes. However, an independent assessment by a medical practitioner found that 57 percent of the drivers were affected by alcohol (Posanau, 1990).

Alcohol was reported to be a factor in 80 percent of motor vehicle fatalities in Santiago, Chile, 35 percent in Peru, 11 percent in Mexico, and 25 percent in Papua New Guinea (Ryan, 1989b, 1990). Such differences among countries may be real, or they may result from lack of testing and variability in reporting.

Alcohol also plays a role in many nonfatal crashes. In Nigeria, alcohol was reported to be a factor in 88 percent of drivers treated in an emergency room. In the small Moslem city of Kaduna, Nigeria, it was estimated that 10 percent of drivers and 24 percent of passengers injured in traffic crashes were drunk (Asogwa, 1980c). In New Delhi, 29 percent of injured motor scooter drivers admitted having consumed alcohol prior to their crash (Mishra et al., 1984). In Taiwan, intoxicated riders accounted for at least 7 percent of motorcycle crashes (Chiang, 1989).

Alcohol and Other Injuries
The role of alcohol in non-motor vehicle injuries is incompletely documented even in many developed countries. Nevertheless, alcohol is known to be associated with many deaths from a variety of different types of injuries. For example, it has been estimated that in the United States in 1980, 35 percent of deaths from drowning, 25 percent from fires, 50 percent from homicide, and 30 percent from suicide were attributable to alcohol (Ravenholt, 1984).

Several studies in indigenous populations in North America have found alcohol involvement in a large proportion of injuries. Among aboriginal Canadians in northwestern Ontario, at least 25 percent of deaths from injuries were considered to be alcohol related (Young, 1983), while in Alberta between 60 and 100 percent of deaths from the most common fatal injuries were attributable to alcohol (Jarvis and Boldt, 1982). In aboriginal communities in northern Québec, a community survey using confidential interviews found that self-reported binge drinking was strongly associated with the incidence of both unintentional and intentional injuries to self and others (Robitaille and Barss, 1994).

A prospective study of deaths among Canadian Indians was carried out in the province of Alberta in 1976 using verbal autopsies, medical examiners' reports, and blood alcohol concentrations (BACs) (Jarvis and Boldt, 1982). It was estimated that over 40 percent of all deaths were a direct result of alcohol. The majority of victims of intentional and unintentional injuries were legally impaired (BAC $\geq$ 0.08 percent), including 71 percent of victims from motor vehicle injuries, 90 percent from fires, 63 percent from other unintentional injuries, 72 percent of suicides, and 100 percent of homicides. Among the Inuit of Greenland during 1968–85, one-third of fatal falls were alcohol-related (Bjerregaard, 1990a). In the same population, the rate of suicide increased more than 10 times between 1962 and 1986 (Thorslund, 1990); the increase was correlated in time with reported increases in alcohol consumption. Information about alcohol was available for about 50 percent of suicides. Of these, only 8 percent had no alcohol in the blood, while 20 percent had BAC's greater than 0.20 percent. Regional and secular trends for deaths from alcohol-related unintentional injuries were similar to those for suicide (Bjerregaard and Juel, 1990). Of all deaths from unintentional injuries, 23 percent were alcohol-related, including 20 percent of all boating fatalities. Alcohol-related deaths comprised a higher proportion of fatal injuries in females than in males, 30 percent versus 20 percent; in the 25–64 year age group, the corresponding proportions were 61 percent versus 34 percent.

Since alcohol is frequently such an important risk factor for so many different types of injuries, it is important to ensure that alcohol-related deaths are correctly certified and coded as such by health providers and coders. Although alcohol is obviously a major risk factor for many types of injuries, information about other personal, environmental, and equipment factors should be obtained even when alcohol is believed to have contributed to the event. Modifications of the environment or equipment to provide automatic protection for the intoxicated, for other high-risk individuals, and for the general public during temporary lapses of behavior or attention are highly desirable.

Tobacco and Other Drugs

The role of tobacco in the etiology of injuries in developing countries must be documented. Nicotine is a highly addictive drug, and tobacco is heavily marketed in developing countries because governments in developed countries are tightening control over this dangerous drug, the leading cause of mortality, morbidity, and disability in many countries.

In developed countries, cigarette smoking is an important risk factor for housefires, especially when combined with alcohol abuse. In the state of Washington in the United States, the risk or odds ratio for fatal or nonfatal unintentional fire injuries was 1.5 times as great (95 percent confidence interval 0.6–4.2) for households whose members collectively smoked 1–9 cigarettes per day, as compared to households with no smokers, 6.6 times as great (95 percent confidence interval 2.5–17.5) for households consuming 10–19 cigarettes per day, and 3.6 times as great (95 percent confidence interval 1.9–7.2) for households consuming 20 or more cigarettes per day (Ballard et al., 1992). Although the consumption of five or more drinks of alcohol per occasion (binge drinking) was also found to be important, multiple regression analysis suggested that smoking was the more significant risk factor.

Cigarette smoking is one of several factors that affect the development of osteoporosis in women. It may do this by lowering estrogen levels (Kelsey and Hochberg, 1992). Smoking is associated with decreased hip bone mineral density among both men and women (Hollenbach et al., 1993). This contributes to an increase in mortality and morbidity from fractures among the elderly. Smoking cessation is beneficial in reducing losses of bone mineral density. Smoking also delays healing of fractures, probably because of impaired circulation to bone ends. Disability from back injury is also associated with smoking.

While data are scarce to establish drugs other than alcohol as a common risk factor for injury, many commonly used medications, including barbiturates and benzodiazepine tranquilizers such as diazepam have an additive or synergistic effect when combined with alcohol (Joscelyn and Maickel, 1975; Moskowitz, 1976). Many antihistamines cause drowsiness and decrease attentiveness to the surroundings (Burns, 1990).

Little is known about the use of drugs in developing countries. However, recent reports suggest that the use of cocaine, marijuana, and solvents is widespread in the Americas, including Mexico and Central and South America (PAHO, 1990). In a small survey of injured vehicle drivers treated in hospital in the Kaduna region of Nigeria, 20 percent were found to be abusers of cannabis and amphetamines (Obembe and Fagbayi, 1988). Although other drugs such as *khat* and *areca* (betel) are used by millions, little is known about their effects on the risk of injury.

Marijuana has been found to affect coordination, tracking, perception, vigilance, and performance during driving simulations and on the road (Moskowitz, 1985). However, it has been difficult to determine risk in non-experimental studies because blood levels of tetrahydrocannabinol decline rapidly. The level of drug in the urine does not correlate with the degree of impairment, and symptoms are often masked by simultaneous use of alcohol. Nevertheless, it has been reported that marijuana, cocaine, and opiates all impair driving performance (Bradbury, 1990). This effect may be mediated by increased risk-taking and impaired judgment, which are not measured by standard tests used by police (Brookoff et al., 1994; Angell and Kassirer, 1994).

Cocaine also causes sudden deaths from cardiovascular toxicity, including strokes and cardiac arrest. Evidence of cocaine use was found in the blood or urine of 27 percent of fatally injured New York City residents (Marzuk et al., 1995).

Inhalation of solvents, including gasoline and other liquid and aerosol products, is common among young people in aboriginal communities in northern Québec (Robitaille and Barss, 1994) and other areas of North America. Chronic exposure to neurotoxic solvents can cause permanent brain damage, and acute inhalation can result in sudden death. Such deaths could be due to cardiotoxicity and sudden arrhythmias attributable to either the solvent itself or to other chemical additives. Solvents sold as aerosols also contain propellants. New propellants have been adopted to replace chlorofluorocarbons, which cause damage to the ozone layer of the atmosphere. Many deaths from abuse of solvents are not reported to poison control centers or hospitals that accumulate data used for surveillance of product toxicity. Solvent abuse often occurs with a background of underlying social pathology, and increases when alcohol is prohibited or unavailable.

Physical and Medical Factors

Epilepsy
Epilepsy is the most common serious neurological condition in every country of the world (Shorvon, 1990; Lancet editorial, 1997). The incidence of epilepsy in the general population of developed countries is about four to ten affected individuals per 1000 population (Shorvon, 1990). In some developing countries, including Central American nations (Acha and Aguilar, 1964) and Irian Jaya (Subianto et al., 1978) the prevalence of epilepsy is higher because of parasitic infections that affect the brain, such as *cysticercosis* (tissue cysts of pork tapeworm).

Epilepsy is an important risk factor for several types of injuries, including drowning, burns, and falls (Canadian Red Cross Society, 1996a; Barss, 1991; Barss and Wallace, 1983; Fallon et al., 1989). Certain village activities are particularly hazardous in the presence of untreated or poorly controlled seizures. Examples include, climbing during tree agriculture, fishing from open canoes, underwater spear fishing, bathing in any open body of water, and cooking and heating with open flames. The probability of serious injury is much greater if persons with epilepsy engage in such activities alone, or if their family and companions are frightened and flee when a seizure occurs.

While people can be affected by epilepsy at any age, many cases begin in childhood or early adulthood. This early onset puts many young and economically productive individuals at increased risk of serious or fatal injury. Unfortunately, in developing countries many individuals with seizure disorders receive no treatment whatsoever, either because of a lack of resources and limited access to health providers and medications, or because of traditional cultural beliefs (Tekle-Haimanot, 1993; Tekle-Haimanot et al., 1991). In rural areas of many of the least developed countries, anticonvulsant medications are completely unavailable. It has been estimated that in the Philippines and Pakistan only 6 percent of patients receive treatment, and in Ecuador, only 20 percent (Shorvon and Farmer, 1988).

Dementia
Impaired central nervous function from organic causes, such as various causes of dementia, particularly among the elderly, increases the risk for certain domestic injuries, such as hot water burns, drownings during bathing, and housefires. People with demenita are obviously also at high risk when exposed to situations such as traffic.

Impaired Vision

Vision is a factor in avoiding some types of injury. A study of taxi drivers in Lagos, Nigeria, found that one–third had serious deficiencies of visual acuity, but only 10 percent were aware of their need for corrective lenses (Alakija, 1981). Compulsory vision tests for drivers have all but eliminated this problem in many countries.

It has been suggested that night blindness resulting from vitamin A deficiency may increase the risk of injury at night. Malnutrition and certain vitamin deficiencies could impair recovery from injuries in a variety of ways, including lowering resistance to infections.

Osteoporosis

Weak bones lower the injury threshold and thereby increase the risk of injuries such as fractures of the hip, vertebrae, and distal radius. Osteoporosis is evident on X-rays as decalcification of bone. However, less obvious changes in cellular and fibrous trabeculae of bones may be even more important than calcium content in altering the risk of fracture during a potentially injurious event such as a fall.

There has been considerable interest, particularly regarding the elderly, in research showing that exercise may strengthen the trabecular structure of bone and thereby increase its resistance to fractures (Ford, 1989; Wickham et al., 1989). Hip fractures appear to be rare among elderly rural inhabitants of some developing countries (Barss, 1985a). This may be because such individuals remain active and walk a great deal, even in old age. Exercise early in childhood and adolescence is important (Kelsey and Hochberg, 1992). On the other hand, cigarette smoking has an adverse effect on bone mineral density.

Occupation

Occupation is frequently an important predictor of risk for both unintentional and intentional injuries. Few examples are presented here, since occupational injuries are discussed in greater detail in Chapter 11.

In developing countries, injury rates for any given occupation are generally higher than in developed countries. For example, factory workers in India have mortality rates 50 percent higher than factory workers in the United States (Mohan, 1984), and Nigerian coal miners had mortality rates seven times higher than miners in England (Asogwa, 1980b).

Certain occupations are particularly hazardous because of frequent exposure to hostile environments. Differences in death rates for specific occupations within an industry may be even greater than differences among industries, yet difficult to discern or prove statistically because of the small numbers of workers in specific job categories.

In the United States, among different industries, there is a tenfold difference in rates of death by traumatic injury. Workers in agriculture and mining and quarrying industries, for example, have high death rates, while those in trade industries have much lower rates (National Safety Council, 1994). At a time when the average occupational injury death rate was about 10 per 100,000 workers per year, fire fighters were found to have mortality rates of 75 deaths per

100,000 (IAFF, 1980). For full-time workers on active oil rigs in 1978, mortality rates were estimated to range from 188 to 283 deaths per 100,000 workers per year (CDC, 1980).

Agriculture has been identified as a hazardous industry, although the highly mechanized farming in many developed countries poses risks different from those faced by illiterate subsistence farmers using small unprotected machines. Rates for construction workers are also high. Occupations that involve the handling of money, especially in small facilities at night, may place workers at high risk of violent death during robberies.

Maritime occupations pose significant hazards (Schilling, 1971). In Greenland, native Inuit mortality rate from boating incidents was 65 times the rate for the general population of Denmark (Bjerregaard and Juel, 1990). Most of the deaths were drownings. The mortality rate in males has decreased over the past century, mainly because changes in occupation require less traditional hunting and fishing from kayaks (Bjerregaard, 1990a). Although studies of occupational drownings from developing countries are rare, it is likely that serious underreporting occurs, since when drownings occur at sea or in other remote locations, the bodies may not be recovered. In addition to drowning, fishers in small open canoes and divers who spear fish are exposed to environmental hazards such as penetrating wounds and marine envenomations (Barss, 1982, 1984a, 1985a; Paux and Bahuaud, 1989; Auerbach, 1991).

In developing countries, economic factors play an important role in occupational injuries in three ways. First, economic necessities encourage workers to take hazardous jobs, second, investment costs induce employers to avoid taking essential safety measures (Mohan, 1987c; Qadeer and Mohan, 1989), and third, oversight costs inhibit the development of appropriate government institutions and trained staff to monitor the safety of worksites. Another special point to be considered in developing countries is the exposure of women and children to injuries by farm animals and by small farm machines with unshielded moving parts. The usual reporting systems tend to miss many farm injuries (Qadeer and Mohan, 1989).

Socioeconomic Status and Education

Social and economic status and education are closely linked. There are exceptions, since in some countries, certain occupations convey relatively high prestige and social standing, but provide low income. The type of housing and its location are environmental factors closely linked to social, economic, and educational status. While socioeconomic status and education are individual personal factors, they are also community environmental factors. These factors can be compared among countries. For some governments, equity is a major consideration, and their policies have a major influence on income differentials and the average level of education in the population.

Although socioeconomic status, education, and housing are important risk factors for many diseases (Bjerregaard and Bjerregaard, 1985; Hobcraft et al., 1984; Brennan and Lancashire, 1978; Hobart, 1976; Berg and Adler-Nissen, 1976), there have been few studies of the effect of such variables on the risk of injury, even in developed countries. Low educational status is a determinant for different types of injuries, but specific educational programs for injury prevention have not been particularly successful.

In Greenland, mortality from injuries was high in low-income groups (Bjerregaard, 1990b). Among the Inuit, suicide rates were found to be a problem mainly of lower income strata, contrary to general opinion. This strata included the unemployed, people with unstable occupations, hunters, and fishers (Thorslund, 1990). Much lower suicide rates were found among white collar workers, the self-employed, housewives, and retired persons.

Among Canadian Indians, a widespread lack of secondary education, resulting in exclusion from meaningful work in the modern world, is the underlying cause of many injuries, including many alcohol associated deaths (Jarvis and Boldt, 1982). Inadequate education often causes unemployment, underemployment, low socioeconomic status, feelings of uselessness and estrangement from society, and alcoholism.

Maoris and Pacific Islanders in New Zealand had age-standardized injury mortality rates of 148 and 128 per 100,000 per year compared with 92 in the rest of the population. If Maori injury death rates had been the same as those for the rest of the population in each social class and age group, these would have been 20 percent less Maori deaths (Pearce et al., 1983, 1984).

Pedestrian and cyclist fatalities are particularly common among persons of low socioeconomic and educational status because wealthier people travel in the protected environment of cars. Male workers doing casual and menial jobs and recent migrants to the city accounted for a significant proportion of pedestrian fatalities in Delhi (Sarin et al., 1990f).

In a report of nonfatal motor vehicle injuries in children and adolescents under 20 years of age in Latin America, the pattern of injury differed. In Brazil, there was a two-and-one-half times and, in Venezuela, a five-and-one-half times greater risk of traffic injury for children from households headed by a person with a university education, compared to children from households headed by a person with only a primary education (Bangdiwala and Anzola-Perez, 1990). On the other hand, in Brazil, children and adolescents in households headed by a person with only a primary education had three times the risk of a home injury, such as a fall or burn, compared to children of highly educated parents.

Children of affluent parents are more likely to sustain nonfatal injuries as passengers inside a vehicle, while children of the poor more frequently sustain fatal injuries as pedestrians or as bicyclists struck by a motor vehicle; they also suffer more injuries in the home.

In São Paulo, Brazil, death rates from traffic injuries were twice as high among industrial and manual workers as among professionals, and homicide rates were five times as high (World Bank, 1989). Homicide rates are substantially higher among the poor than among the middle class in both Rio de Janeiro and São Paulo. In the United States, adults of low socioeconomic status also appear to be at increased risk of violent death, as discussed in Chapter 13.

Poverty is often the underlying factor for many injury hazards. The high injury rates observed among the poor suggest that targeted educational approaches to injury prevention may fail unless basic environmental and societal improvements are also made. This includes improvements in equity and general education, and reductions in violence and neighborhood hazards. Reducing poverty and socioeconomic gradients and improving education requires greater commitment from governments and society.

Interpersonal Skills

Impaired interpersonal skills and low self-esteem can lead to depression and suicide attempts. While injuries arising from such personal impairments may appear as isolated events indicative of individual pathology, they are often a manifestation of pervasive problems affecting families, communities, or entire cultures. This is particularly evident in indigenous communities in developed countries, where suicide and substance abuse are epidemic because of external assaults on the integrity of entire cultures.

Skills in interpersonal communication, assertiveness, and the ability to seek help for psychological crises are important to avoid isolation, depression, and substance abuse that can lead to violence such as suicide or suicide attempts. Significant deficiencies in these basic communication skills were found among Zuni aboriginal adolescents in the United States who had attempted suicide or who had ideas about committing suicide, compared to those never attempting suicide (Howard-Pitney et al., 1992). Adolescents need to receive life skills training to prevent suicide and improve the ability to cope with other areas of life.

Training in life skills is particularly important for children from broken homes, homes where there is alcoholism, and otherwise disturbed families. Better communication skills for parents would help reduce interpersonal family violence.

Other Personal Risk Factors

For children or dependent adults, the characteristics of any caretaker can determine risks of injury. The age, educational level, alcohol use, and smoking habits of siblings or parents may affect the risk of certain injuries. Family size may also affect injury risk, particularly if small children are left in the care of young siblings.

EQUIPMENT FACTORS

The inherent design of equipment, including motor vehicles and other devices, can substantially affect the risk of injury. In addition, special safety equipment can be used by individuals or incorporated into vehicles to reduce the risk of specific injury if a crash or other incident occurs. Thus, certain products pose an inherent risk for injuries, by virtue of poor design or by encouraging participation in unsafe activities. On the other hand, many products have been developed specifically to reduce the risk of injury.

Special safety equipment that reduces the risk of injury during a hazardous incident includes devices such as helmets for cyclists, personal flotation devices for boaters, hypothermia suits for travel in northern climates by boat and over ice by snowmobile, safety belts, and air bags in automobiles. Impact-absorbing vehicle interiors and bumpers help to reduce the severity of injuries even if a crash occurs.

Better lighting, improved road signs, anti-lock brakes, reflective materials, and bright colors to increase the visibility of pedestrians, cyclists, and motor vehicles are innovations that reduce the probability of collisions. These are primary preventions that require no sustained or repetitive efforts by individuals. Examples of equipment to reduce other types of injuries include enclosed stoves and lamps to prevent burns from open fires and harvesting of fruit by devices on long poles to prevent falls from trees.

Devices that provide automatic protection are preferable, since they do not require constant vigilance by individuals. Safety equipment that is repeatedly put on or attached must be carefully adapted to the needs and tastes of consumers, ensuring that it is light, comfortable, attractive, inexpensive, and quick and easy to use.

Many products have been improved to reduce an inherent risk of them causing injury. Nevertheless, new products and chemicals are being released constantly, and their potential for harm must be monitored. Canada and the United States have been monitoring these risks in networks of emergency rooms. In the United States, reports are made to the Consumer Product Safety Commission. (It is unfortunate that injuries caused by two of the most dangerous products in the United States, cigarettes and firearms, are not included in the mandate of this commission.) Agencies empowered to regulate the safety of consumer products exist in many developed countries but are rare in developing countries.

Specific equipment or vehicle changes intended to prevent various types of injuries are discussed in more detail in chapters on specific injuries.

ENVIRONMENTAL FACTORS

The environment consists of physical and psychosocial elements. Both are substantially affected by poverty, rural-urban residence, and development. The environment can become more hazardous after dark and during weekends. Pedestrian traffic injuries to children are affected by crowded streets and inadequate play areas in poor urban neighborhoods, as discussed above. Substandard housing may also increase the risk of death from housefires and from disasters such as earthquakes and cyclones.

Certain aspects of hazardous physical and psychosocial environments in poor neighborhoods can be altered or compensated for, if the specific problems can be documented and the relevant decision makers influenced to make the necessary changes. Many inhabitants of these neighborhoods share certain personal risk factors that place them at higher risk for various types of injuries (Bagley, 1992b).

Rural Versus Urban Environment

Rural-urban differences in unintentional injuries often reflect underlying differences in exposure to occupational and environmental hazards. High rural rates of intentional injuries, such as suicide, may be a result of specific social and cultural features of village life, the impact of rapid development, and the effects of isolation on the lives of women and adolescents.

In rural areas of some developed countries, a lack of timely access to good medical and emergency care, because facilities are over-centralized, is believed to contribute to higher rates of fatal injury (Bentham, 1986). Much more serious problems of communications, transport, and access to health care are found in rural areas of many developing countries.

In industrialized countries such as Canada, the United States, and New Zealand, rural residents have higher rates of fatal unintentional injuries than urban residents (Borman and Leiatua, 1984; S.P. Baker et al., 1992). Rural-urban differences persist even when adjustment is made for the per capita income in the residential area. In rural areas, travel tends to be on open roads at high speeds, speed limits are often unenforced, roads may be less safe, exposure to farm machinery and firearms is widespread, and medical care is generally less accessible.

Data on rural–urban differences in developing countries are limited, but the patterns are expected to vary significantly depending upon the local environment. For example, in a rural area of Nepal, traffic injuries were not among the top nine listed causes of injury during an 18 month period in 1985–86. However, in an urban hospital in Kathmandu in 1987, traffic injuries were the second most common type of injury leading to hospital admission, casualty department visits, and death in the casualty department (Thapa, 1989). In Taiwan, the rate of traffic fatalities is relatively high in the mountainous country-side, but is twice as high in the flat urban areas (Chiang, 1989).

In some remote areas, aboriginals often travel over water in small boats and have high drowning rates (Health Canada, 1998; Choinière et al., 1993; Bjerregaard, 1992; Muir, 1991). Among the Inuit of Greenland, the rate of maritime injuries is higher in smaller communities (Bjerregaard, 1990b; Bjerregaard and Juel, 1990). The majority of fatal injuries, including drownings, burns, hypothermia, and unintentional firearm injuries, are related to traditional lifestyles, which are most common in the less affluent settlements and remote areas.

In China, rates of suicide and drowning are much higher in rural than urban areas; death rates from falls in the elderly, on the other hand, are much higher in urban areas (WHO, 1991). In the highlands of Papua New Guinea, rates of suicide among women and of drowning among men are significantly higher in remote rural villages than in periurban villages (Barss, 1991).

Thus, the relative importance of particular types of injury may vary widely from one place to another. While suicide, drownings in open bodies of water, falls from trees, burns from open fires, and high speed car crashes are important causes of death for many rural residents, for city residents, the greatest likelihood of dying from injuries may be as a pedestrian, a cyclist, or a passenger in the back of an open vehicle or hanging on to the outside of a bus.

Development

The process of development brings about exposure to many new hazards; however, there may be concomitant decreases in other hazardous exposures from everyday village life, such as those related to subsistence farming and fishing. Even if the overall injury mortality rate does not change significantly during development, different patterns of causes occur. Some changes are due to differences between life in rural and urban environments, while others are caused specifically by the rapid introduction of new occupations, motor vehicles, hazardous machinery, cutting tools, and other technology. Development of large gradients by social class can lead to high rates of violence.

Increased exposure to alcohol marketing and consumption together with social instability may contribute to violence in the home and suicide. Employment in factories or on plantations with hazardous, poorly shielded machinery may replace the traditional high-risk activities of fishing from small canoes and clearing forests for gardens. With large amounts of energy concentrated in the form of machinery and motor vehicles, the potential for severe, permanently disabling injury may increase. On the other hand, injuries sustained during subsistence activities, such as penetrating wounds from sticks and deep lacerations of extremities from simple tools such as machetes, can cause permanent disability or death if basic first-aid and treatment are unavailable.

When modern industry is transferred to developing countries, safety features are often omitted. This is done to save on costs, since regulations and enforcement are less stringent in developing countries. Outdated technology and banned products, such as hazardous pesticides and other chemicals may be imported. Thus, an increase in hazards may be built into the way technology is transferred to developing countries. The gas-leak disaster at the Union Carbide plant in Bhopal, India was a dramatic demonstration of the risks of introducing modern technology to a developing country without the usual safeguards (Melius and Binder, 1989; Bertazzi, 1989; Mohan, 1987b).

Motor vehicle injuries are obviously related to development in various ways. At low levels of development, there are generally small numbers of motor vehicles and relatively low per capita rates of motor vehicle fatalities. However, the fatality rates per vehicle tend to be high. This is because of poor roads, unprotected road users, such as bicyclists and pedestrians, sharing the road with motor vehicles, open vehicles that offer little protection to passengers, overloading of vehicles, poor vehicle maintenance, and inadequate driver training and licensing.

As development progresses and the number of vehicles increases, the population-based fatality rate may increase, but the rate per vehicle decreases. At high levels of development, the per capita rate may level off or even fall. One study, however, questions the theory that injury mortality from motor vehicles is a disease of development (Wintemute, 1985). The author found no relationship between the per capita gross national product and the rates of motor-vehicle injury reported to the World Health Organization for 46 developing and industrialized countries. However, the highest injury mortality rates were reported from developing or transitional countries. This raises questions about how rapid changes in the level of development affect injury mortality, as opposed to the level of development per se. Unfortunately, injury mortality data from the poorest countries were not available.

Some of the adverse effects of development causing a variety of injuries among remote aboriginal populations can be discerned by reviewing the literature on indigenous Canadians, indigenous Americans, and Greenland Inuit, as already discussed under various sections above. There may, however, be beneficial compensating factors of development for some aboriginals in developed countries, benefits that are unavailable to indigenous populations in countries that possess far fewer resources. These include improved housing, transportation, education, and health care.

It is unfortunate that the harmful effects of development, including injuries, often arrive before sufficient local knowledge, education, management skills, bureaucratic structures, legal expertise, and technology have been established to prevent them or deal with the consequences. The negative impact of development can be seen in the high rates of injuries, alcoholism, solvent abuse, nicotine addiction, lung cancer, obesity, and diabetes among many aboriginal Canadians (Muir, 1991). Greater efforts are needed to anticipate the harmful effects of development, many of which are highly predictable on the basis of current epidemiologic knowledge.

Day of Week and Time of Day

Injury rates often vary dramatically in relation to the day of the week and time of day (S.P. Baker et al., 1992). It was suggested at an international meeting on injuries in the circumpolar environment that the most effective method of reducing the injury rate in Greenland would be to abolish Saturdays! (P. Bjerregaard, personal communication, 1992) Of course, the underlying determinants for such temporal risk factors are often other risk factors that are associated with certain days, times, or seasons, including excessive alcohol consumption, fatigue, reduced visibility from darkness, or an increase in hazardous activities.

In developed countries, weekends are often a time for travel, socializing, and recreation, and, unfortunately, also for the consumption of alcohol. Thus the risk of a number of types of severe or fatal injuries, especially those related to driving, is significantly higher on Fridays and Saturdays. Although travel is less at night, nighttime alcohol use contributes to higher motor vehicle death rates at night. Night travel also affects visibility.

In New Delhi, fatalities of pedestrians and bicyclists were more frequent in the morning between 6 A.M. and noon, while fatalities of motorcyclists were more common in the afternoon and evening between noon and midnight (Mohan and Bawa, 1985). Differences among days of the week were less pronounced than in many developed countries (Mohan and Kumar, 1989).

Among Canadian Indians in the province of Alberta during 1976–77, Friday and Saturday were found to be the most deadly days for deaths from injury, and the early hours of the morning the most deadly time (Jarvis and Boldt, 1982). Alcohol-related deaths from fire were 27 times more frequent among aboriginals than among other Canadians. Almost half of these deaths from fire occurred on Saturday night and 83 percent during sleep. Similar patterns have been observed among the Greenland Inuit, with increased fire deaths also observed around the time of Christmas festivities (Bjerregaard, 1992).

Season and Climate

Seasonal changes also affect the risk of injury. Seasonal and climatic factors are important determinants of disasters, such as floods in low-land deltas and landslides in deforested regions.

In the United States, the number of police-reported traffic crashes with property damage is highest during the cold winter months, but the number of crashes with severe or fatal injury is higher during the summer. Rates of drowning and electrocution are high in the summer. Fatal housefires are most common during the coldest winter months at night.

Cold weather increases the risk of drownings complicated by hypothermia. Immersion hypothermia is most evident during spring, autumn, and winter. Snowstorms impair visibility and, together with darkness, alcohol, and high speed, increase the risk of drowning in holes in the ice during travel by high-powered snowmobiles (Canadian Red Cross Society, 1996).

INTERACTION OF MULTIPLE DETERMINANTS

Combinations of risk factors and other determinants of injury may have either additive or multiplicative effects on the probability of injury. Multiplicative effects imply a synergistic interaction of risk factors (Rothman, 1986). For example, the probability of a motor vehicle fatality, given the combination of several factors such as an inexperienced, immature, male teenage driver, alcohol, fatigue, darkness, an unfamiliar road, and excessive speed, may greatly exceed the sum of the individual probabilities of injury for each factor taken separately. The combination of cigarette smoking and alcohol abuse substantially increases the risk of residential fires (Ballard et al., 1992). Among children from poor families, the adverse physical environment in crowded urban neighborhoods may interact with risk-taking behaviors related to psychosocial personal factors so as to greatly increase the risk of pedestrian injuries (Bagley, 1992b).

The effects of certain exposures can differ depending upon the sex of the person exposed. Although males tend to abuse alcohol and engage in binge drinking more often than females, women who do drink appear to be more sensitive to the effects of alcohol than male drinkers (Waller, 1992). For a given quantity of alcohol based upon body weight, blood alcohol levels in females rise higher and the alcohol is eliminated more slowly than in males, and performance in driving and other tasks is more impaired among females than among males. Women have an increased crash rate at lower levels of alcohol. Moderate chronic consumption of alcohol has also been reported to increase the risk of hip and forearm fractures among women by dissolving calcium from bones. The adverse impact of alcohol on women's fractures may be greater because of their smaller bone size.

The interaction between personal risk factors and environmental hazards may be an important determinant of injury. For example, in villages where open cooking fires are still the norm, untreated people with epilepsy often sustain severe burns when they fall into fires during seizures. Nonfatal burns are sometimes so severe that they necessitate amputation of an arm or leg (Barss and Wallace,

1983). Thus, the synergistic interaction of a personal risk factor, untreated epilepsy, and an environmental exposure, an open cooking fire, leads to a severe injury. However, the probability of such an injury in the presence of only one of these factors would be much less than the probability in the presence of both.

Often it is not necessary to eliminate all of the risk factors to achieve a substantial reduction in injury. Regular treatment of an individual patient's epilepsy with anticonvulsants can reduce the risk of injuries associated with sudden loss of consciousness during seizures. Unfortunately, such treatment is not always feasible in remote areas of poorer countries, and even when it is, compliance with long-term drug therapy tends to be poor.

One alternative approach is a population-based intervention to reduce the hazards of open cooking fires in the household environment by promoting the use of simple enclosed stoves throughout the entire community or region. This approach would have other desirable features, such as fuel economy and a reduction in lung damage and respiratory infections from smoke (Nation's Health, 1992), as well as prevention of burns among the general population, including women, children, and the elderly. A program introducing simple enclosed stoves significantly reduced the incidence of burns in one area of Nepal (Thapa, 1989). Education targeted to people with epilepsy is another approach to preventing burns. Families of affected persons would be instructed either to use an enclosed stove or never to leave the epileptic individual alone near an open fire.

Each of these three policies would have certain positive and negative aspects, and a combination of approaches might be appropriate. The environmental approach of enclosing the hazard would provide a more permanent solution by reducing the need for continuous vigilance by the affected individual and the family.

chapter 7

Traffic Injuries: Introduction

There has been a rapid increase in exposure to motor vehicles in many parts of the world. Nevertheless, traffic injuries need not be an inevitable consequence of development, since motor vehicles are a man-made hazard and subject to control or modification. Unfortunately, few countries, in both the developed and developing world, have made deliberate efforts to favor alternate methods of transport (Lowe, 1989). In the absence of explicit government policy to favor safer methods of transport, rapid motorization can be expected to continue as demand is stimulated by local pressure from users, by external marketing activities of vehicle exporting countries, and by policies of international lending institutions (Replogle, 1991; Orski, 1990; J. Wong, 1994b).

Control of traffic injuries is a multidisciplinary undertaking that has stimulated innumerable books and articles in many fields. It is not possible to consider all aspects of this vast topic in this book. However, this chapter should provide the reader with an overview of traffic injuries, an awareness of some of the important differences between the issues that face developed and developing countries, and an idea of where one might begin to describe and address specific problems of traffic injuries in a country or community. The next chapter considers specific determinants of injuries for different road user types.

Traffic injuries are considered from several perspectives, with special consideration for the needs of unprotected or vulnerable road users—those who do not have the protection afforded by the metal frame of a closed vehicle compartment. Pedestrians, bicyclists, motorcyclists, passengers in the rear of open-backed trucks, and persons boarding and leaving buses are all highly vulnerable to injury compared to vehicle occupants.

Intercountry or regional differences in patterns of injury by road user type have significant implications for prevention policies. Advisors and policymakers who ignore such differences and base their decisions mainly on data from developed countries risk promoting costly and relatively ineffectual policies for prevention of traffic injuries.

IMPORTANCE OF TRAFFIC INJURIES

Traffic injuries are undeniably an important cause of lost life and limb in most countries today. The global impact of traffic injuries on mortality and morbidity has been estimated at about 300,000 deaths and 10–15 million persons injured per year (Transport and Road Research Laboratory, 1991). A different source estimated that there are 500,000 traffic deaths per year and that 350,000 of the deaths occur in developing countries (World Bank, 1990). Each traffic fatality means, on average, a loss of about 30 person-years of life expectancy (PAHO, 1986).

Traffic injuries are also a leading cause of hospitalization and disability. There are between 10 and 25 times more injuries than deaths from motor vehicles, with about half of the injured requiring hospitalization (Feachem et al., 1992). The number of persons left permanently impaired after traffic injuries is estimated to be about equal to the number of fatalities. Brain and spinal cord injuries have a particularly devastating long-term impact on victims, their families, and society (Miller et al., 1989).

The number of traffic fatalities per vehicle is many times higher in developing than in developed countries (Fig. 7.1).

While traffic injuries in developed countries are still an important cause of mortality and hospitalization, various interventions have contributed to substantial reductions in recent years even as traffic has increased. In developing countries, there have been marked increases in the numbers of traffic fatalities (Fig. 7.2). However, in certain countries, as the number of cars has increased, there has been an improvement in the number of fatalities per vehicle, even as the death rate per 100,000 inhabitants rose (Downing et al., 1991). This could reflect improvements in traffic safety, but other possible explanations include slower speeds due to urban congestion, fewer occupants per vehicle, and greater protection to travelers, as a large proportion became vehicle occupants, instead of more vulnerable types of road users.

Figure 7.1

Traffic deaths per 10,000 vehicles per year, selected countries, 1985-1986.
Source: UK Transport and Road Research Laboratory, *Towards Safer Roads in Developing Countries,* 1991. Copyright Controller of HMSO 1991. Reproduced with permission of the Controller of HMSO.

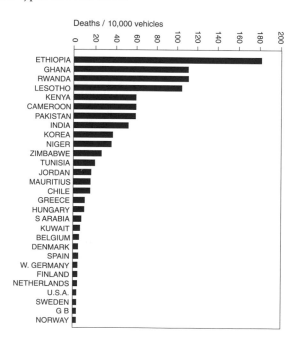

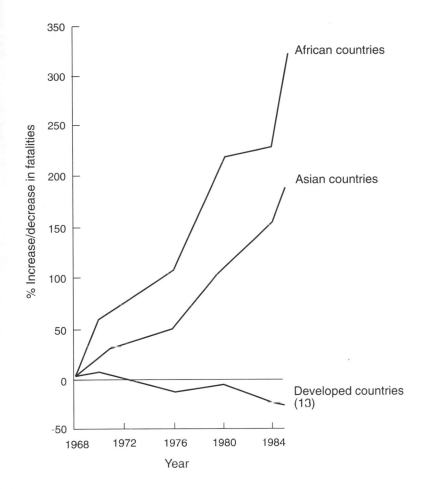

Figure 7.2

Change in number of traffic deaths in Africa, Asia, and developed countries, 1968-85. Source: UK Transport and Road Research Laboratory, *Towards Safer Roads in Developing Countries,* 1991. Copyright Controller of HMSO 1991. Reproduced with permission of the Controller of HMSO.

In many developing countries, traffic injuries have a significant economic impact. This has been estimated to range between 1 and 3 percent of the gross domestic product (GDP), with the average probably at least 1 percent (Transport and Road Research Laboratory, 1991; Mackay and Petruccelli, 1990; WHO, 1987; Fouracre and Jacobs, 1976). In Kenya, for example, traffic injuries have been conservatively estimated to cost the national economy about 2.5 percent of GDP (Gekonge, 1990). In Iran, traffic crashes were estimated to cost about 1.5 percent of GDP (Ayati, 1990), and in Thailand, close to 2 percent (WHO, 1987).

If the average cost of traffic crashes for all countries with a GDP per capita of less than $3,500 US dollars were 1.0 percent of GDP, then the total annual costs for those countries would be about $25 billion (Downing et al., 1991). This is a tremendous waste of resources that developing countries can ill afford, and is a serious drag on improvements in the standard of living.

SPECIAL FEATURES OF TRAFFIC INJURIES IN DEVELOPING COUNTRIES AND INDIGENOUS COMMUNITIES

In developed countries, occupants of private automobiles comprise the majority of traffic injury victims, but this is not the case in many developing countries. Pedestrians, bicyclists, motorcyclists, and passengers who ride in buses and open trucks are often the majority of victims (Dessie and Larson, 1991; Mohan, 1990a, 1990b; Desai et al., 1990a, 1990b; Jacobs and Sayer, 1983). The low proportion of automobile occupants as victims in some densely populated developing countries, such as India, may be because of both a different vehicle mix and overcrowded roads that have few areas where significant speed can be achieved (Mohan and Bawa, 1985).

In developed countries, the vast majority of victims are drivers or front seat passengers in automobiles (U.S. Dept of Transport, 1990), so most resources for prevention of traffic injuries are focused on this category of road user. Different research and prevention priorities are needed for many developing countries and indigenous communities.

Nearly 80 percent of the world's automobiles are owned by the 15 percent of the world's population who live in North America, Western Europe, and Japan. In these regions, each family on average owns one or more cars. However, in India and China, less than 1 in 60 families own a car (Mohan, 1990a, 1990b).

Unimaginable as it may seem to urban commuters in developed countries, the bulk of the world's population travel primarily by means other than as occupants of automobiles. Many children in developed countries are provided with bicycles for recreational purposes, while in

Table 7.1 Percentage of fatalities by road-user class

	Pedestrians	Cyclists	Motorcyclists/ Scooterists	Drivers/ Passengers	Year
Ethiopia	84	1	1	13	1980
Tripoli, Libya	66	0	0	32	1987
Swaziland	55	5	0	40	1976
Sri Lanka	51	10	10	28	1980
Thailand	47	6	36	12	1987
Jordan	47	1	2	50	1979
Guyana	45	13	10	28	1977
Kenya	45	9	2	40	1972
Jamaica	41	5	17	37	1978
Zambia	40	8	3	49	1977
Zimbabwe	36	9	2	47	1979
Nigeria	35	3	20	42	—
Delhi, India	32	10	20	2	1985
Indonesia	23	15	31	30	1980
West Malaysia	22	13	33	32	1979
Hong Kong	70	4	7	19	1980
Kuwait	55	2	2	41	1978
United Kingdom	32	5	19	44	1980
United States	15	2	9	74	1987

First group of countries all had per capita GNP <US$2500; second group included for comparison. Adapted from Jacobs GD, Sayer I. *Accid. Anal. and Prev.* 1983;15:34 and Mohan D. *J Traffic Med* 1990;18:153–155

some developing countries, a bicycle may be a luxury for most people and is used for essential transportation rather than recreation.

As a result of such differences in principal modes of transport, there are great disparities in the proportions of traffic fatalities as pedestrians, bicyclists, motorcyclists, drivers, and passengers (Table 7.1). Passengers often greatly outnumber drivers in developing countries. These data significantly underestimate the importance of injuries to pedestrians and bicyclists, since injuries to these road users tend to be markedly underreported by police (Sayer and Hitchcock, 1984). This could account for the relatively low percentage of pedestrian involvement reported for some of the developing countries included in Table 7.1.

In New Delhi, India, during 1985, 77 percent of the victims of motor vehicle crashes were unprotected road users (Mohan and Kumar, 1989). In 58 percent of cases, the victims were struck by buses or trucks. Only 1.5 percent of victims were occupants of cars, and cars were involved as the impacting vehicle in only 6 percent of cases. Pedestrians, bus passengers, and users of two-wheelers, including bicycles and motorcycles, constituted the majority of traffic victims. Figure 7.3 provides a comparison of the types of road users killed in traffic injuries in New Delhi and Montréal, Canada. This illustrates how the proportion of vulnerable road users differs between metropolitan areas in a developing country and a developed one.

These different injuries reflect the types of vehicles involved in crashes, which differ considerably between developed and developing countries. The percentage of traffic fatalities that involved trucks and buses ranged between 25 and 44 percent in Botswana, Egypt, Ghana, Pakistan, Papua New Guinea, and Zimbabwe, as compared to 21 percent in the United Kingdom (Downing et al., 1991). Similarly, in Beijing, China, about 30 percent of victims were bicyclists, 20 percent were pedestrians, and the remainder were motor vehicle occupants (Ryan and Ukai, 1988).

Developing countries face other problems that are unfamiliar in developed countries, such as combinations of the newest modes of transport with some of the oldest in the world. Roads designed in the West, mainly for automobiles, carry both human and animal powered vehicles, as well as most types of modern transport. For example, in Delhi, India, road traffic includes hand carts and cycle rickshaws, along with large numbers of different types of motor vehicles (Deputy Commissioner of Traffic Police, Delhi, 1989).

The relative importance of traffic injuries compared to other injuries and diseases can vary significantly among countries and regions within a country, depending, among other factors, upon the degree of motorization. While traffic injuries, particularly of pedes-

Figure 7.3

Urban road user fatalities: New Delhi, India and Montreal, Canada.
Source of data: Choinière R. et al. *Profil des Traumatismes au Québec: Disparités Régionales et Tendances de la Mortalité (1976 à 1990) et des Hospitalisations (1981 à 1991)*. Québec, Québec: Gouvernement du Québec, Ministère de la Santé et Services sociaux, 1993, and Mohan D. Vulnerable road users: an era of neglect. *Journal of Traffic Medicine 1992; 20: 121-128.*

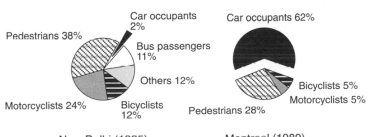

Pedestrians 38%
Car occupants 2%
Bus passengers 11%
Others 12%
Motorcyclists 24%
Bicyclists 12%

New Delhi (1985)

Car occupants 62%
Bicyclists 5%
Motorcyclists 5%
Pedestrians 28%

Montreal (1989)

trians, are generally a leading cause of unintentional injury deaths in urban areas of developing countries (Dessie and Larson, 1991), they are of secondary or even minor importance in rural areas with few roads, as in Nepal and Bangladesh (Thapa, 1989; Fauveau and Blanchet, 1989). In Nepal, for example, much of the terrain is so mountainous and the country so poor that, in many areas, goods and people are moved on the backs of animals or other people.

This is not always the case, and rural roads in some developing countries can be more dangerous than urban ones, as they are in the United States (McShane and Roess, 1990; Baker et al., 1987). Important rural risk factors include speed, two-way traffic, and lack of enforced speed limits.

The actual physical condition of the roads can be important. In some countries, narrow dirt roads that are frequently damaged by erosion from heavy rainfall are used by high speed vehicles. On the other hand, in India, modern national highways appear to be more dangerous than urban roads because of problems in design and a diverse mixture of vehicle types that move at varying speeds (Sarin et al., 1990e).

In rural areas of some developing countries, the use of hazardous open-backed vehicles for transporting passengers is widespread. During a crash, several unprotected individuals can be ejected from the rear cargo compartment of an open truck.

While rural roads are particularly dangerous for occupants of open trucks, many urban streets are lethal for pedestrians and lack the most basic facilities for pedestrians, including sidewalks and footpaths, as well as stop signs and traffic lights (Dessie and Larson, 1991).

The proportion of traffic victims who are children varies among countries, due to the demographic composition of the population and the degree to which they are exposed to traffic as pedestrians. In Botswana, Egypt, Ghana, Pakistan, Papua New Guinea, and Zimbabwe, the percentage of fatalities that were children below 16 years of age ranged from 11 to 28 percent, as compared to 9 percent in the United Kingdom (Downing et al., 1991). While pedestrian injury rates of children remain high per kilometer walked in the United Kingdom, the risk per child is believed to have fallen because more children are now transported by buses and cars.

Males are at particularly high risk in some developing countries, which may reflect both greater male exposure on urban streets as vulnerable road users and the personal and behavioral characteristics of males. In Addis Ababa, Ethiopia, male mortality rates from traffic injuries were four times greater than for females, 29 per 100,000 population per year versus 7; nearly all were pedestrians (Dessie and Larson, 1991).

Indigenous communities in northern climates have many motor vehicle deaths and injuries resulting from travel in off-road vehicles, including snowmobiles and all-terrain vehicles. Injuries occur from off-road collisions, overturnings, crashes, and drownings when vehicles go through the ice, as well as from collisions with cars and trucks when crossing or traveling on highways.

MULTIDISCIPLINARY NATURE OF TRAFFIC INJURY CONTROL

The prevention of traffic injuries is a multidisciplinary collaborative undertaking. Ideally, public health agencies, traffic engineers, vehicle designers, urban planners, police, agency regulators, economists, and community leaders and politicians should be involved. Unfortunately, most professionals work in isolation and tend to concentrate their expertise on the protection of vehicle occupants rather than on the more vulnerable road users.

Public health professionals, including injury epidemiologists and demographers, conduct injury surveillance as part of overall monitoring of the health impact of injuries and other conditions. They can regularly reassess the relative importance of traffic injuries as a cause of death and hospitalization in different demographic subgroups of the population. Public health professionals can also provide interregional comparisons of rates of traffic deaths and hospitalizations between rural and urban areas, and sometimes between rich and poor neighborhoods.

Coroners can play a useful public health role in investigating traffic fatalities, particularly if they concentrate upon preventable environmental, equipment, and personal factors in their investigations and summarize their findings in regular reports circulated to agencies that have the power to implement recommended changes. Coroners are sometimes able to provide accurate data concerning the importance of alcohol in local traffic fatalities.

Increasingly, epidemiologists and other members of the public health community with a special interest in injury control have begun to analyze and interpret police and transport data on traffic injuries. This is often done in collaboration with other professionals in an attempt to reduce the public health impact of traffic injuries on the community. In some areas, professionals such as university demographers and geographers have made useful contributions to traffic safety analyses (Adams, 1988).

Traffic engineers concentrate mainly upon designing a traffic environment that is not only efficient, but also as safe as possible for all categories of road users. An important goal is the design of "forgiving highways" that allow drivers time and space to recover from errors and incorporate features to minimize the consequences if a crash does occur. It is possible to design these roads by knowing where collisions are most likely to occur (McShane and Roess, 1990). Traffic engineers also search for and correct hazardous locations or "blackspots" in existing traffic networks. The design and installation of unambiguous road signs and signals is an important function of municipal and regional traffic engineers.

Urban planners can design residential neighborhoods, public parks and playgrounds, and traffic flow patterns that provide safe environments for pedestrians and cyclists and for children's play. Company engineers focus upon equipment factors, designing safer vehicles and protective equipment, such as helmets, for vulnerable road users. Politicians, agency personnel, and insurance companies can implement regulations, adjust fees, and make other changes to address environmental and equipment hazards and to modify dangerous behavior. Economists can estimate the direct and indirect costs of past, present, and future traffic injuries and alcohol-related crashes and assess the costs of alternative preventive solutions.

Police are responsible for the collection of the individual crash data that make it possible to identify hazardous environments. The police also have an important and often difficult role in the enforcement of regulations.

While some advances in the prevention of traffic injuries can be transferred to developing countries, it is necessary for injury prevention programs in developing countries to focus on identifying and modifying local hazards and risk factors for vulnerable road users (International Conference on Traffic Safety, 1990). Certain hazards may be unique to a particular environment and unfamiliar to safety experts in developed countries. The ideal is to prevent injuries by eliminating collisions. This is not always possible, so a reduction in the number and severity of injuries is also a worthy and achievable goal (West-Oram, 1990).

RISK OF INJURY BY TYPE OF TRANSPORT

In most countries private independent transport is the most hazardous means of travel, although in some developing countries certain forms of public transport are also excessively dangerous. In general, however, decreasing the number of miles traveled by hazardous personal transport, such as motorcycles, by shifting to safer modes could considerably reduce the risk of injury per mile traveled.

Unfortunately, although the occupants of large vehicles such as buses are relatively well-protected, buses and large trucks cause the death of many pedestrians, cyclists, and car occupants (Adams, 1988). In Great Britain in 1985, the average bus or lorry was about five times more likely to kill someone than the average car, and about 69 times more likely than the average bicycle.

Vulnerable road users, such as motorcyclists who travel at high speed without the protection of a vehicle compartment, are at greatest risk (Table 7.2). In developed countries, the risks for motorcyclists are extremely high, and in West Germany, the death rate per kilometer of travel is 44 times higher than for vehicle occupants (Appel et al., 1986).

Table 7.2 compares deaths per billion kilometers for different forms of transportation between the city of New Delhi and the countries of Great Britain and the United States. (The reader is reminded that death rates for motorized transport tend to be higher in rural areas than in cities, where speeds are usually lower, and that caution

Table 7.2 Fatality rates by mode of road travel, per billion passenger kilometers for the city of New Delhi, Great Britain, and the United States

Mode of travel	Deaths per billion km		
	New Delhi	Great Britain	United States
Bus	3.4	0.4	0.4
Automobile	3.5	5	9
Bicycle	11	64	155
Pedestrians*	nd	78	nd
Motorcycle	17	131	335
Percent non-urban population	0	10	24

Sources: Mohan, 1986b; West-Oram, 1990 (1987 data); Baker et al., 1992, 1993 (1986–90 data); World Almanac, 1993; Note: * nd = no data

is needed in comparing an urban population with an entire country.) Although motorcycle travel is the most hazardous mode in all three environments, the differences among modes are less extreme in New Delhi. One reason could be that motorcycle operators in New Delhi tend to be older, about 25 to 50-years-old. However, congestion and slow speeds could also contribute to low rates among both motorcyclists and bicyclists.

The substantially higher rate of fatalities for buses relative to automobiles in New Delhi, as compared to the United States and Great Britain, can be attributed to extreme overcrowding, which results in people hanging onto the outside of buses and falling off during entry and exit, and to the fact that buses in Delhi have no doors and a platform that is higher than the road.

Because there are such large differences in mortality and morbidity rates for various forms of transport, it is important that the rates for each category of road user be examined separately. To do otherwise could mean that an overall improvement in rates might mask a significant increase in, for example, pedestrian deaths (West-Oram, 1989, 1990, 1991). This has been identified as a problem in Great Britain, and similar limitations in the reporting of traffic data in other countries are probable. As discussed later, the completeness of reporting also differs for different modes of transport, with underreporting of injuries to vulnerable road users a great problem (Odero et al., 1997).

A method of comparing road safety among countries by adjusting for different proportions of road user and vehicle groups, using a "relative safety index", has been suggested. The index would be used to compare external situations in developing countries with those in industrialized countries, and for comparisons internally within a country (Nelson and Strueber, 1990).

When advocating changes in modes of transport, planners must remember the risks that many individuals are willing to assume to travel by relatively unsafe transport. People often assume significant personal risk in exchange for a reduced travel time or greater convenience. A careful consideration of such factors should remind planners that it is important to maximize both convenience and safety in cities and in their associated transport systems for the inhabitants.

It is unfortunate for vulnerable road users that most measures to improve road safety and reduce travel time have been directed to vehicle occupants. Motorists have gained improved performance through the development of safer vehicles and road environments; this allows them to travel faster at lower risk (Adams, 1988). Safety measures for vulnerable road users, on the other hand, often penalize performance and efficiency. For example, many pedestrian barriers and footbridges slow or lengthen pedestrian travel and are, therefore, greatly underutilized. Only recently has anyone questioned the assumption that vulnerable road users must always fear and defer to the least vulnerable users.

DATA SOURCES AND DATA QUALITY FOR TRAFFIC INJURIES

Data have several different functions in the prevention of traffic injuries. It is necessary to assess the severity and relative importance of traffic injuries as a cause of death, hospitalization, disability, and economic losses at national, regional, and community levels. Environmental, equipment, and personal risk factors need to be described. Hazardous regions, neighborhoods, and specific road sites or black spots must be identified. The efficacy of interventions must be evaluated.

Information needed to study the impact of traffic injuries and trends is derived from two general sources of routinely collected data. Health staff and police complete the records and reports that are the basis of the two data sources.

The first source includes data on mortality, morbidity, and disability derived from records of health professionals, including death certificates and coroners' reports for fatalities, and hospital discharges for severe nonfatal injuries. Other potential sources are special questions about injuries included in community health interview surveys.

The second general source of data on traffic injuries includes crash reports prepared by police; these are often entered and stored in special computer databases by other sectors, such as the Department of Transport. Urban planners and traffic engineers may make extensive use of such records. Some public health injury epidemiologists are also beginning to use crash data.

Unfortunately, in the past, there tended to be little or no communication between public health professionals, who carry out surveillance of deaths and hospitalizations using health data, and professionals working in other sectors, who rely upon databases prepared from police crash reports. This lack of communication has begun to change as epidemiologists have come to appreciate the tremendous impact of traffic injuries on mortality and morbidity and the possibility of preventing many of these injuries. Recognition that traffic injuries are a public health problem has helped to improve collaboration with other sectors.

INDICATORS OF EXPOSURE AND SEVERITY

There are a number of different indicators available to study the severity of the problem of traffic injuries in a country or a region (Bangdiwala et al., 1985; Jacobs and Sayer, 1983; Haight, 1980, 1983). Appropriate use and interpretation of such indicators requires considerable knowledge and good judgement.

Many indicators are rates, which are calculated using various numerators and denominators. The numerators include the events counted in a geographic area, and may include deaths, minor or severe injuries, and/or collisions or crashes. Deaths and injuries should be recorded separately for different categories of road users.

The significance of the number of traffic deaths, serious injuries, and/or crashes in a geographic area can be assessed relative to a number of different denominators, which then can be grouped into two general categories (McShane and Roess, 1990). The first includes the numbers of events during a standard time period (usually one year) per unit of persons, vehicles, or road surface, as, for example, deaths per 100,000 population, per 10,000 registered vehicles, or per 1,000 miles of highway. The second category includes the number of events per unit of exposure for a given type of road user, for example, per 100 million automobile, truck, motorcycle, bicycle, or pedestrian kilometers, or per 10 million vehicle hours (West-Oram, 1989, 1990, 1991). However, while exposure-based rates are often preferable, the necessary data are not always available to calculate them, unless special transport surveys have been undertaken in the geographic area of interest.

To obtain a more complete understanding of the significance and impact of road traffic events in an area, the numerator and denominator of the indicators used ideally should reflect the specific category of event divided by the unit of exposure for the specific type of road user. In practice, such data are not always available, and data for different types of events and different road users are sometimes combined, which can be highly misleading (West-Oram, 1989, 1990, 1991; Adams, 1988).

Police generally count crashes and injuries and record their findings as collision or accident reports. The police definition of what constitutes a traffic injury can have a major impact on traffic injury data. For example, the definition of "slight injuries" in Great Britain is highly subjective, the definition of a "serious injury" is very broad, and the degree of underreporting increases greatly as the severity of the injury decreases (Adams, 1988). Apparently only one-quarter of the casualties classified by police crash reports as seriously injured were actually seriously injured, and many of those classified as slightly injured were actually seriously injured.

Thus, the completeness and accuracy of police reporting is good for deaths, moderately good for serious injuries, and usually poor for less severe injuries. Misreporting of serious injuries as slight injuries by police may be a greater problem among vulnerable road users than among vehicle occupants. Reporting is generally relatively good for severe crashes involving a motor vehicle, but may be poor for less severe crashes or collisions involving vulnerable road users.

The completeness and validity of reports vary substantially depending upon the number of police officers in the area and the time they have available to investigate crashes (Adams, 1988). If high-quality health facility data are used to count injuries, much higher numbers and more accurate classification of severity may be obtained than from police reports. Unfortunately, the quality of routine hospital data is often poor. In order to obtain more accurate counts of severe traffic injuries than police reports, hospital discharges must be consistently coded by External Cause of Injury codes. Otherwise, data can be collected by special surveys of hospital emergency departments for a period of several weeks or months (Dessie and Larson, 1991).

Vulnerable road users may be taken to hospitals before police arrive, or police may not be called to the scene. Thus, in both developed and developing countries, underreporting of nonfatal injuries by police has been found to be much greater for road users other than vehicle occupants, such as bicyclists and pedestrians (Sayer and Hitchcock, 1984; Stutts et al., 1990; Harris, 1990; Agran et al., 1990).

The injury to fatality ratio can vary substantially between different areas of a country. Factors that affect the ratio include the definition of an injury, whether police or hospital reports are used, the number of police in an area, the traffic mix and speed on different types of roads, and the availability of appropriate treatment. In Great Britain in 1985, for example, the injury to fatality ratio ranged from 103:1 in London to 23:1 in more rural areas (Adams, 1988).

In Addis Ababa, Ethiopia, in 1988, the injury to fatality ratio was 16:1; injuries included only victims treated either as outpatients or inpatients at hospitals (Dessie and Larson, 1991). The authors believed that there would have been a greater proportion of fatal injuries if the study had been carried out in a non-urban area with higher speeds. In this study, 82 percent of traffic injury victims were treated as outpatients, 12 percent were hospitalized, and 6 percent died. About one-half of all fatalities occurred on the scene and another one-third within minutes of arrival at hospital.

Deaths and injuries may be inversely related on different types of roads (Adams, 1988). In congested urban areas where traffic moves slowly, there may be many injuries and few deaths of motor vehicle occupants, whereas on high speed motorways, the number of injuries may be relatively low but the number of deaths high because the severity of injuries increases with the velocity of impact. There may also be larger numbers of severe injuries and deaths of vulnerable road users on urban roads simply because there are so many more road users present to be injured.

In developed countries, the severity level of injuries is increasingly being quantified by the use of measures such as the Abbreviated Injury Scale (AIS) and Injury Severity Score (ISS) (Petrucelli, 1990, Waller, 1985, Baker et al., 1974), and, most recently, the New Injury Severity Score (NISS) (Osler et al., 1997). This allows comparison of the impacts of different injuries, and the evaluation and comparison of interventions in different populations. For persons who need to use these measures, special short training courses in the use of injury scales are available from the Association for the Advancement of Automotive Medicine in Des Plaines, Illinois, United States.

The severity of disability does not appear to correlate well with AIS or ISS injury severity scores (Bull, 1985). Multiple injuries, including chest and abdominal trauma, contribute to a high injury score; however, it is generally a single injury, such as a limb fracture, that results in disability.

Thus, the validity and comparability of data on nonfatal injuries can be affected both by reporting biases, when events are counted incompletely, and by problems in recording levels of severity of injuries. The severity of some serious internal injuries and other conditions with a delayed presentation, such as whiplash injuries of the neck, may not be obvious initially to the police, whereas other minor external wounds such as scalp lacerations could initially appear to be quite serious because of profuse bleeding.

The relative importance of the traffic problem with respect to other causes of death, including diseases and other injuries, can be determined by calculating the proportion of deaths from all causes represented by traffic deaths, if reliable information is available for other leading causes. This figure is affected by the completeness of reports regarding different causes of death and by the fact that deaths of vulnerable road users tend to be undercounted as compared to those of vehicle occupants.

Traffic deaths can be compared with other unintentional injuries (Table 7.3) or to all injuries to ascertain their relative importance among other injuries. Other important indicators of the severity and adverse impact of traffic crashes include economic aspects and morbidity, including disability, all of which were discussed in Chapters 4 and 5.

Table 7.3 Reported unadjusted motor vehcile mortality rates expressed as a percent* of deaths from all injuries and all unintentional injuries for various developing countries, with other countries for comparison

	Motor Vehicle Death Rate per 100,000 pop.		Motor Vehicle Deaths as a percent of All Injury Deaths		Motor Vehicle Deaths As a percent of All Unintentional Injury Deaths		
	m	f	m	f	m	f	Year
AFRICA							
Mauritius	27	5	38	25	56	34	1991
SOUTHEAST ASIA							
China, rural	20	9	22	13	32	27	1994
China, urban	16	7	33	22	41	30	1994
Sri Lanka	4	1	4	3	8	6	1986
Thailand	21	6	20	21	41	36	1981
EASTERN MEDITERRANEAN							
Egypt	11	3	22	10	43	26	1987
AMERICAS							
Ecuador	31	9	31	32	41	39	1988
Mexico	25	7	24	29	39	37	1993
Panama	28	6	35	29	53	39	1987
Colombia	22	7	10	21	38	38	1991
El Salvador	20	7	11	21	32	37	1984
Costa Rica	21	5	35	30	49	39	1991
Paraguay	14	5	23	26	35	35	1987
Argentina	14	5	19	16	32	24	1991
Uruguay	18	7	19	20	26	25	1990
Chile	18	5	17	17	46	33	1992
Peru	10	3	22	21	28	27	1986
Guatemala	2	1	2	4	7	9	1984
COMPARISON							
Venezuela	33	8	33	36	55	45	1989
Kuwait	28	6	61	46	66	56	1987
United States	22	10	26	31	47	44	1992
Sweden	9	4	14	12	26	19	1993
Russian Fed.	38	11	9	11	17	18	1994
Australia	16	6	28	29	46	39	1993

Source: *World Health Statistics Annual 1986–1995* (WHO, 1986–1996)

*Percents calculated from exact rates, therefore figures may differ slightly from results obtained by using rounded rates from Table 3.1.

Three of the indicators most widely used when assessing the importance of traffic injuries include the motorization index or ratio of vehicles per 1000 population, the death rate per 10,000 vehicles per year, and the death rate per 100,000 population per year. One serious limitation of using indicators such as these is that they are not based upon exposures for specific categories of road users.

The rate of traffic deaths per 100,000 population provides a measure of the impact of traffic on a population relative to other causes of death. However, comparisons of such rates among countries can be misleading as an indicator of the relative safety of the roads in the countries (Andreassen, 1991). At best, traffic deaths per unit of population should only be compared among countries with similar vehicle ownership ratios and population densities, and even then such comparisons can be misleading as an indicator of the relative efficacy of different road safety policies (European Conference of Ministers of Transport, 1984).

Another indicator is the severity index. This index is defined as the number of fatalities per crash, and has been used to describe the relative severity of crashes (McShane and Roess, 1990), but may need an adjustment to accommodate the larger numbers of passengers per vehicle in some developing countries.

Improvements in overall traffic casualty rates may reflect a shift from vulnerable modes of travel to travel in enclosed vehicles. Such improvements in overall rates may conceal a deterioration in risk for vulnerable road users, such as bicyclists and pedestrians, with no improvement or even a deterioration in the risk for vehicle occupants (West-Oram, 1989, 1990, 1991). If adequate records are available at health facilities, they may be used to calculate rates of killed and seriously injured persons by road-user type. Unfortunately, records at many health facilities, if available at all, often lack even such basic information.

In the absence of estimates of the number of kilometers walked by all pedestrians, it has been suggested that the fatality rate of 10–14 year old pedestrians in traffic per 100,000 population can be used as a substitute for monitoring trends in pedestrian fatalities. In Great Britain, this group has not changed its walking patterns substantially over time (West-Oram, 1989, 1990, 1991).

There are often much lower levels of motorization, that is, vehicles per 10,000 population, in developing countries, and thus it is necessary to use an indicator of risk that is based on the number of vehicles. An even better indicator of exposure to risk is the death rate per person-kilometer traveled; however, this information is not available for most countries, and thus the number of deaths per 10,000 vehicles is usually used for comparison. The numerator is the number of deaths during a fixed period of time, usually one year. The denominator is the average population of motor vehicles in the country during the period of interest, rather than the population of people.

Many developing countries have motor vehicle fatality rates per 10,000 vehicles far exceeding those of developed countries (Fig. 7.1), although there have been improvements in some developing countries (Downing et al., 1991; Transport and Road Research Laboratory, 1986; Jacobs and Sayer, 1983). Mortality rates per vehicle were about 50 times higher in Ethiopia and Nigeria than in Great Britain or the United States.

The National Safety Council of Singapore used the indicator of deaths per 10,000 vehicles to compare their own 1987 rate with the situation in other countries. The Singapore rate was 4 deaths per 10,000 vehicles (including motorcycles and scooters), as compared to rates of 274 in Sri Lanka, 67 in Pakistan, 61 in India, 13 in Indonesia, 12 in Hong Kong, 9 in West Malaysia, 9 in the Philippines, 6 in Thailand, 3 in the United Kingdom, and 3 in Japan (National Safety Council of Singapore, 1988).

Such comparisons of mortality data for densely populated urban areas to country-wide data could provide an unfounded basis for complacency. Although crash rates are generally high in urban areas with many vehicles, death rates per vehicle tend to be lower than in rural areas because of slower speeds resulting from speed limits and urban congestion. Urban centers with similar population and traffic density should be included in such comparisons.

An example of the relative values of different indicators of mortality from traffic injuries is provided for Papua New Guinea, a country with a relatively low motorization index of 0.015, i.e., 15 vehicles per 1000 population or about 1 vehicle per 60 inhabitants (Nelson and Strueber, 1991; Trinca et al., 1988). In 1987, there were 60 deaths reported per 10,000 vehicles and 9 deaths per 100,000 population (G.A. Ryan, 1989b). By comparing the data in this paragraph with Table 7.3 and Figure 7.4, it is evident that although the Papua New Guinea death rate per 100,000 population from traffic injuries is relatively low, the death rate per 10,000 vehicles is high.

Recent large increases in motorization in many developing countries are one of the reasons motor vehicles have such a major

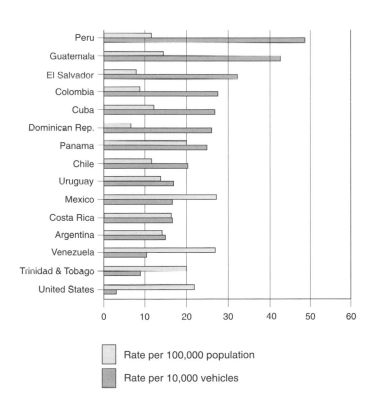

Figure 7.4

Death rates from motor vehicle traffic injuries per 100,000 population and per 10,000 vehicles, 1980.
Source: Pan American Health Organization, *Health Conditions in the Americas 1981-1984, Volume 1*. 1986. Reproduced with permission.

Rate per 100,000 population

Rate per 10,000 vehicles

impact on health. In 17 countries of the Americas, between 1969 and 1980, increases in the numbers of registered vehicles ranged from 13 percent to 324 percent (PAHO, 1986). The range of increases in the motorization index was from 12 to over 800 percent (Table 7.4).

In India, the population of motor vehicles has been increasing at about ten percent per annum for the past four decades (Kadiyali et al., 1990). In Delhi, the number of vehicles on the road increased 170 percent between 1980 and 1988 (Deputy Commissioner of Traffic Police Delhi, 1989).

One important factor that the ratio of motor vehicles per 1000 inhabitants does not incorporate is an increase in the number of vehicles with respect to the available roads. If there are rapid increases in both the number of vehicles and the population while the length of the road network remained unchanged, each inhabitant would experience a substantially increased exposure to motor vehicles on the more crowded roads, even if there was no increase in the motorization index. However, if traffic density increased enough to substantially reduce the average speed of travel, the risk to the population could decrease.

This effect of speed has been observed in India. While Delhi, Bombay, and Calcutta are cities of similar size, Delhi has about 1600 traffic deaths as compared to about 400 each in Bombay and Calcutta, where rates are similar to those of London and New York. This difference is attributable mainly to higher speeds in Delhi where there is less congestion; however, an increase in the number of vehicles in Delhi is resulting in lower speeds, and the death rate is predicted to fall.

Table 7.4 Trends in vehicles per 1000 population in selected countries* in the Americas between 1969 and 1980

Country	Vehicles/1000 pop.		
	1969	*1980*	*Percent Difference*
Group 1			
Dominican Republic	4	39	854
Mexico	31	95	207
Costa Rica	32	98	206
Chile	27	76	182
Guatemala	11	27	146
Colombia	13	31	139
Argentina	76	60	111
Panama	39	76	95
Uruguay	82	92	12
Group 2			
Trinidad and Tobago	85	187	120
Venezuela	86	182	112
United States	500	728	46

* First group of countries all had per capita GNP <US$2500; second group included for comparison.
Adapted from Pan American Health Organization, *Health Conditions in the Americas 1981–1984,* 1986.

CRASH REPORTS

Crash reports are generally prepared by the police. When studying crashes, secondary data contained in data bases derived from such reports must be used, because crashes occur too infrequently to be studied directly by observation in the same manner as other aspects of road traffic.

Reports are generally more complete and detailed for severe crashes and for crashes involving motor vehicles. However, if deaths that occur after hospitalization are never reported back to the police, those deaths may not be included in police reports. Unfortunately, minor crashes and injuries to vulnerable road users, particularly bicyclists and pedestrians, often go unreported or are poorly documented. In Colombo, Sri Lanka, completeness of police reporting was 26 percent for hospitalized bicyclists and 75 percent for pedestrians (Sayer and Hitchcock, 1984).

Another factor affecting the completeness of police reports is the desire of drivers to avoid notifying the police, perhaps to escape a rise in insurance premiums. In Nigeria, when there are nonfatal injuries, the drivers commonly come to mutual agreement as to the guilty party and negotiate payment for hospital care and repairs (Asogwa, 1992). Single vehicle crashes are often not reported by mutual agreement with passengers.

Some of the potential biases and other limitations of police data were discussed in Chapters 3, 4, and 6. Police selection of victims for alcohol testing can also be biased (Öström et al., 1992).

The utility of crash reports for research and planning may be improved if developing countries use standardized police report booklets and computer software prepared by the Overseas Unit of the UK Transport and Road Research Laboratory. The address is provided at the end of the chapter (Downing et al., 1991; Transport and Road Research Laboratory, n.d.). The precise location of each crash must be specified in a standardized manner so that all crashes at any given location can be aggregated at periodic intervals. On numbered highways, map mercators are sometimes used to describe the precise location for a crash. In urban areas, two street names are generally used to localize crash sites, since mercators may be too far apart to localize crashes. A certain amount of "cleaning" of data may be necessary to correct slight variations in the way police record street names. Environmental, equipment, and personal factors and specific hazardous activities that contributed to the crash should all be recorded.

BLACKSPOT ANALYSIS

The location and other details of individual crashes are important to traffic engineers (McShane and Roess, 1990). In the aggregate, they help to identify hazardous locations that can often be corrected in a cost-effective manner by straightforward engineering changes. Such data are increasingly being computerized by traffic authorities. In addition, crash maps that use colored pins to denote individual events are often maintained to locate blackspots, locations with higher than expected crash rates. Unfortunately, studies of blackspots are based upon the use of crash data, and these may be subject to a high degree of underreporting (Adams, 1988).

Using the information from crash reports, detailed diagrams can be prepared of blackspots. These diagrams include a condition diagram, that maps the environmental conditions at the blackspot, and a collision diagram, that represents the nature and location of all of the collisions at the blackspot during the period studied (McShane and Roess, 1990). By analyzing these two diagrams, corrective strategies can be developed. The changes required may be as simple as improved signs or signals.

In developing countries, blackspot analyses may be especially valuable if injuries and deaths involve vehicle occupants. If the problem is pedestrian fatalities, too often the solution recommended is to construct a fence in the middle of the road, preventing pedestrians from crossing. This may simply cause migration of pedestrian casualties to another location.

Readers with a statistical background may be interested in some of the more complex methods that have been used to evaluate the effect of improvements to blackspots. Traditionally, the significance of observed changes in crash rates has been assessed using statistical analyses based upon the Poisson distribution. However, it has been suggested that in certain circumstances, other distributions, such as the binomial or negative binomial, should be used, since they provide a closer approximation to reality (Nicholson, 1985; Mountain and Fawaz, 1991).

The natural tendency for regression to the mean of unusually high or low crash frequencies for different locations must be considered when evaluating statistical changes in crash frequency after blackspots have been modified (Adams, 1988; Maher and Mountain, 1988). Such tendencies can also give rise to erroneous impressions of crash migration from corrected locations to other sites.

In view of the importance of pedestrian injuries in cities, areawide problems such as high-speed traffic in residential areas and the lack of sidewalks, footpaths, stop signs, and crossing signals may warrant extra attention, in addition to focal hazards that contribute to vehicle crashes. The advice of an experienced statistician before interventions and evaluations is desirable. However, many of the environmental road hazards in developing countries and at notorious locations in industrialized countries may be sufficiently severe that both the problem and the effects of intervention will be evident without sophisticated statistical modeling.

HEALTH SECTOR AND CORONER DATA

General applications of health data and indicators of mortality and morbidity were discussed in Chapters 3 and 4. A few specific considerations for traffic injuries are briefly mentioned here.

Mortality data from the health sector and coroners' reports can be used to compare traffic death rates between countries and regions. Because deaths are somewhat rare events compared to hospitalizations, the population groups to be compared should be relatively large and the time period sufficiently long, usually a year or more.

If there is extensive travel between regions for work or other purposes, it may be useful to compare death rates by place of residence and place of death to see whether there are substantial differences, since this would need to be considered when planning target areas for interventions. Motor vehicles often kill children, women, and the elderly when they are walking in their home neighborhoods. Men sometimes travel long distances to work in other neighborhoods and cities or reside temporarily in other regions as migrant laborers. Men could be injured as passengers or cyclists en route to work, as pedestrians in their neighborhood of work, or in their home neighborhood. Intoxicated males are also sometimes injured near bars or while returning home.

The utility of hospitalization data for surveys of traffic injuries depends on whether hospital discharges are coded using an External Cause code and whether health providers include this as part of their diagnoses, as discussed in Chapter 4. In addition, most physicians do not include acute alcohol intoxication as one of their discharge diagnoses for injured patients. If this were done consistently, perhaps by modifying discharge forms to request this information as a routine, coders could then code alcohol intoxication as an associated diagnosis.

Another factor in the utility of hospital data is access to care in different regions. If variables such as these can be reasonably compared among regions, it may be possible to use hospital discharge summaries to compare regional rates of hospitalization for traffic injuries. In urban areas, hospitalization rates can be compared for different high-density or large population neighborhoods. As for mortality data, it may be necessary to consider location of residence as well as location of injury; however, location of injury may not be available in routine hospital discharge summaries. Patterns of transfer to or between hospitals could also complicate hospitalization data in some regions.

The costs of permanent disabilities from head, spinal, and extremity injuries need to be considered. The high costs of life-long care for victims of spinal cord injuries in developed countries (Miller et al., 1989; Ziedler et al., 1993) differ in developing countries because many victims die soon after injury in locations that lack personnel and other resources for chronic care of spinal cord injuries.

Potential biases in data must be carefully considered. At present, routinely collected health data are inadequate to study traffic injuries in many developing countries. Nevertheless, as coding, access, and computerization of data improve, such applications may become more feasible.

SPECIAL RESEARCH STUDIES

Where essential data are unavailable in standard databases, special studies must be developed to collect new data or to apply experimental epidemiology to existing databases. Examples of simple studies that can be done rapidly at selected locations are observing the behavior of different road user types, such as if they use safety belts in cars or observing the behavior of bus commuters (Mirza et al., in press).

Case-control studies on traffic injuries have assessed the association between various personal and environmental factors and the risk of injury. A classic study by Haddon et al. (1961) in New York city demonstrated an association between pedestrian fatalities and high levels of blood alcohol.

Simple observational studies can provide rapid assessment of local hazards for traffic injuries.

Venezuela is a country with many automobiles. One of the authors (P.B.) conducted a simple study of the level of seatbelt use by occupants of vehicles on a main road passing through the center of a town in the Sierra Nevadas near Merida. The survey was completed in one hour while waiting for a local bus. The only equipment necessary was a pencil and a scrap of paper.

In only 4 vehicles out of 100 observed were any of the occupants wearing a seatbelt. Most vehicles contained several occupants. The vehicles that were counted included automobiles, small pick-up trucks, and jeeps. In many of the vehicles shoulder belts were noted hanging unused.

More recent case-control studies have focused on issues such as the association between child pedestrian injuries and traffic volume, speed, high density curb parking, and physical separation of driveways from children's play areas (Roberts, 1995; Roberts et al., 1995a, 1995b). By using cases as their own controls, it is possible to compare the risk of injury at sites with different characteristics. This is known as the case-crossover approach (Mittleman et al., 1997; Roberts et al., 1995a). An example of pair-matching is a study that compared characteristics of drivers judged responsible for two-car collisions to the drivers of the other car (Perneger and Smith, 1991). Drivers responsible for crashes had higher blood alcohol concentrations, as well as greater probability of previous alcohol-related traffic violations.

Data obtained by interviews may differ from direct observation. When there is a differential recall bias between cases and controls, the odds ratio for injury may be invalid (Roberts, 1994). When the conditions for measurement of exposure differ for cases and controls, this may also bias the evaluation of risk (Roberts and Lee-Joe, 1993).

EXAMPLES OF OVERALL MORTALITY FROM MOTOR VEHICLES

In many developed countries motor vehicles are the largest single cause of injury death. Similarly, in urban areas of developing countries, motor vehicles are usually either the leading cause or second only to homicide as a cause of death, especially for young adults.

Overall rates for all motor vehicle fatalities and hospitalizations by age and sex are useful for comparison of the overall traffic injury problem to other injuries or diseases. They are inadequate to reveal important differences between developed and developing countries or indigenous communities in injury risk for different road user categories.

Motor vehicle mortality rates per 100,000 population vary widely by country, with many having lower rates than Sweden and the United States, and some greater (Table 7.3). In some of the oil-rich countries of the Middle East, motor vehicle injuries are the leading cause of all deaths (Bayoumi, 1981). In Thailand, motor vehicle injuries have been the leading cause of death since 1968 (Jadamba, 1991; National Epidemiology Board of Thailand, 1987).

In the 19 countries of the Caribbean subregion, traffic injuries were found to be the leading cause of loss of potential life before age 65 years (YPLL). When comparing rates of traffic deaths between countries, it is worth verifying whether similar definitions were used to classify a death as traffic related. Some countries include the deaths of all victims within 30 days after the crash, while others include only deaths that occur within one day of the crash (Bezzaoucha et al., 1988).

Countries with limited motorization may have low motor vehicle mortality rates per 100,000 population but extremely high mortality rates per vehicle (Fig. 7.4).

Trends in Mortality

Death rates have increased rapidly in some countries and declined in others, as shown by the following examples (PAHO, 1986; Bangdiwala and Anzola-Pérez, 1987). The striking differences in injury mortality between countries should generate many useful questions as to why there have been such remarkable differences in secular trends.

Between 1969 and 1980, the mortality rates per 100,000 persons showed increases ranging from 10 percent to 167 percent in Cuba, Costa Rica, Ecuador, Uruguay, Panama, and Guatemala.

The worst traffic injury situation in the world is reported from countries in Africa, with Nigeria, Ethiopia, and Malawi reported to have the highest crash and fatality rates (Asogwa, 1992). In Nigeria during the three decades between 1960–89, the number of traffic deaths increased five times from the first to last decade, while the annual death rate per 100,000 population rose from 4 to 8 to 11 during these periods (Oluwasanmi, 1993). An economic oil boom in Nigeria in the early 1980s led to a rapid increase in private ownership of vehicles with a corresponding rise in crashes and fatalities. More recently, severe recession has led to crashes from other factors such as an inability to obtain replacement parts and poor vehicle maintenance (Asogwa, 1992). Many taxis have been replaced by more hazardous commercial motorcycles, while crashes of overloaded poorly maintained buses often result in multiple deaths.

Recently, death rates from traffic fatalities have increased more slowly in some of the wealthier developing countries, including Venezuela, Barbados, and Malaysia (Feachem et al., 1992). Although it was suggested that prevention programs and use of safety belts in these countries were better than average for developing countries, the use of safety belts was observed to be very low, at only 4 percent, in at least one area of Venezuela. Large old American cars and cheap gasoline were widely available so that many persons traveled by automobile (P Barss, unpublished data, 1992).

The slower than expected increase in traffic fatalities in the wealthier developing countries may reflect the fact that a much greater proportion of the population travel as vehicle occupants rather than as vulnerable road users. As discussed elsewhere, a similar trend in mode of travel was shown to have accounted for a fall in pedestrian fatality rates in the United Kingdom at a time when the environment had actually become more dangerous for pedestrians.

In some countries, there have been reductions in traffic deaths. Traffic death rates per 100,000 population have fallen between 4 and 26 percent in Argentina, Dominican Republic, El Salvador, and Colombia. There were reductions in mortality per 10,000 vehicles between 55 and 74 percent in Argentina, Costa Rica, El Salvador, Colombia, the Dominican Republic, and Chile.

As legislation, roads, vehicles, and drivers have improved in many developed countries, and as people have gradually shifted from being pedestrians to relatively more protected vehicle occupants, death rates per 10,000 vehicles have fallen markedly. Death rates per 100,000 population have fallen to a lesser extent, or even increased, as the number of vehicles and miles traveled have increased. However, as discussed above, such improvements in overall rates can mask a serious deterioration in fatality rates for vulnerable road users, unless individual rates are also calculated for different categories of road users. If nothing is done to protect vulnerable road users, their risk of death may rise substantially with increasing motorization, as they are exposed to ever increasing numbers of motor vehicles.

An analysis of trends in some of the richer developing countries, including Libya, Kuwait, Bahrain, and Trinidad and Tobago, showed that the rate of fatalities per 10,000 vehicles was inversely related to the number of vehicles per unit of population—the motorization index (Makky, 1985). In countries where increase in motorization was more rapid, the decrease in the rate of fatalities per 10,000 vehicles was slower than in countries where motorization proceeded more slowly. It was suggested that when motorization is very rapid, the system does not have time to learn or adapt to the negative aspects of the changes, to develop ways of dealing with traffic congestion and injuries. When the rapidity of change in motorization is not matched by an appropriate response, the system operates in an inefficient and hazardous state. However, as the situation improves and fatality rates per vehicle become very low, marginal returns from improvements to the system may decrease.

The impact of congestion on injury rates may differ between rural areas and cities. In cities, severe congestion may lower speeds and result in a decrease in casualties. In rural areas without separated highways, congestion can lead to frustrated drivers and dangerous overtaking.

When considering secular trends in motor vehicle injury death rates, it is important to recall that they may be affected by demographic changes in populations, such as the recent rapid increase in the proportion of young adults in the population of Taiwan, where age-adjustment reduced an apparent increase in YPLL from motor vehicle injuries of greater than 500 percent to about 400 percent (Baker and Mackinney, 1990).

In many developed countries, the motor vehicle mortality rate per unit of travel has decreased dramatically over time since 1940 (Vulcan, 1995) due to a variety of factors including, among others, improved vehicle crash-resistance, better highway designs, speed restrictions, increased use of safety belts and air bags, and decreases in alcohol consumption. However, another factor that could account for some of the decline is the decreased proportion of vulnerable road users at high risk of death (West-Oram, 1989, 1990, 1991). A model for this decline has been developed by Haight (1980), who compared the state of many developing countries with that of the United States in 1920.

Similarly, as development increases beyond a certain point the mortality per unit of travel begins to decrease in many developing countries. Thailand experienced increases in motor vehicle mortality rates of nearly 30 percent per year, but these have now begun to level off. In Delhi, India, road crashes decreased from 80 per 10,000 vehicles in 1980 to 48 in 1988, while the number of vehicles on the road increased from 535,129 to 1,441,961 during the same period (Deputy Commissioner of Traffic Police, Delhi, 1988). Traffic deaths in Brazil continue to be a major cause of death; however, death rates have been constant during the 1980's, whereas they more than doubled in some areas during the 1960's (World Bank, 1989).

Some road improvements may actually have an adverse effect on traffic safety, especially when they increase travel speeds. Improved high speed roads in Nigeria were associated with increases in traffic fatalities (Asogwa, 1992).

Motor vehicle fatality rates also remain disproportionately high in many aboriginal communities in developed countries. This may reflect in part the hazard of open rural roads, where high travel speeds, poor road design, low use of safety belts, older vehicles, small trucks, and binge drinking together make a deadly combination (Young et al., 1992; May, 1992; Muir, 1991). It would be more appropriate to compare traffic death rates in indigenous communities to other rural communities, rather than to aggregate population data that include major urban areas.

EXAMPLES OF MORBIDITY FROM MOTOR VEHICLE INJURIES

Motor vehicles are also an important cause of serious nonfatal injuries. As many as 40 percent of the adult surgical beds in some urban teaching hospitals in developing countries are devoted to the treatment of motor vehicle victims. In Thailand, it was estimated that 30 percent of beds in hospitals outside Bangkok and 30 percent of doctors, nurses, and other health personnel have been used to care for the victims of traffic crashes (Jadamba, 1991).

Length of hospital stay is often highly correlated with the severity of traffic injuries. In Colombo, Sri Lanka, only 5 percent of minor (AIS 1) patients stayed three or more nights, whereas 84, 95, and 94 percent of severe, serious, and critical (AIS 3, 4, and 5) patients did so (Sayer and Hitchcock, 1984). Similar results were noted from the United Kingdom.

Average hospital stays are longer for traffic injuries than for many other conditions. In one Nigerian study at Ile-Ife, 25 percent of patients were hospitalized for more than two months (Balogun and Abereoje, 1992). The latter data were from a tertiary hospital where one would expect a greater concentration of severe cases, and should not be taken as typical of all hospitals. Long stays were attributed in part to closed management of fractured femurs and other bones, in order to avoid the risk of infection and other complications of internal surgical fixation.

In urban areas where the majority of victims are pedestrians, multiple injuries are most common, followed by head and lower extremity injuries. In Addis Ababa, Ethiopia, 44 percent of injuries seen at hospital as outpatients and inpatients involved multiple body parts, 22 percent the head, 20 percent the lower extremity, and 6 percent the upper extremity (Dessie and Larson, 1991).

In rural Haryana, India, a survey of injuries was carried out by visiting 3,365 households with a population of 22,883 persons every two weeks for a year (Varghese and Mohan, 1990a, 1990b). Injuries that disabled the victim for more than 24 hours were studied. Of 2059 injuries, 18 percent were transportation-related. Of these, 35 percent involved pedestrians, 25 percent bicyclists, 18 percent riders of scooters and motorcycles, and the remainder drivers or passengers of motor vehicles (including tractors).

Traffic injuries are an important cause of hospitalization in many aboriginal communities in developed countries (Muir, 1991). They are the leading cause of hospitalization for injuries in many communities with road access. In northern communities such as Arctic Alaska, snowmobiles and all-terrain vehicles sometimes account for greater numbers of severe injuries and deaths than automobiles and trucks (Johnson et al., 1992).

Permanent disability is an important consequence of nonfatal injuries. In developed countries, serious disabilities occur in about 3 percent of inpatient hospital cases and in about 1 percent of all casualties (Bull, 1985). In developing countries, where treatment is often delayed or inadequate, the prevalence may be much higher. An exception is spinal cord injuries, since survival time tends to be short due to lack of resources for long-term care. Hence, while the incidence may be high, the prevalence is low.

Serious long-term disability results from spinal cord injuries; about 75 percent of spinal cord injuries were due to motor vehicles in Zaria, Nigeria (Iwegbu, 1983) and 47 percent in São Paulo, Brazil (Sposito et al., 1984). The direct and indirect costs of head and spinal injuries and other disabilities from traffic injuries need to be quantified for developing countries as they have been for developed countries (Miller et al., 1989; Guria, 1993; Ziedler et al., 1993), since a severe disability can be much more expensive to society than a death.

REGULATORY APPROACHES FOR PREVENTION OF TRAFFIC INJURIES

Appropriate regulations can have a major impact on traffic injuries, particularly if enforcement is effective and the regulations are acceptable to a majority of the public. Regulations can affect the following:

- Behavior, such as use of alcohol while driving, observance of speed limits, use of seatbelts or helmets;
- Equipment, such as modified front ends of vehicles, seatbelts and airbags, lights on motorcycles and vehicles that turn on with the ignition, protective covers to prevent passengers from falling out or being ejected from open-backed vehicles during crashes;
- The environment, through regulations governing the design of roads and the roadside environment, including, in areas with many pedestrians, protected sidewalks and footpaths, together with stop signs and traffic lights.

Taxation can also affect the traffic mix by ensuring that the full costs of inefficient and environmentally harmful transport, such as private automobiles, are passed on to the users. High taxation and/or large registration fees for hazardous modes of transport, such as motorcycles, can be implemented. Similarly, taxation of gasoline and other vehicle fuels can serve as a valuable means of shifting transportation preferences.

Taxation and vehicle registration fees can also be used as a source of revenue to subsidize less dangerous modes of transportation, and to serve as a user tax to pay for the cost of improved medical and rescue services for victims of motor vehicle crashes. High taxation of alcoholic beverages, such as wine, can decrease consumption among young adults and help to recover costs of treatment for victims of drunk drivers.

Many developing countries still have no laws that authorize police to test individuals involved in road crashes for alcohol in breath or blood, and in others, no legal level has been established for intoxication. Not all politicians welcome such legislation, perhaps because they too will be subject to testing. More stringent alcohol regulations are warranted for drivers of large commercial vehicles. In areas where young drivers are a risk, the legal drinking age may need to be raised (Jones et al., 1992).

The laws of kinetic energy apply without discrimination to both developed and developing countries. Thus, reductions in speed limits should result in reductions in casualties in crashes in developing countries, as they have in developed countries, but only if they are enforceable. When road improvements are planned that allow vehicles to travel at higher speeds, the added costs of enforcement of speed limits need to be included in cost estimates.

In roadways shared by pedestrians and motor vehicles, speed limits need to be substantially lower because of the vulnerability of the unprotected human body to injury. In a collision of a car with a pedestrian, the probability of death for the pedestrian is about 20 percent at 30 kilometers per hour, and about 80 percent at 60 km/hr (Schweig, 1990). For this reason, experimental speed zones of 30 km/hr were introduced into some German cities, first on an experimental basis, and later permanently after the passage of appropriate legislation. In other traffic-restricted areas, wheeled traffic must keep to a walking pace of 4 to 7 km/hr.

Even on major motorways, the reduction of speed limits from 65 to 55 miles per hour in the United States was effective in substantially lowering fatalities, as well as severe and moderate injuries. Where such limits have been raised due to public and political pressure, increases of 40 percent in serious injuries and of 20 percent in mortality have been observed (Wagenaar et al., 1990). Speed limits may need to be reinforced by technical devices to ensure compliance.

Obviously, regulatory approaches may fail if the resources that are made available for enforcement of regulations are inadequate. More attention needs to be directed toward the enforcement of penalties for violations that endanger the lives of pedestrians, such as ignoring pedestrian crossings and red lights, and excessive speed in areas where pedestrians must coexist with motor vehicles.

Medical insurance is another potential area of injury control. By requiring full liability and personal injury coverage for hazardous vehicles, such as motorcycles or unsafe cars, governments can discourage their use and encourage a shift to safer forms of road transport (O'Neill, 1990). Premiums can be adjusted to reflect the extent of public funding of the treatment of injured victims and the maintenance of the disabled. Although the general public is often unaware of the relative hazards of various modes of transport, this is not the case for insurance actuaries, whose specialized knowledge can be conveyed to the public indirectly but in a very tangible manner by establishing insurance and taxation rates at levels appropriate to the risks of different modes of transport.

Urban spaces in virtually all countries urgently need redesign. To safely accommodate pedestrians and cyclists on city streets and to provide safe neighborhoods requires reordering of transportation priorities. A major principle of such designs is to make motorized traffic move with less variation in speed, using measures generally classified as "traffic calming". Reducing speeds to a 30 kph maximum in residential areas through street design is an important element of traffic calming. On heavily traveled roads, attention needs to be given to the needs of cyclists and pedestrians through cycle lanes, pedestrian

> **Control of traffic injuries should include long-term planning and system-wide countermeasures.**

International organizations should promote long-term solutions to the traffic injury problem to help countries and communities prevent road traffic incidents from occurring, rather than simply promoting efforts to improve existing defective systems. Long-term prevention would include developing and encouraging alternatives to rapid motorization, such as appropriate urban planning to reduce the need for long distance travel for work, shopping, and recreation (Replogle, 1991; Downing et al., 1991). This should decrease the need for motorized personal transport. Another long-term consideration could be planning to eliminate high speed traffic in residential areas and to develop regional hierarchies of traffic flow and speeds.

crossing facilities, and other engineering measures to reduce traffic speeds and give pedestrians and cyclists priority over motor vehicles (Vahl and Giskes, 1990; Federal Office of Road Safety, 1994).

ORGANIZATIONAL ASPECTS OF TRAFFIC INJURY PREVENTION

Since even in urban areas of developing countries, the majority of traffic victims often die either on the scene or within moments of arrival at hospital (Dessie and Larson, 1991), primary prevention is essential. This requires an organized multisectoral approach. Efforts by the clinical health sector to improve prehospital care and treatment can be helpful for a proportion of traffic victims, but should not be allowed to divert attention from the complex issues of planning fundamental intersectoral interventions for the control of proximate determinants of injury.

Each country and region needs to carefully consider its own particular problems and develop the most appropriate policies for its own traffic mix and environment. Since it is generally easier and less expensive to incorporate environmental safety features into roads and neighborhoods as they are constructed, rather than trying to add them later, planning should preferably be proactive, rather than merely reactive.

Specific policies and interventions obviously need to be adapted to the prevailing mix of vehicle types and road users at greatest risk. Thus, each country needs a national road safety committee and reporting system to address its specific problems and needs (Bangdiwala and Anzola-Pérez, 1987). Regions may also have similar requirements. Others have suggested that a specific traffic safety agency is needed to provide an institutional infrastructure through which research can be conducted, data collected, policies developed, and programs implemented and evaluated (Mackay and Petrucelli, 1990). Independent peer-reviewed research needs to be funded, and health professionals should be involved.

Many organizations are involved in traffic safety and prevention of traffic injuries. Developed countries have often suffered from the lack of a central national authority with the ultimate responsibility for traffic safety (West-Oram, 1990). Such organizations may be ineffective, however, unless they are adequately funded (Asogwa, 1992). In such cases, alternative approaches need to be considered.

Injury control epidemiologists based in public health units may be helpful in surveillance of mortality and morbidity from traffic injuries. They can help to construct linked databases that combine data from vital statistics, coroners, hospitals, police, and transport (Ferrante et al., 1993). Epidemiologists and demographers can follow secular trends and assess the relative importance of traffic injuries with respect to other health conditions and may be able to provide interregional and inter-neighborhood comparisons of rates of death and hospitalization that could be useful in considering area-wide system changes. Public health agencies that have developed their capability to conduct basic injury surveillance may also be able to collaborate with traffic engineers, police, and urban planners to search for and correct specific high-risk black spots on highways and poor neighborhoods.

It would also be helpful to include the expertise of health economists in assessing the community impact of injuries as measured in various types of costs, as discussed in Chapter 5. The validity of their cost estimates should be improved by access to reliable epidemiologic incidence data from injury surveillance.

The Pan American Health Organization has developed a systematic and in-depth epidemiological approach for evaluation and intervention for traffic injuries in developing countries of the Americas (Bangdiwala et al., 1990a). National workshops provided suggestions for the establishment of national road safety committees, intersectoral collaboration, adoption of uniform reporting categories, and improved uniform statistical information systems. Obviously, a commitment from governments will be needed for such organizational changes to be financed and implemented.

The need for a coordinated approach to the control of traffic injuries is exemplified by the situation in India, where there are at least nine separate acts that deal with regulatory aspects of traffic and transportation (Gupta, 1990). However, since safety problems were inadequately addressed through the existing acts, a comprehensive act was proposed to address the issue. This involved the creation of an appropriate authority to provide physical and fiscal planning; coordination, integration, evaluation, and monitoring; implementation of projects; and management and operation of various traffic systems.

> **Creative public policy could encourage human-powered transport modes.**

International development and economic policies have tended to favor growth of high-cost energy-intensive, and nonsustainable transport at the expense of human-powered modes (Replogle, 1991). Bikeways provide a transport capacity much greater than many automobile freeways and close to that of buses in mixed traffic. Rather than simply adapting to intense pressure to favor automobiles at the expense of other modes, creative public policy could encourage other methods of transport by providing both safety and economic incentives.

LITERATURE ON TRAFFIC INJURIES

A review of current literature can be helpful in obtaining a rapid overview of progress in the field and some of the research indicators and innovative solutions that have proven useful elsewhere. New interventions are gradually being developed in a number of developing countries, and the reader is advised to consult the current journals to keep up with advances in this area. A few examples include *Accident Analysis and Prevention, Injury Prevention, Journal of Traffic Medicine, Transportation Quarterly,* and *Traffic Engineering and Control,* which occasionally include papers from developing countries. Authors of textbooks on traffic engineering are now beginning to devote entire chapters to the analysis and prevention of road crashes, as well as including consideration of such factors throughout the texts (McShane and Roess, 1990). Other books include those by Evans (1991) and Ogden (1996).

Publications that are particularly appropriate to the needs of developing countries include many articles and books by the Overseas Unit of the UK Transport and Road Research Laboratory (TRRL), Old Wokingham Road, Crowthorne, Berkshire, England RG11 6AU. The books include *Towards Safer Roads in Developing Countries, A Guide for Planners and Engineers* (1991) and *Costing Road Accidents in Developing Countries* (1994). TRRL has also developed a Microcomputer Accident Analysis Package (MAAP) and standardized police crash report forms for developing countries.

chapter 8

Traffic Injuries:
Determinants by Road User Type

This chapter considers the nature and determinants of traffic injuries for different major user categories focusing on vulnerable road users, including pedestrians, bicyclists, motorcyclists, occupants of open-backed vehicles, and users of off-road vehicles. Determinants of traffic crashes in general are also considered.

INJURIES OF PEDESTRIANS

There are generally more pedestrians in developing than in developed countries, as discussed in Chapter 7. In surveys of developing countries by the Overseas Unit of the British Transport and Road Research Laboratory, it was found that pedestrians represented up to 70 percent of all traffic fatalities (Downing, 1990).

In urban areas, pedestrians comprise a larger proportion of traffic injuries than on rural roads, since vehicle occupants are relatively well-protected at slower urban speeds. In Addis Ababa, Ethiopia, pedestrians accounted for 91 percent of all traffic injury victims who reached a hospital emergency department or died before reaching hospital (Dessie and Larson, 1991). In a study of traffic fatalities in New Delhi, India, pedestrians comprised 42 percent of victims (Mohan and Kumar, 1989).

The impacting vehicle is often a bus or truck rather than a car. In a Delhi casualty hospital, all injured pedestrians in severe or critical condition, including cases in Abbreviated Injury Scale (AIS) categories 4 and 5, had been hit by buses or trucks (Dave and Rastogi, 1990). Most of the less serious cases, including patients in AIS category 3, had been struck by cars. However, in Addis Ababa, taxis accounted for over one-half of all motor vehicle injuries (mainly of pedestrians) followed by buses.

Personal Factors
Males are generally at substantially higher risk of pedestrian injuries in all age groups except toddlers. The age distribution of injured pedestrians may differ considerably among countries, as shown in a

study that compared pedestrian fatalities in Rio de Janeiro and Baltimore. Age-specific death rates also differed; in children up to age 10, similar rates of pedestrian fatalities were found in the two cities, but above this age the fatality rates in Rio de Janeiro far exceeded those in Baltimore (Figure 8.1) (Baker, 1977).

In the United States, pedestrian death rates are highest above age 60, with lower peaks for children and teenagers. Nonfatal injury rates are highest for children ages 5–14 (Baker et al., 1992). On the other hand, in Addis Ababa casualty departments, injury rates were high in males in all age groups between the ages of 10 and 65+ years of age, with the highest injury rates in the 20 to 29 and 50 to 64 year age groups (Dessie and Larson, 1991).

Lack of awareness of appropriate behavior in traffic and of the potential hazard of motor vehicles may be important contributors to pedestrian injuries in developing countries. In Pakistan about one-half of pedestrians surveyed were unaware that they should walk facing traffic, especially at night; over one-half were actually observed to walk with their backs to the traffic flow. Virtually no one was aware of the importance of wearing bright clothing (Downing, 1990).

In other developing countries, many children were unaware that they should stop and look before crossing, and many failed to look to the side while crossing (Jacobs and Sayer, 1983). In Jordan, 48 percent of pedestrians crossing a road did not check for oncoming traffic even once before or during crossing (Kandela, 1993). In a study from Visakhapatnam City, India, only 0.5 percent of pedestrians possessed a high knowledge level of road safety (Rao and Venkataram, 1990). Children in developing countries were found to receive much less advice on road safety than in the United Kingdom (Downing, 1990).

In a number of developing countries, drivers are poorly trained,

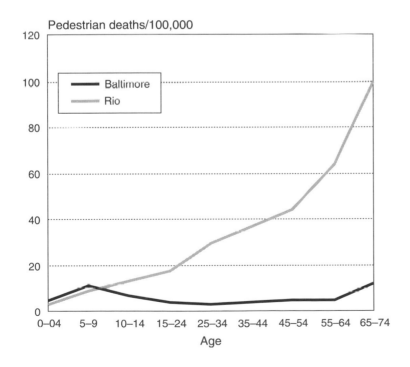

Pedestrian deaths/100,000

Age

Figure 8.1

Rates of pedestrian deaths by age in Rio de Janeiro, Brazil, and Baltimore, United States. Source: Reprinted from *Accident Analysis and Prevention* Vol. 9: Baker SP. Pedestrian deaths in Rio de Janeiro and Baltimore. pp 113-118. Copyright 1977, with kind permission from Elsevier Science Ltd., The Boulevard, Langford Lane, Kidlington OX5 1GB, UK.

and law enforcement is inadequate. Thus drivers tend to stop for pedestrians in designated, marked, crossing sites far less often than in many developed countries (Jacobs and Sayer, 1983); similar findings were noted for failure to stop at red lights. Only 17 percent or less of drivers in developing countries stopped for pedestrians at crossings, as compared to 72 percent in the United Kingdom (Downing, 1990).

In India, an integrated program of road safety education has been recommended, including components in pre-school, primary, middle, and high school, and also for license applicants (Malini, 1990). It has been suggested that in view of the frequency of injury to pedestrians and cyclists and to groups of low socioeconomic status and low levels of education, programs of traffic education should be developed for them (Sarin et al., 1990c, 1990f). A case-control study of urban pedestrian injuries in Montreal, Canada, revealed that if a child did not clearly understand traffic rules, the risk of injury was increased by a factor of five (Joly et al., 1990).

Although pedestrians are often trained in road safety in developed countries, motor vehicle drivers are given relatively little training to prepare them to cater to the safety of pedestrians. Enforcement of laws that prohibit violations of the rights of pedestrians by motorists is generally poor (West-Oram, 1990). In Finland, for example, it was found that young drivers failed to appreciate the importance of the risk of injuring pedestrians and other vulnerable road users (Hatakka et al., 1990). Their training appeared inadequate to render them aware of the risks and of potential dangers.

In Paris, France, immigrant children were greatly overrepresented among victims of severe traffic injury (Tursz et al., 1990). Since about one-half of the injuries among children occured close to the child's home, special educational programs were recommended. Environmental changes would provide a more permanent solution, although they might initially be more costly and difficult to implement.

Similarly, in Great Britain, Asian minority children aged 0–4 and 5–9 years were found to be twice as likely to be injured as non-Asian counterparts (Lawson and Edwards, 1991). The excessive risk of the Asian children was attributed to the masking effect of parked vehicles in the crowded inner city streets where they lived, that is, to their environment, rather than to their ethnic origin per se.

Socioeconomic status and level of education can be important factors for injury risk in children, although the most important underlying determinants of injury risk may relate to the child's environment. In Montreal, Canada, the risk of pedestrian injury was 2.5 times as high for children of parents who had not completed secondary education (Joly et al., 1990). Lack of supervision while on the way to school increased the risk of injury three times, and lack of supervision after school, 11 times. Increased risk-taking related to cognitive impairments and stress was found among children in poor neighborhoods in Calgary, Canada (Bagley, 1992b). This behavior, together with an adverse environment, was believed to be a contributor to the high injury rates observed among poor children.

In New Delhi, India, low levels of income and education were said to be associated with pedestrian fatalities. Most of the families of the victims were unaware of their legal right to compensation for the

death of the victim (Sarin et al., 1990f). Many male fatalities occurred among workers doing casual and menial work, while most female pedestrian casualties involved housewives. About a third of
road fatalities were among road users who had migrated to the city
within the previous five years. Heavy vehicles were responsible for 80
percent of the fatalities of pedestrians and cyclists.

Alcohol has been implicated as an important factor in many
adult pedestrian injuries. Thus walking in areas with motorized
traffic after alcohol consumption should be considered a high-risk
activity. In developed countries, while there has been some improvement in lowering the association of alcohol with fatalities of
vehicle drivers, there has been no improvement in pedestrian intoxication.

Equipment Factors

High visibility is important for pedestrians. This can be achieved
through bright and light-colored clothing and reflective vests or carrying bags, as advocated for cyclists (Mohan and Bawa, 1985). Shopping bags for stores can be manufactured with bright yellow or orange colors that are highly visible both day and night (Patel and
Mohan, 1990b).

The front ends of motor vehicles can be modified to prevent
many of the pedestrian injuries that occur at lower speeds (Bly,
1990). The Transport and Road Research Laboratory in Great
Britain has estimated that such injuries could be reduced by up to 25
percent by changes in vehicle design. The front ends of buses and
large trucks need to be fitted with energy-absorbing devices to protect not only pedestrians, but also cyclists and the occupants of
smaller vehicles.

The type and severity of pedestrian injuries are related to the
height of the bumper, to the location of the leading edge of the
hood, and to their rigidity (Cesari, 1990). The addition of a second
easily deformable bumper below the standard bumper was more effective in preventing injuries in cadaver studies than were modifications of standard bumpers (Schroeder et al., 1990). Smooth frontal
structures of cars have a significant impact on reducing the frequency and severity of pediatric injuries, but not of adult injuries of
the thighs and pelvis (Otte, 1990). However, bumpers that are integrated into the vehicle cause fewer open and complicated fractures,
and often prevent injury of the lower legs. Newer vehicles with
frontal design improvements were found to cause less severe injuries
than older vehicles, especially at low impact speeds below 50 km/hr.
For pedestrians struck by newer vehicles, there were fewer head and
lower limb fractures, particularly comminuted leg fractures
(Schuller et al., 1990). Other modifications in the design of trucks
have been developed so that pedestrians or cyclists are pushed away
from the vehicle when they are struck, rather than under the wheels
(Middelhauve and Appel, 1990).

Motorcycles cause many injuries to pedestrians. A study of traffic
injuries at a Delhi casualty department found that 16 percent of victims had been struck by motorcycles (Varghese, 1990). In view of the
increasing number of motorcycles in developing countries, and of
their frequent involvement in collisions with pedestrians, it has been
suggested that consideration may need to be given to modifying the

front ends of motorcycles to reduce pedestrian injury in collisions (Varghese, 1990).

Although many motorcycles in developing countries are imported, designs of locally made vehicles also need to be made safer. An example of how this can be achieved is the use of crash modeling software to simulate impacts of three-wheeled scooter taxi crashes in India (Mohan et al., 1997). The results show that simple changes such as the addition of padding and alteration of surfaces should result in a reduction in fatal and non-fatal injuries.

Environmental Factors
In motor vehicle crashes, certain hazardous locations or "blackspots" often account for a substantial proportion of crashes. Treating blackspots associated with repeated motor vehicle crashes often provides good return on money spent in developed countries. This appears to be the case less often for collisions affecting pedestrians and cyclists, at least in developed countries.

Pedestrian injuries may be related to a general area. In developed countries, many injuries occur mid-block as well as at intersections (Snyder and Knoblaugh, 1971; West-Oram, 1990; Joly et al., 1990). System-wide measures that alter traffic flows, including engineering changes to direct traffic away from residential areas, and innovative layouts of road networks within neighborhoods, have been developed to prevent pedestrian injuries (Malek et al., 1990). Measures such as urban "beltways" are being introduced to cities such as Guangzhou, China, to reroute high-speed traffic away from residential neighborhoods (Thomas et al., 1992). Other factors include the proximity of housing to busy streets in poor neighborhoods and the lack of safe play areas close to children's homes (Bagley, 1992b, Dougherty et al., 1990).

While many injuries of child pedestrians occur when they run out between parked vehicles at mid-block locations, intersections with signals are highly dangerous locations for both children and adults because the lights and pavement markings often engender a false sense of security. Unfortunately, motorists often speed up rather than slowing down as they approach a traffic light, in order to avoid having to wait at a red light. About 80–90 percent of severe injuries and deaths of pedestrians at intersections in Canada are inflicted by vehicles travelling straight through or turning left (P. Barss, unpublished data, 1994). Vehicles turning right from the right-hand lane usually turn at a tighter angle and must slow down. Thus, pedestrian injuries from right-turning vehicles are less frequent and less severe.

Intersections that force all motorists to slow down while simultaneously eliminating the possibility of vehicles passing straight through or turning left are of great potential interest for preventing pedestrian injuries. The modern roundabout intersections that are widely used in Europe allow continuous movement of vehicles, but do achieve these objectives. Speeds of vehicles can also be reduced at intersections by raising pedestrian crossings 100–150 mm above the road surface.

In the United Kingdom, the Transport and Road Research Laboratory Urban Safety Project attempted to reduce collisions that occured in scattered locations by applying low-cost safety measures on an area-wide basis in five communities (Lines, 1990). The objectives were to facilitate a safer use of main routes by traffic, to discourage the use of residential roads for through traffic, and to create safer conditions in residential areas.

Collisions and flow in each area were analyzed and a road hierarchy established. Engineering measures were then implemented to ensure that only the appropriate traffic mix used each type of road and to reinforce compliance with low speed limits in residential areas. The measures used included control of right turns, installation of speed bumps, controlled parking, central refuges for pedestrians, speed tables, raised junctions, road closures, pedestrian closures, pedestrian crossings, road pinches, and junctions controlled by mini-roundabouts. Evaluation showed an overall reduction of collisions of 13 percent.

Vehicle speed is an important determinant of the severity of pedestrian injury. In Germany, the risk of a pedestrian fatality rises from 20 percent to 80 percent when vehicle speed increases from 30 km/hr to 60 km/hr (Schweig, 1990). Thus, speed limits of 30 km/hr or less are suggested for locations where there are many pedestrians at risk, including residential, shopping, and school areas. Since the effects of improved vehicle front end design are most beneficial at low impact speeds, the combination of modifications to these two factors could offer greater benefits than expected from adding the separate effects of interventions; that is, there would be a multiplicative interactive effect.

Comprehensive area-wide speed management should be implemented and include speed control devices to improve compliance by drivers (Jørgensen, 1992). In Turkey, a device known as a heavy vehicle shaker was placed before stop or yield right-of-way signs; it was constructed of concrete in such a way that it shook only heavy vehicles such as trucks (Orer, 1990).

Improved street lighting is another example of an environmental measure to prevent traffic injuries. Lighting offers other benefits as well, such as deterrence of crime (Downing, 1990).

To be effective, so-called zebra crossings for pedestrians must be conspicuous and their proper use by motorists enforced by police. Jaywalking by pedestrians is a common problem, particularly if legal crossings are inconveniently located or are difficult to use. For example, between 11 and 84 percent of persons were observed jaywalking at 10 pedestrian crossings in Madras, India (Malini and Victor, 1990); median fences were found to be effective in preventing jaywalking on major roads.

Many road projects are undertaken without any provision for adequate sidewalks or safe, easy to use pedestrian crosswalks. In Addis Ababa, the absence of sidewalks forces pedestrians to walk in the streets with motor vehicles (Dessie and Larson, 1991). Sidewalk maintenance is also important to prevent falls. In crowded areas, rails or barriers help to prevent pedestrian flow from spilling over onto motorways.

Although area-wide solutions should be considered for pedestrian safety, there may be specific high-risk locations or short stretches of road with heavy use by vulnerable pedestrians where corrective measures can be applied with good results. In New York city during a 5 year period, 22 pedestrian deaths and another 18 presumed deaths occurred along a busy 2.5 mile boulevard (Retting et al., 1989). All 20 victims for whom ages were available were at least 60 years of age. A number of environmental modifications to the street were implemented, including increased pedestrian crossing time at stop signals, improved road markings, and oversized speed limit signs. Other measures included increased police enforcement of speed limits and safety education presentations at senior citizen centers. The average annual number of pedestrian fatalities on the boulevard fell by more than 50 percent during a two-year follow-up, compared with a four percent decrease in pedestrian fatalities in the city as a whole.

INJURIES OF BICYCLISTS AND MOTORCYCLISTS

Bicycles and motorcycles share a number of features, but there are also important differences. Common to both are a lack of occupant protection in crashes, low visibility relative to four-wheeled vehicles, and high lateral mobility that often results in the operator darting in and out of traffic. The major difference is the greater speed of motorcycles, which may result in high energy crashes and gives motorists less time to react after detecting the presence of the cyclist. Another important difference, more so in some countries than others, is that bicycles may be used by women and children, whereas the use of motorcycles is more common by male adults. There are exceptions, such as entire families riding together on a motorcycle.

The combined presence in mixed traffic of two- and four-wheeled vehicles presents serious problems because of important differences in speed, visibility, lateral mobility, and vulnerability. For example, a study of five dangerous locations in Hyderabad, India using time-lapse photography revealed serious problems because of high lateral mobility and low visibility of two and three-wheeled vehicles such as bicycles and rickshaws (Chari and Nath, 1990). This gave inadequate reaction time for the less mobile four-wheeled vehicles, such as buses, trucks, and cars, with the result that there were frequent frontal and rear-end collisions. Collisions of motor vehicles with cyclists often occur in scattered locations rather than repeatedly at black spots (Lines, 1990).

Bicycles

Throughout most of Asia, bicycles and rickshaws are a major mode of transport. In Asia alone, bicycles transport more people than do all of the world's automobiles (Lowe, 1989). In Africa and Latin America, bicycles are somewhat less common, since, with the exception of Nicaragua and Cuba, the use of bicycles has generally not been fostered by government policies. Unfortunately for the average person in many countries, transport systems favor motorized traffic. The percentage of trips represented by bicycles varies a great deal among cities (Table 8.1).

The world's 800 million bicycles outnumber cars by two to one and are the only alternative to walking that many people can afford. In addition to serving as a convenient and inexpensive means of personal transport, in some countries, unpowered cycles also provide an important means of transporting goods. For example, in Asia, heavy-

Table 8.1 Bicycling trips as a percent of all daily passenger trips in different cities

City Country	% of trips by bicycle
DEVELOPING COUNTRIES	
Tianjin, China	77
Beijing, China	48
Dhaka, Bangladesh	40
New Delhi, India	22
DEVELOPED COUNTRIES	
Groningen, Netherlands	65
Tokyo, Japan	25
Moscow, Russia	24
Copenhagen, Denmark	20
Manhattan, United States	8
Toronto, Canada	3
Sydney, Australia	1

Source: Lowe MD. The Bicycle: Vehicle for a Small Planet, Washington, DC: Worldwatch Institute, Worldwatch Paper 90, 1989.

duty tricycles are used to carry loads of up to half a ton, and in Bangladesh, such tri-shaws are reported to transport more tonnage than all motor vehicles combined.

China is one of the few developing countries where public policy has deliberately favored bicycle commuting (Lowe, 1989). In Beijing, it was reported in 1981 that there were 3 million bicycles, 180,000 motor vehicles, and 20,000 mopeds and scooters. By 1985, among a population of 10 million, there were 6.3 million bicycles in Beijing, as compared with 90,000 trucks and 93,000 cars (Ryan and Ukai, 1988). There were estimated to be about 300 million bicycles in all of China. More than one in four Chinese owned a bicycle, while only 1 in 74,000 owned an automobile.

In some developed countries, gasoline and automobile sales taxes are deliberately set at high levels to discourage the use of motorized transport and to force users to pay for the environmental damage caused by their vehicles. For example, in Denmark in 1987, the gasoline sales tax was 355 percent, while in the United States it was only 45 percent (Lowe, 1989).

As urban gridlock and air pollution worsen in many industrialized countries, the bicycle is increasingly seen as an important alternative to motorized transport in countries such as the Netherlands and other western European nations. However, there are major disincentives to widespread use of the bicycle as a primary means of transport in both developed and developing countries. These include the hazard and discomfort of sharing roadways with ever increasing numbers of larger and heavier motor vehicles emitting foul-smelling and toxic fumes.

Bicycle injuries are an understudied and unrecognized problem in most developing countries (Mohan, 1990a, 1990b), perhaps because the victims are often from lower socioeconomic groups. In view of the widespread use of the bicycle in many developing countries, together with its recognized importance as a source of serious injury in developed countries, it is surprising to find relatively few published articles on bicycle injuries in developing countries.

Where information is available, it suggests that injuries to bicyclists pose a serious problem in developing countries. In Beijing, China, about one-third of all traffic deaths occur among bicyclists (Ryan and Ukai, 1988). In Wuhan, China, bicycle helmet use is nonexistent although bicyclists comprise 45 percent of all traffic fatalities (Li and Baker, 1997). Studies from New Delhi, India, report that bicyclists constitute 12 to 21 percent of the fatalities among road users, second only to pedestrians at 33 to 45 percent (Sarin et al., 1990b; Mohan and Kumar, 1989; Mohan and Bawa, 1985; Mishra et al., 1984).

Researchers who rely upon only police data may seriously underestimate the relative importance of bicycling injuries, since in police data, bicycle injuries are frequently underreported in both developed and developing countries (Stutts et al., 1990; Harris, 1990; Agran et al., 1990). In Colombo, Sri Lanka, 92 percent of children and 54 percent of adults who were hospitalized for bicycling injuries were not included in police reports (Sayer and Hitchcock, 1984). Reporting was much worse than for pedestrian injuries.

Personal and Behavioral Factors

In many developed countries, bicycles are available to most children as a recreational item or toy, and a large proportion of bicycling fatalities occur among children. The situation differs in many developing countries where a bicycle is used mainly for adult transport to work. In Delhi, India, 85 percent of bicycling fatalities involved individuals between the ages of 15 and 59 years, while only 10 percent were children less than 15 years of age; only 5 percent of victims were females (Mohan and Bawa, 1985; Mishra et al., 1984). On the other hand, in the United States in 1989 about 42 percent of bicycling fatalities involved persons under age 16 (Baker et al., 1992). Nevertheless, there have been rapid increases in bicycling death rates in adults in the United States during the past decade because of increased recreational cycling by adults.

Bicycling is a common activity in Holland. Most serious injuries occur while approaching or crossing intersections (Brookhuis et al., 1990). After establishing normative rules of cycling behavior based on legal safety standards, the behavior of bicyclists was recorded by unobtrusive cameras mounted on other bicycles. Many of the actions based upon normative behavior were not used by bicyclists, even at intersections. In a survey in Visakhapatnam City, India, it was found that only about 10 percent of cyclists had substantial knowledge of road safety (Rao and Venkataram, 1990). In Indonesia, where there are many thousands of cycle rickshaws, drivers and passengers are placed at great risk not only by their vulnerability, but also because rickshaw drivers frequently ignore all traffic rules and regulations (Jacobs and Sayer, 1983). While these studies do not provide evidence for a causal association, they do suggest that bicyclists and rickshaw cyclists have little understanding of the rules of the road, and that this may place them at risk.

Alcohol can be an important risk factor for bicyclists, although its importance is seldom investigated unless a bicycle collides with a motor vehicle. In Finland, alcohol was involved in 25 percent of adult fatalities involving collisions and 63 percent with no collision; only 4 percent of non-injured controls were under the influence of alcohol (Olkkonen, 1990, 1993). In the United States, 32 percent of fatally injured bicyclists age 15 or older had been drinking and 23 percent had BACs of 0.10 percent or higher (Li and Baker, 1994).

Equipment Factors

Major issues with respect to equipment include increasing the visibility of bicycles and cyclists to avoid collisions and the use of appropriate helmets to reduce the risk of severe head injuries in falls or collisions.

High visibility of bicycles and cyclists is important at all times, especially during darkness. In Australia during 1981–84, 90 percent of night-time fatalities resulted from cyclists being struck from behind, whereas in the daytime only 40 percent of victims were hit from behind (Hoque, 1990). Adults were the most frequent victims after dark, whereas children were most often injured between 8 and 9 A.M. Bicycles need to be made much more conspicuous. This can be achieved by legislation that requires that bicycles be sold only in highly visible colors, such as bright yellow or orange (Mohan and Bawa, 1985). The use of multiple reflectors on the wheels and reflective tape on the fenders and frame are relatively inexpensive. Bright-colored and reflective vests for the cyclist are also useful, as is reflective material on helmets.

Since in developed countries most bicycle fatalities are a result of head injuries unassociated with other major injuries, the proper use of appropriate bicycle helmets could considerably reduce fatalities to bicyclists. For example, a review of all fatal bicycle injuries from 1985–87 in Ontario, Canada, in children from 0 to 15 years of age, reported that 67 percent of the injuries were unsurvivable; of these, 95 percent were head/neck injuries (Dykes et al., 1989). Collisions with motor vehicles accounted for 96 percent of the deaths, and none of the victims was wearing a helmet.

A 20 percent reduction in head injuries to bicyclists was observed following a promotional campaign to increase the use of bicycle helmets in the state of Victoria in Australia during 1982–85 (Wood and Milne, 1988). In Seattle, Washington, helmet use was associated with an 80 percent reduction in head injuries (Thompson et al., 1989). Bicycle helmets have been found to be protective of all age groups and in collisions with motor vehicles as well as under other circumstances.

Many cyclists cannot reach the ground with their feet; bicycles with lower saddle heights could reduce the chance of unstable bicyclists falling into the path of other vehicles (Mohan and Bawa, 1985).

Certain bicycle-related injuries in developing countries may differ from those seen in industrialized countries. For example, in Sangli, Maharashtra, India, it was found that amputation of the right toe by an unguarded chain was the most common non-crash bicycling injury. This injury occurred in children who were riding as passengers on the rear carrier (Subrahmanyam, 1984; Subrahmanyam et al., 1980). There is a local law to prohibit the carrying of children on the rear carrier, but enforcement was difficult.

Protection of vulnerable road users is a public policy priority for effective control of traffic injuries in developing countries.

In developing countries, special attention needs to be focused on the protection of pedestrians, bicyclists, motorcyclists, and users of public motor vehicles. This suggests that specialized divisions of government departments or ministries, as well as private organizations, should be established to investigate and lobby for the safety and rights of vulnerable road users, often the poor and illiterate who may be unable to lobby effectively for their own special needs.

Environmental Factors

In view of the scattered location of many collisions between bicycles and motor vehicles, system-wide improvements should be considered. In some urban areas of Great Britain, for example, low cost area-wide engineering measures to control traffic flow and reinforce low speeds have reduced injuries to all vulnerable road users, including cyclists (Lines, 1990).

In addition to promoting personal protective equipment such as helmets, much more should be done to provide a safer environment for bicyclists. Traffic separation and bicycle lanes are eminently feasible in many localities. However, their effectiveness needs to be monitored, since poorly designed lanes could even increase the risk to cyclists. In Finland, 66 percent of bicycling fatalities occurred at intersections (Olkkonen, 1993). Similar data are needed for developing countries.

In more remote rural areas, poorly built and badly maintained bicycles used over rough narrow trails are also likely to be a cause of injuries, but further studies are needed to document this. Waller (1985) reports that bicycle injuries are a serious problem at night on unlit rural roads, where injured cyclists are often not discovered until daybreak. The use of bicycles to transport cargo was also mentioned as a hazard.

In the United States, about 90 percent of bicycling fatalities involve collisions with motor vehicles (Baker et al., 1992). In New Delhi, only 8 percent of bicyclists were struck by cars, while 77 percent were hit by buses and trucks (Mohan and Bawa, 1985; Mishra et al., 1984).

Further study of the epidemiology of bicycle crashes in both rural and urban areas of developing countries is needed to define high risk groups, causes, circumstances, and types of injuries to determine the most suitable preventive interventions.

Motorcycles

Motorcycles are rapidly being introduced into many developing countries as low-cost transportation with little thought given to their hazardous nature, much greater than that of other forms of transport.

In China, high registration fees, equivalent to about 10 months salary, have been imposed on motorcycle users, and this has helped to restrict the use of motorcycles (Ryan and Ukai, 1988). In Guangzhou, China, the traffic situation became so serious, after an increase of 4,000 percent in the number of motorcycles between 1980 and 1990, the city government had to place a limit on the number of new motorcycle licenses to be issued each year (Thomas et al., 1992).

However, in many other developing countries, the use of motorcycles is not restricted, and is growing very rapidly. The number of motorcycles in Taiwan has increased faster than that of any other type of motor vehicle, and in 1988 motorcycles accounted for 76 percent of all motor vehicles (Chiang, 1989). Motorcycles were rare in 1961 in Taiwan; by 1986 there were about 3800 per 10,000. During the same period, the number of automobiles increased from near zero to about 800 per 10,000 (Baker and MacKinney, 1990). In Taiwan in 1987, 61 percent of all traffic crashes involved motorcycles; 88 percent of the riders and 95 percent of the passengers were not wearing safety helmets (Chiang, 1989). In Indonesia in 1988, there were nearly five times as many motorcycles as trucks and cars (Radjak and Agustiono, 1989).

Motorcycles will probably remain a popular choice in congested urban areas because of thier low cost and ability to bypass traffic jams consisting of larger vehicles. Although the risk of fatality may be lower in low-speed situations than on high speed open roads in developed countries (see Table 7.2), all appropriate measures need to be taken to reduce the risk to a minimum.

Personal and Behavioral Factors

Most motorcycle users are poorly trained. In Taiwan, 18 percent of the motorcyclists injured in crashes did not even have a license (Chiang, 1989). In the United States, the situation may be worse; in California, 67 percent of motorcycle operators killed or severely injured in crashes during 1985 and 1986 did not have a valid motorcycle license (Insurance Institute for Highway Safety, 1990c).

In Hong Kong, a case-control study of injured motorcyclists showed that the risk of injury decreased with years of experience (T. W. Wong et al., 1990). It was suggested that motorcyclists should receive more intensive training on special circuits before licensing. In a study of injuries among motorcyclists in Malaysia, Australia, Singapore, and Japan, it was found that the highest risk of injury was among motorcyclists operating on a learner's permit, followed by those in their first year of riding (McLean et al., 1990). However, off-road training of riders in Japan and Singapore did not appear to have been effective in reducing the risk of injury. It was suggested that more effective methods of rider training needed to be developed. In view of the high risk of crashes among novices, it was felt that they should be prohibited from carrying passengers.

Equipment Factors

It is important to increase the visibility of motorcyclists. Motorcyclists are highly vulnerable when they are approaching from the opposite direction towards a motor vehicle commencing a left turn. The multiple head movements and visual detection required of the motorist during such turns, together with the low visibility and high speed of a motorcycle, greatly increase the risk of a collision (Hancock et al., 1990). Interventions to increase the visibility of motorcycles have included mandatory use of headlights at all times and much larger and wider taillights and signal lights.

Head injuries are the major cause of death for users of motorcycles, scooters or mopeds. Thus, their use of safety helmets is very important. It has been recommended both in Indonesia and in Taiwan that every buyer of a motorcycle should be supplied with an appropriate helmet as part of the purchase (Radjak and Agustiono, 1989; Chiang, 1989). Unfortunately, some countries which require helmets for motorcycle drivers do not do so for passengers.

In Malaysia, it was estimated that the introduction of a helmet law resulted in a 30 percent reduction in fatalities (Supramanian, 1984). This is similar to the results observed in the United States where helmet laws have been implemented (Robertson, 1992).

When not required by law to do so, most motorcyclists do not wear helmets. Helmet use declines in the evening in New Delhi when enforcement is less strict (Mohan, 1986c). Passengers in New Delhi are not required to wear helmets and less than one percent do so. Unfortunately, some countries, such as Nigeria, that had helmet laws have repealed them (Asogwa, 1992).

Even in countries where helmets are widely worn, they may not always provide adequate protection. This was attributed to improper use in a study in Nigeria (Asogwa, 1980a, 1992), but other factors could also be important. In India, it has been found that helmets secured by chin-cups are unsafe, since the helmet tends to come off during impact (Mohan, 1986c). The strap needs to be affixed firmly behind the chin. A helmet has been developed in India that provides improved side protection against impacts and has better ventilation for tropical climates (Patel and Mohan, 1990a).

In Taiwan, brake failure and overloading with too many passengers were identified as important causes of motorcycle crashes that need to be addressed (Chiang, 1989). A major need is leg protection for motorcyclists, such as the energy absorbing devices under development by the Transport and Road Research Laboratory in Great Britain, which reportedly have the potential to protect the motorcyclist's legs and prevent about 40 percent of serious injuries (Bly, 1990).

The development by Japanese companies of ultra high speed motorcycles, known as "bullet bikes", has created a serious hazard in some countries. Their use is severely restricted in Japan because of safety concerns, but they are exported in large quantities to other countries. Their extreme hazard may be unrecognized until large numbers of young people have been sacrificed.

In the long run, public policies to shift users away from hazardous forms of transport such as motorcycles may be most useful in preventing fatalities and permanent disabilities from head, spinal cord, and lower-extremity injuries.

OPEN-BACKED VEHICLES AND PUBLIC TRANSPORT

In some developing countries, travel by public transport such as buses and open trucks is common as well as hazardous. Equipment or vehicle factors are important in the etiology of injuries in these conveyances. Special attention needs to be directed to public vehicles and their drivers for other reasons, since buses, trucks, and taxis also cause many injuries of vulnerable road users.

Equipment Factors

A major problem in India is overcrowded buses with large numbers of passengers clinging to the outside. In New Delhi India, bus passengers accounted for 10 percent of all traffic fatalities and 52 percent of motor vehicle occupant fatalities, while buses represented only 4 percent of all three or four wheel registered vehicles. Most of the fatalities were a result of falls from the buses while getting on or off or from being crushed while riding on the footboard, not from crashes (Mohan and Bawa, 1985; Mohan and Kumar, 1989). A change in bus design so that passengers cannot ride on the outside of the bus and can easily be seen by the driver as they enter and exit might help to prevent such fatalities. All buses must be equipped with automatically closing doors.

The situation differs somewhat in other developing countries where many passengers are carried in the backs of open trucks; the cargo compartments of such vehicles were not designed to carry passengers safely and they offer little protection. In oil-rich countries such as Bahrain, pickup trucks and lorries were reported to have the highest casualty rate per 100,000 registered vehicles; severe injuries were sustained by passengers who fell out or were ejected (Ruehsen and Abdul-Wahab, 1989).

A similar situation prevails in poorer rural countries that have developed basic road networks, but where traffic density is relatively low and much of the travel is in crowded open-backed vehicles. In Papua New Guinea, a mainly rural country, the risk per vehicle of a crash is relatively low; however, when a crash occurs, the risk of fatalities is very high (Nelson and Strueber, 1991). Open-backed vehicles were not involved in more crashes than expected for their numbers, but many more casualties per crash occurred than for automobiles. While small pickup trucks made up about 35 percent of all motor vehicles and were the primary vehicle in 38 percent of all crashes, passengers in pickup trucks accounted for 65 percent of all motor vehicle casualties (Nelson and Strueber, 1991). In crashes, passengers in the rear of both pickup trucks and larger trucks were found to be at much higher risk than the drivers, since passengers were frequently ejected from the vehicles.

In 1987, pedestrians and occupants of utility vehicles and trucks combined comprised 90 percent of victims of death and injury (Ryan, 1989b). Single vehicle crashes were more common than they are in developed countries. The capital, Port Moresby, was the only area of the country where cars were a significant source of injuries. Even so, 45 percent of traffic fatalities in Port Moresby were passengers, 34 percent pedestrians, and 18 percent drivers (Sinha and Sengupta, 1989).

Similarly, in Kenya, where trucks represented only 5 percent of registered vehicles, they accounted for 16 percent of occupant deaths (Jacobs and Sayer, 1983). This excess mortality may reflect greater mileage by the average truck, more passengers per vehicle, and the exposed position of many truck passengers. In rural areas, most vehicle crashes involved single vehicles (Gekonge, 1990), whereas in built up areas the main victims were pedestrians.

A switch to buses or enclosed rear vehicle compartments could help to reduce the number of such deaths.

OFF-ROAD VEHICLES

Off-road vehicles include snowmobiles and all-terrain vehicles (S. M. Smith and Middaugh, 1989). In some northern aboriginal communities, they are the leading cause of motor vehicle injury and cause more serious injuries than do cars and trucks (Johnson et al., 1992; Damestoy, 1994). All-terrain vehicles are also sold in some developing countries, but relatively few persons would be able to afford them.

Personal Factors

Snowmobiles contribute to drowning deaths when an intoxicated driver travelling at high speed at night or during a snowstorm fails to see a hole in the ice when crossing a lake (Canadian Red Cross Society, 1996; Eriksson and Björnstig, 1982).

Most deaths from all-terrain vehicles occur among children. If an adult-sized vehicle overturns, it is too heavy for a child to control, and he can be crushed. Some jurisdictions are using legislation to prohibit children from using adult-sized all-terrain vehicles.

Equipment Factors

To boost lagging sales, manufacturers of snowmobiles and all-terrain vehicles have made them faster and more powerful. Riders are unprotected in high speed collision. Since lower extremity injuries are common and often result when riders fall from their machines, redesign may be needed.

Three-wheeled all-terrain vehicles are particularly unstable and have been banned, but are still in use in many villages. Helmets are promoted to protect riders of off-road vehicles. They can prevent head injuries, but not crushing injuries that occur when such vehicles overturn onto children. Helmets with face shields can help to protect against blinding, perforating eye injuries from branches when traveling through the forest. Snowmobile suits that provide flotation and hypothermia protection can prevent drowning and immersion hypothermia.

Since many injuries occur after dark, more powerful lighting systems would improve visibility at high speeds. Reduced maximum speeds could also be helpful (Rowe and Bota, 1991; Hamdy et al., 1988).

Environmental Factors

Collisions can occur with motor vehicles when off-road vehicles are crossing or travelling on roads. Off-road, the machines are now so powerful that it is questionable whether they should be used at full-speed, since hazards are unpredictable, and the riders are in a situation of vulnerable exposure.

The situation is worsened by impaired visibility from darkness, snowstorms, or blinding snow. In the fall and spring, ice over lakes and rivers is less stable and the risk of drowning increases (Canadian Red Cross Society, 1996b; Rowe and Bota, 1991).

DETERMINANTS OF MOTOR VEHICLE CRASHES

A few examples of risk factors specific to motor vehicles such as cars and trucks are presented here. General determinants of injuries were discussed in Chapter 6.

While the majority of road crashes tend to be attributed by police to driver error, it is generally unproductive to focus on blaming the victims of crashes. Thus, while personal factors must be considered, they should not be overemphasized, since this could delay the implementation of more efficacious system-wide interventions based upon modifications of equipment and/or the environment.

In some developing countries with high motor vehicle injury rates among vulnerable road users such as pedestrians, there are relatively few drivers and vehicles, and it is feasible to focus interventions on both drivers and vehicles. In Addis Ababa, Ethiopia, for a population of about 1.6 million in 1988, there were approximately 60,000 registered drivers and 48,000 registered vehicles (Dessie and Larson, 1991).

Personal and Behavioral Factors

Driver age and sex are important contributing factors in traffic crashes in developed countries, with male teenage drivers and, to a lesser extent, elderly drivers, at higher than average risk. The importance of driver age may vary among different developing countries. It is often less important than in developed countries, since in many countries most teenagers and elderly individuals do not have access to a motor vehicle. However, the situation differs in wealthy countries such as Saudi Arabia that are undergoing rapid development; young drivers and poorly educated drivers were frequently involved in crashes in the Riyadh area (Al-Zahrani and Bener, 1990). Even in Addis Ababa, drivers less than 26 years of age had a risk of involvement in a motor vehicle injury nearly 15 times the average, compared with controls; this high risk for young drivers could be attributable, at least in part, to inexperience (Dessie and Larson, 1991).

In China, driving a motor vehicle was a profession, and six months of training was required to obtain a license (Ryan and Ukai, 1988). In Papua New Guinea in 1987, about 30 percent of the vehicles involved in crashes were owned by a government agency or a company (Ryan, 1989b), while in Addis Ababa 37 percent of vehicles involved in crashes were owned by government and another 9 percent by international organizations. However, even among professional drivers, age is often a significant risk factor. In Hong Kong, a study of bus drivers showed that older drivers had a dramatically lower crash rate than younger ones (Evans and Courtney, 1985). The largest differences were between the oldest (58–60 years) and the youngest (22–27 years) groups. There is little information from developing countries on gender differences in crash rates, although high rates in young males appear to be a worldwide phenomenon.

In situations where professional drivers must work long hours, fatigue is a contributor to injury risk. For example, in the study of Hong Kong bus drivers mentioned above, it was found that some drivers had to work for periods exceeding 8 or 9 hours. The crash rate rose after about 7 hours on duty; this was attributed to fatigue. In many developing countries, drivers may have to work substantially longer shifts. In Addis Abiba, drivers with a taxi license accounted for 48 percent of all motor vehicle injuries, light bus and truck drivers for 19 percent, and heavy bus and truck drivers for 9 percent (Dessie and Larson, 1991).

Visual acuity may affect the risk of crashes. In Lagos, Nigeria, one out of three of taxi drivers was found to have serious visual deficiencies, but only one in ten was aware of the need for corrective lenses (Alakija, 1981). In addition to static visual acuity, kinetic visual acuity appears to be important for drivers. Visual acuity is measured using relative motion between the test subject and the object being viewed. It has been suggested that this parameter should be tested in applicants for liscences to drive major vehicles such as trucks and buses.

In a study of men in Australia, it was found that low socioeconomic status, low level of education, and a history of juvenile offenses were associated with an increased risk of road crashes

(O'Toole, 1990). Nevertheless, attempts to identify such high-risk individuals have not been very productive compared to system-wide environmental improvements.

Limited understanding or non-observance of the rules of the road and of appropriate driving behavior in traffic has been suggested as a factor in many crashes in developing countries (Downing, 1992). The situation may differ from that in more developed countries such as the United States, where it was found that high school driver education programs actually led to increased fatality rates by putting more young drivers on the roads (Robertson, 1980). Such programs tended to increase exposure to injury by encouraging more young people to become licensed at earlier ages. However, in New Zealand, experience with driver education programs is reported to have been more positive (Kirkwood, 1990). Low socioeconomic status and lack of education are associated with a low rate of use of safety belts in developed countries (Shinar, 1993). Rates of use of safety belts are low in many developing countries and indigenous communities (Oluwasanmi, 1993; Robitaille and Barss, 1994).

The results of a survey of 24,000 road injuries in Calcutta provide an example of some of the knowledge and behavioral problems in a developing country (Sen and Ghosal, 1989). High-risk behaviors that were identified included unsafe overtaking by buses competing to get more passengers on the same route, overtaking near bus stops, lack of awareness by road users of traffic rules and regulations, parking of vehicles on the sides of congested roads, failure to dim headlights when passing, and non-use of helmets by motorcycle passengers.

Studies comparing drivers in Reading and London, England with those in a number of cities in developing countries reported that fewer drivers in developing countries stopped for pedestrians at crossings and at red lights (Jacobs and Bardsley, 1977). However, the inexperience that some rural pedestrians and urban migrants have with traffic may also contribute to their increased risk.

Many drivers in developing countries, including professional bus drivers, have had little or no training and a poor understanding of the characteristics of their vehicles, such as stopping distances. This may be because of a lack of funds for training and testing drivers, a low level of general education among the public, and the use of bribery to obtain licenses without tests (Asogwa, 1992).

In a study of 720 road users in Visakhapatram City, India, it was found that 65 percent of motor vehicle drivers had obtained their driving license through middlemen (Rao and Venkataram, 1990). Their knowledge of traffic symbols and signs, turns, and intersections was rated at about 60 percent and of pedestrian crossings at about 40 percent. Only 20 percent of motor vehicle drivers, 10 percent of cyclists, and 0.5 percent of pedestrians had a high knowledge level about safety. Although respondents with high knowledge levels were not immune from crashes, many of their crashes were attributed to other road users.

In view of the fact that trucks account for nearly 30 percent of road crashes in India, a survey was conducted of 755 truck drivers operating on a national highway into Delhi (Sarin et al., 1990d). They were shown ten road signs and five sketches of different traffic violations. Only about 10 percent of the drivers understood at least 50 percent of the road signs, and only 1 percent understood 75 percent or more. About 15 percent of truck drivers had a greater than 50 percent knowledge of the road traffic rules, and less than 1 percent had more than 75 percent knowledge. Older age, better education, and licensing through a driving school were associated with slightly higher knowledge levels. The limited knowledge of road signs was felt to be particularly disturbing, since before licensing, truck drivers in India are supposed to pass tests on their knowledge of road signs.

While knowledge may be a necessary condition for safe driving, it is not sufficient to bring about desired changes in behavior. Effective enforcement of regulations is also necessary.

The use of alcohol is a major risk factor for traffic injuries and in some developed countries it is important in up to one-half or more of all traffic fatalities (Evans, 1990). Alcohol not only impairs drivers and increases the risk of a crash, but also increases the risk of death in a crash, with a doubling of risk at 0.1 percent BAC and a tripling at 0.25 percent (Evans and Frick, 1993). It has been noted that even in countries with a low prevalence of drinking drivers on the roads, the level of impaired drivers among traffic fatalities remains high, suggesting a chronic "hard core" of dangerous alcohol abusers who are resistant to control (Ross, 1993). It is unknown whether these findings apply to developing countries and indigenous communities, and it is possible that a greater proportion of their fatalities result from sporadic binge drinking and inexperience.

Alcohol as a risk factor for injuries was discussed extensively in Chapter 6. The effects of drugs other than alcohol have been difficult to document, in part because they are often used in combination with alcohol.

In the United States, one-third of fatally injured truck drivers tested positive for alcohol and/or other drugs, including methamphetamines, over-the-counter medications and, more rarely, marijuana and cocaine. Personal factors associated with drug-positive drivers included a suspended or revoked license, prior alcohol or other drug history, and violation of federal hours of service regulations.

It has been recommended that a zero level of alcohol be established as the legal limit for commercial drivers. Police were authorized to impound a vehicle for 24 hours if there was any evidence of alcohol at all, and the license of the driver could be revoked for one year if he tested at a blood level of 0.04 percent (Voas, 1990). Some jurisdictions have established zero tolerance levels for alcohol for commercial drivers, and, increasingly, for young drivers.

The association of alcohol with traffic injuries is even more serious among many aboriginal populations in developed countries. Among indigenous populations in the United States, it was estimated that 65 percent of traffic deaths were related to alcohol abuse (May, 1992).

Better data from developing countries should become available as individual countries move to establish legal blood alcohol levels (BAC) for intoxication and to make testing for alcohol by police or health providers mandatory in all cases of suspected intoxication of drivers and at the time of traffic crashes. The few available data show that a serious problem already exists in some countries (Downing et al., 1991). Among traffic fatalities in Trinidad in 1988, 41 percent of drivers and 41 percent of pedestrians were found to have BACs greater than 0.08 percent.

Interventions that prevent collisions by improving visibility of vehicles and pedestrians.

Mandatory use of vehicle front and rear lights at all times increases visibility, and is probably even more important for smaller vehicles such as motorcycles than for cars. Daytime lighting is now required by law in some countries for motorcycles and is also being introduced for cars. Automatic lighting should be particularly effective in countries where drivers avoid or forget to turn on their lights at dusk.

Visibility of bicycles and cyclists can reduce crash involvement. New bicycles should be manufactured, imported, and sold only in highly visible colors such as orange or yellow and with appropriate reflectors and lights. The added protection of motorcycle drivers and passengers by appropriate helmets, clothing, and conspicuous lighting such as headlights that automatically switch on with the ignition are other proven interventions.

Roadside alcohol surveys of drivers in Papua New Guinea were carried out between 10 P.M. and 2 A.M. on weekends; 24 percent of drivers had levels exceeding 0.08 percent, which is the legal limit in the United Kingdom. The comparable figure for drivers tested in Great Britain was 2 percent over the limit. In traffic fatalities in Zimbabwe in 1979, 56 percent of drivers and 72 percent of pedestrians tested positive for alcohol. These were nearly double the comparable figures for Great Britain. In Ankara, Turkey, a random sample of drivers were tested for alcohol. The results were as follows: 82 percent had any amount present, >0.00 percent BAC; 54 percent, ≥0.05 percent BAC; 34 percent, ≥0.08 percent BAC; and 14 percent, ≥0.15 percent BAC (Vural and Saygi, 1991).

In a study of traffic victims seen at hospital emergency departments in Kaduna, Nigeria, of 50 drivers, 14 percent were drunk and another 30 percent were abusers of cannabis or amphetamines known as *kwaya* (Obembe and Fagbayi, 1988). Of 128 non-drivers, 18 percent were drunk and 16 percent were abusers of cannabis or amphetamines.

Equipment Factors

The development of safer vehicles and roads has often required energetic, well-organized, and sustained public lobbying of governments to induce them to draft legislation to overcome the reluctance of manufacturers to include essential safety features in the designs of their vehicles (Nader, 1991). Safety features that add to the cost of a vehicle are incorporated voluntarily only when large numbers of consumers become sufficiently sophisticated and affluent to choose vehicles with such features over those that lack them.

Design problems can also be critical in public vehicles. In areas where buses and trucks cause many injuries of vulnerable road users, impact-absorbing front ends are needed (Bly, 1990; Mohan, 1986c). Vehicle problems identified in a Calcutta study included a lack of highly visible front and rear turn and stop signals (Sen and Ghosal, 1989).

Poor vehicle maintenance has also been identified as a problem in some countries (Waller, 1985); the most effective solution for this still needs to be worked out for developing countries since the problem sometimes is an economic one and/or relates to scarcity of essential spare parts. In a study of Delhi buses, it was found that brake lights did not work in 90 percent of buses, turn signals in 47 percent, and speedometers in many (Jacobs and Downing, 1982). Over one-half had improperly or unevenly inflated tires. In a study on the main highway between Delhi and Bombay, it was found that one-quarter of fast-moving vehicles did not have a proper brake/stop light (Desai et al., 1990a, 1990b). Even worse problems have been described in Nigeria and were attributed to economic factors (Asogwa, 1992).

Environmental Factors

Poorly designed roadways can lead to repeated vehicle crashes and/or injuries to vulnerable road users (Transport and Road Research Laboratory, 1991; Downing et al., 1991). Environmental factors can be critical in certain high risk locations or blackspots that result in repeated crashes, and also in more generalized system-wide problems that contribute to crashes at multiple and often unpredictable locations.

As an example of the importance of localized hazards, a study by a community health department of the highways in one region of Québec, Canada, identified 28 priority sites or black spots (Brown et al., 1991). These represented only 6 percent of total highway length, but accounted for 53 percent of deaths, 30 percent of serious injuries, and 32 percent of minor injuries that occurred on numbered highways.

In Hyderabad, India, a study of the five worst black spots was carried out using time-lapse photography at one-second intervals. This showed that the amber period at intersections with traffic signals was inadequate to allow for clearing of the intersection, unless it was at least six seconds (Chari and Nath, 1990).

A number of important environmental features of roadways affect the risk of crashes and of severe injury. Fixed roadside obstacles are an important source of severe injuries to vehicle occupants. Overall, and especially in rural locations, these are trees (Mintsis and Pitsiava-Latinopoulou, 1990). Protective barriers or breakaway features in "road furniture" such as signs and lampposts are needed. Transitional curves are another important environmental hazard. Such curves do not have a constant curvature, and this misleads drivers into misjudging their approach speed. It is relatively inexpensive to correct transitional curves to a constant curvature, with highly cost-effective results (Stewart and Chudworth, 1990).

Physical or environmental factors identified as contributing to the risk of injury in a Calcutta study include inadequate width and maintenance of roads and paths, unauthorized occupation of footpaths by shops and vendors, and poor design and/or faulty installation of traffic signs and signals on the roads (Sen and Ghosal, 1989).

In some developed countries, major controlled highways with limited access, such as the interstate system in the United States, are safer than most other roads. However, in Great Britain, death rates are similar on major motorways and more built-up roads (West-Oram, 1990). The relative scarcity of vulnerable road users on major roads can result in low overall death rates for such roads, but with rates for vehicle occupants similar to those for other types of roads.

The situation may differ in developing countries. The National Highway System in India is about 34,000 km long and constitutes only about 2 percent of the total road system in the country. However, it accounts for 25 percent of crashes, 34 percent of traffic fatalities, and 28 percent of traffic injuries (Sarin et al., 1990e). One stretch in the state of Gujarat experienced a 100 percent increase in crashes between 1981–86. Some of the factors that were believed to contribute to the high crash rate on this stretch included large differentials in speed due to the mix of traffic, a high volume of traffic, shoulders of inadequate width, straightness and continuity, monotonous conditions, poor driving practices, and lack of law enforcement. It was observed that the highway had good structural features, but lacked important design safety elements in the road and roadside features. The National Highway between Delhi and Bombay is one of the most important highways in the national road network of India; however, it is a frequent location of crashes (Shah et al., 1990).

In Nigeria, improvements of roads sometimes led to increased death rates from traffic crashes. The improvements facilitated travel at higher speeds, and there was inadequate enforcement of speed limits (Asogwa, 1992).

Since road junctions and intersections are the location of about 20 to 25 percent of all road crashes in many developed and developing countries, their appropriate design is a subject of considerable importance (Ranganathan et al., 1990; Aggarwal, 1990). In Great Britain, such locations appear to be especially hazardous, with 70 percent of road crashes reported to occur at road junctions (West-Oram, 1990). In developing countries, intersections are needed that provide maximum protection to pedestrians, bicyclists, and motorcyclist, and not simply a false sense of security.

Urban speed management is being approached in a comprehensive systematic area-wide manner in some countries (Jørgensen, 1992). Specific technical measures such as "speed breakers" are frequently used in urban areas, and provide a physical means of inducing vehicle drivers to slow down. These have to be developed carefully, however, so that they will be safe, effective, and acceptable to motorists (Sarin et al., 1990a). Special designs have been developed that affect only large heavy vehicles (Orer, 1990).

Crash rates as well as the proportion of different road user types often differ between rural and urban areas. The control of traffic fatalities in rural areas has been generally neglected, and overall rural traffic fatality rates tend to be higher than in urban areas in both developing and developed countries (Transport and Road Research Laboratory, 1986; Baker et al., 1987).

In West Malaysia during 1977, 61 percent of traffic fatalities occurred on roads in non-built-up areas, 26 percent in villages, and only 12 percent in towns; in the same year, in Great Britain, 44 percent of fatalities occurred in non-built-up areas. In Taiwan in 1986, motor vehicle mortality rates were highest in areas with mountainous terrain and poor road conditions, including unpaved roads (Wu and Malison, 1990). In Iraq, the number of fatalities per crash in rural areas was about 2 to 4 times that in urban areas (Razouki, 1990). Speeds commonly exceeded the legal limits on rural roads.

chapter 9

Unintentional Injuries: Drownings, Falls, and Burns

Drownings, falls, and burns are the major causes of fatal or severe unintentional injury, after traffic injuries. In isolated or mountainous areas with few roads, and even in certain cities, their health impact exceeds that of traffic injuries. Falls and burns are leading causes of mild and moderate injuries in the home and elsewhere.

This chapter examines the importance of each of these injuries, special circumstances pertaining to developing countries and indigenous communities leading to these injuries, and the classification, data sources, examples, and determinants for each type of injury. Each of these three types of injuries includes several subcategories that may have quite different determinants and risk groups. Careful classification and specific analyses of circumstances relating to the subcategories most common in a particular area are essential to determine the most appropriate interventions.

DROWNING AND OTHER WATER-RELATED INJURIES

Drowning by immersion is by far the most important of the unintentional water-related fatalities. Drownings happen to people who are in the water for the following reasons:

- Bathing, washing, swimming, fording rivers, wading;
- Recreational boating or travel by boat or ferry;
- A fall.

Drownings also result from the following:

- Motor vehicles leave the road and plunge into water;
- Snowmobiles hit an unseen hole in the ice;
- Aircraft crash into water.

Drownings occur during different types of activities, including the following:

- Daily living activities;
- Recreation;
- Subsistence or paid employment.

Other external causes of water-related injuries include the following:

- Collisions of boats;
- Lacerations by propellers;
- Diving or jumping into water, with head, neck and perforating injuries from submerged branches and rocks;
- Underwater diving using compressed air;
- Immersion hypothermia;
- Envenomations and physical injuries from marine creatures in coastal areas.

Importance of Drowning

Drowning rates in most developing countries and indigenous communities, especially in rural locations, are generally higher at all ages than in developed countries. In special risk groups, such as toddlers and the elderly, rates in developing countries can be several times higher (Table 9.1).

Drowning often ranks second to traffic injuries as a cause of fatality from unintentional injury, particularly among males. In rural areas of some countries or regions, such as Sri Lanka, China, and the deltas of Bangladesh, drowning is the leading cause of fatality from unintentional injuries, exceeding even traffic injuries. Data are rarely available for countries that lack mortality reporting systems, but since drownings tend to be common in rural populations, high rates would be expected in some of the least developed countries. By comparing drowning rates in Table 9.1 with traffic death rates in Table 7.3, it can be seen that even in many of the more motorized Latin American and Asian countries, where motor vehicle fatalities have surpassed drownings, drowning rates remain much higher than in developed countries. Drowning rates published by WHO do not include boating-related drownings, which in some countries are the leading source of drownings (in Canada, 40% of all drownings).

Drowning is the leading cause of death among small children, such as toddlers, in some areas of Bangladesh and south China (Zimicki et al., 1985). Drowning is also the first or second most common cause of death from unintentional injuries in many northern aboriginal communities of North America and Greenland (Bjerregaard, 1992; Muir, 1991), where it happens primarily to adult males.

Rates of drowning reflect frequent exposure to unprotected bodies of water, personal characteristics of local populations, and, in boating-related fatalities, equipment factors. Rural residents who are exposed daily to open water often have much higher rates of drowning than city-dwellers. Studies among various groups of Canadian aboriginals have found their standardized mortality ratios for drowning to be 4 to 26 times greater than for Canadians as a whole (Khatter, 1990; Health Canada, 1998), although the relative importance of traffic injuries is increasing rapidly in some communities as their exposures to development change.

The public health significance of drowning is often underestimated by local health providers who work in clinics and hospitals since they seldom see the victims. Recorded rates of drowning are affected by both the completeness of reports and the types of drowning included.

Accurate information about drowning is particularly difficult to obtain in remote areas of developing countries, since most victims never reach hospital and the event may not be recorded. At times, the body is never recovered. For these reasons, underreporting is often more severe for drownings than for other injuries, at least in areas where certification of deaths is incomplete.

Special Circumstances in Developing Countries and Indigenous Communities

For rural residents of developing countries, drowning is associated with exposure to natural bodies of water such as lakes and rivers, and, for children, ponds, irrigation ditches, water-storage cisterns or tanks, and wells. Drownings often occur during activities of daily living, such as bathing in or crossing rivers, subsistence vocations, such as fishing from small boats, and, for small children, playing near unprotected bodies of water near the home. In deltas, floods and cyclones are periodic sources of mass drownings.

In urban environments, rates of drowning tend to be lower. Artificial man-made collections of water, such as pools and tubs, in the domestic or peridomestic environment, may be of greater importance than natural sources. In some cities, unprotected canals and drainage ditches pose a risk, particularly during heavy rainfall and flooding. However, if urban residents venture into rural environments for water-related recreational activities, they may be at high risk of drowning during boating, fishing, and swimming.

In indigenous communities in cold climates, travel by small boat or canoe, or over ice by snowmobile or on foot are activities associated with drowning (Health Canada, 1998). Nearly all of the victims are adult males. Immersion hypothermia is often a major contributor to such deaths and occasionally is the sole cause. Swimming and bathing are relatively unimportant, since low water temperatures make such activities unattractive during most or all of the year. Drownings of toddlers occasionally occur when they are allowed to play without adult supervision near open natural bodies of water or unprotected building excavations.

In developed countries, most drownings involve adult males engaged in recreational activities such as swimming, fishing, or other outings in small motorboats or canoes; alcohol intoxication and failure to wear a personal flotation device are commonly associated with such deaths (Canadian Red Cross Society, 1994a, 1994c, 1996a, 1996b, 1997). In many developed countries, drowning is the major cause of recreational and sporting fatalities. Domestic drownings involve 1 to 4–year-old toddlers who fall into unfenced swimming pools, ponds, or bathtubs (Barss, 1998b), or the elderly in bathtubs. Recreational boating accounts for about a third of drownings in some developed countries, but is less important in many developing countries. In warm regions of countries with many domestic swimming pools, hospitalization for near drownings among toddlers often outnumber fatal drownings.

Table 9.1 Age-specific mortality rates per 100,000 population for non-boating drowning*

	Sex					Deaths per 100,000 per year						
		<1	1–4	5–14	15–24	25–54	55–64	65–74	75+	all ages	year
AFRICA											
Mauritius	M	0	12	5	6	8	14	20	0	8	1994
	F	0	5	4	0	0	0	0	8	2	
SOUTHEAST ASIA											
China, rural	M	7	62	28	9	7	8	12	35	15	1994
	F	13	46	13	4	4	4	12	25	9	
China, urban	M	4	13	11	5	2	2	4	9	5	1994
	F	1	9	3	1	1	2	2	8	2	
Sri Lanka	M	4	6	5	9	9	8	12	27	8	1986
	F	3	7	3	3	2	2	5	9	3	
Thailand	M	1	15	7	7	17	7	7	15	7	1981
	F	2	11	5	2	6	1	2	4	4	

AMERICAS

	Sex										Year
Ecuador	M	11	10	5	10	28	11	10	17	8	1988
	F	2	6	2	2	3	2	2	3	2	
Uruguay	M	0	7	4	13	7	5	5	2	7	1990
	F	0	3	2	1	0	2	3	0	1	
Mexico	M	1	7	3	9	7	7	9	13	6	1993
	F	2	4	1	1	1	1	1	2	1	

COMPARISON

	Sex										Year
United States	M	2	4	2	3	2	2	2	3	2	1992
	F	2	3	1	0	0	0	0	1	1	
Sweden	M	0	2	2	2	2	4	4	3	2	1993
	F	5	1	0	1	0	0	1	1	1	
Russian Federation	M	2	10	11	18	30	25	14	9	22	1994
	F	1	5	4	3	3	4	3	4	4	

Sources: World Health Statistics Annual 1990–1992, 1995 (WHO, 1991–1993, 1996.

*Does not include drownings related to boating or land or air transport

Near drownings occur when an immersion is not immediately fatal. However, since under normal conditions the central nervous system cannot withstand more than a few minutes of hypoxia, some victims of near drowning who are resuscitated after a delay sustain permanent brain damage and remain disabled. Others die of delayed complications that develop as a result of aspiration of water into the lungs. Hospitalizations for near drownings appear to be far less common than fatalities by drowning in many developing countries and northern indigenous communities, perhaps because the remoteness of the communities causes delays in rescue and resuscitation from large natural bodies of water.

Classification and Coding of Drownings

There are several major categories of drownings; the high-risk groups, determinants, and many of the preventive interventions can be quite different for each of them. Detailed information about the risk groups and circumstances of specific types of drownings is key to developing effective prevention.

When defining and classifying the circumstances of different types of drownings, the major categories noted above should be considered with related activities and personal, equipment, and environmental factors. The circumstances of boating drownings should be described separately, since equipment factors are often an important component. Classification by location of the incident is helpful for planning possible interventions. It is useful to consider the sites of toddlers' drownings separately from those of older children and adults. The location of drownings can be sub-classified under natural and man-made bodies of water. It should also be noted if the drowning occurred in a peridomestic location, since open bodies of water in residential areas should be either eliminated or enclosed.

When studying drowning rates, it is important to know the standard rubrics under which deaths from drowning are classified. While many drownings are coded under the International Classification of Diseases rubrics specific for drownings from swimming, wading, and falls into natural bodies of water, bathtubs, and swimming pools, drownings that occur during travel by boat are separately coded under water transport. Although boating drownings are often grouped with "Other Transport Deaths" in World Health Organization country reports on mortality, it is important to tabulate these deaths separately in countries or regions where travel in small boats is widespread. In the Solomon Islands, for example, boats and canoes are widely used for travel; in a recent year, marine transport losses accounted for at least 20 deaths, whereas road crashes only caused about 6 deaths (Ryan, 1989a). In other countries or localities where motor vehicles are more common, drownings in vehicles that plunge into water from bridges or roads may be relatively frequent (Wintemute et al, 1990). These incidents are normally coded as motor vehicle deaths and may require special searches to locate. There are no specific ICD codes for drownings in motor vehicles.

Drownings on snowmobiles are an important problem for northern indigenous peoples. Unfortunately, there are no specific ICD codes for snowmobile drownings and other snowmobile injuries, so these deaths are often coded under land transport deaths from all-terrain and other off-road vehicles (Bracker, 1989; Damestoy, 1994). However, coders do sometimes classify these deaths as drownings. Thus, in northern regions where such deaths are an important cause of mortality, it is necessary to check for snowmobile drownings under both categories.

Immersions with hypothermia are another classification problem for northern indigenous populations. In near drownings, the presence of hypothermia is assessed by core body temperature measurements, with levels less than 35°C (95°F) indicative of hypothermia (Lloyd, 1989). It is often impossible for a coroner to decide whether a person died from drowning or hypothermia. There is no specific code for such deaths, and it has even been suggested that they should all be diagnosed simply as "immersions" (Golden and Rivers, 1975). It has also been proposed that hypothermia is a symptom rather than a diagnosis (Lloyd, 1989). Possible solutions to coding such deaths could be the consistent use of the appropriate drowning code for external cause of death, together with the separate nature of injury code for hypothermia, or alternatively, the use of two separate External Cause codes.

Drownings that result from seizures are sometimes classified under the rubrics for epilepsy as the underlying cause of death, with drowning listed only as an associated cause. Other drownings may be classified and coded in categories for suicide, homicide, or undetermined intent. When working with hospital records, it is important to be aware of the separate classification code for near drownings.

Other water-related injuries are coded separately from drownings. Injuries other than drownings that occur during boating transports, such as collisions, are classified using subcodes under the general rubric of boating transport injuries. Injuries from jumping and diving into water are coded as a specific type of fall. Injuries from marine creatures are classified either in subcategories of exposure to animate mechanical forces or of contact with venomous animals and plants, and are discussed in Chapter 10.

Drowning codes in the World Health Organization's International Classification of Diseases need to be modified to make them more appropriate to the environmental conditions in developing countries. For example, in the ninth revision of the ICD (WHO, 1978b), drowning from water-skiing was the first rubric listed for codes of drowning deaths, while there was no specific code for drowning in rivers. Many improvements are evident in the Tenth Revision (WHO, 1992), but further refinements are possible as more detailed data on the circumstances of drownings become available from developing countries and northern indigenous communities (Barss, 1991).

Bathtubs and swimming pools have replaced water-skiing as the first-listed external causes of drowning in ICD 10, but there is no specific listing for man-made sources common in villages, such as ponds, irrigation ditches, cisterns, and wells. A generic heading of man-made bodies of water would be more appropriate to the needs of developing countries, and could include subcategories as shown above, as well as the bathtubs and swimming pools that are so important in developed countries.

Because of the limitations of standard coding systems and data sources, a national surveillance system for water-related fatalities was

> **Special surveys or surveillance systems are needed to identify circumstances of drownings.**

Since few drowning victims survive to reach a health facility, special surveillance systems or surveys are needed to define local and national risk factors for drowning. These sources include village surveys using verbal autopsies, ongoing collection and analysis of newspaper clippings, and special surveillance systems based upon systematic abstraction of data from many coroners' reports.

The Canadian Red Cross Society, in cooperation with the Coast Guard, the Life Saving Society, the National Association of Coroners, and public health staff, has developed a national surveillance system for abstracting details of drownings from records at each of the ten provincial coroners' offices (Canadian Red Cross Society, 1994a, 1994b, 1994c, 1997). Data are used as a basis for planning provincial and national prevention programs.

By pooling data from many remote communities in different provinces and territories, national surveillance has been helpful in obtaining adequate data to identify the special circumstances of drownings among remote indigenous populations in Canada. Similar surveillance systems could be useful in selected developing countries where drownings are a significant cause of mortality investigated by coroners.

developed in Canada to obtain accurate numbers and circumstances for all categories of drownings. This involved the collaboration of several organizations, 12 provinces and territories, and the National Association of Coroners. It provides an example of a structured approach to the problem of collecting and organizing data on specific determinants of different types of drownings (Canadian Red Cross Society, 1996a, 1996b, 1997). The costs of such a surveillance system are low in relation to the total costs of even one death, since existing data sources are an important component. Drowning categories and questionnaires for abstraction of data can be tailored to local priorities, while maintaining the major categories of the ICD for international comparability.

Data Sources for Water-Related Injuries

Sources of mortality data, such as coroners' reports and vital statistics, are important in ascertaining the significance, risk groups, and determinants of drownings. The quality of such data will vary depending upon whether coroners routinely include information about activities associated with drownings and the determinants for each activity, including the following:

- Personal factors, such as alcohol abuse, epilepsy, swimming ability, and whether a toddler was alone, with another child, or with an adult;
- Equipment factors, such as type of boat or vehicle, use of personal flotation devices, and overloading; for child drownings, presence and type of protective barriers and gates around the body of water where drowning occurred;
- Environmental factors, such as type and location of water where drowning occurred, whether natural or man-made, and, where relevant, air and water temperatures and duration of immersion.

Hospital records are not very useful for data on drownings. However, the importance of hospitalization for near drownings can be assessed. Other water-related injuries may also be studied using coroners' reports or hospital records, if specific requests are made for the appropriate categories of records. Where relevant, drownings associated with motor vehicles, off-road vehicles, and aircraft also must be specifically requested, since they are not routinely grouped with drownings.

In remote areas where drownings are seldom reported, special surveys may help to determine drowning rates, the importance of the problem, types of drownings, and major determinants. In some countries, newspapers (Rainey and Runyan, 1992) and various organizations such as water safety divisions of the Red Cross, life-saving societies, coast guards, departments of transport, sporting organizations, physical education staff in government or universities, and boating clubs may provide supplementary or alternative sources of information on drownings.

Examples of Mortality from Drowning

Age and sex specific mortality rates for drowning, reported from several developing countries in Table 9.1, illustrate some of the subgroups of the population that are at highest risk, as well as differences in drowning rates among countries. The following examples illustrate some of the characteristics of drowning and its relative importance in specific areas of developing countries.

The highest reported rates of drowning have been from the deltas of rural Bangladesh, where drownings are among the leading causes of death for toddlers. The annual drowning rates were 215 per 100,000 population for children aged 1–4 years, and 546 per 100,000 in 1-year-old males (Zimicki et al., 1985). These extraordinary drowning rates are due to the deltaic nature of the country and frequent flooding. Water is in close proximity to many dwellings, and much travel is by water. Although rates are much lower among adults, drownings are still an important cause of death. For example, in women of childbearing age (15–44 years), drowning accounted for about one-third of all deaths from unintentional injuries (Fauveau and Blanchet, 1989). In remote subsistence villages in the mountainous Tari Basin of the highlands of Papua New Guinea during 1971–86, the drowning rate was unusually high among adult males, 17 per 100,000 per year (Barss, 1991), a rate higher than reported among adult males in Bangladesh. Most of the deaths occurred in fast-flowing rivers, where it was necessary to wade across due to a lack of bridges or, in some cases, to use rudimentary suspension bridges. Rates in adult women were much lower, probably because they travel about less than men.

The overall age-adjusted drowning rates for males of all ages in the rural Bangladesh and Papua New Guinea study populations discussed above were 37 and 20 times greater, respectively, than the 1987 rates for Sweden; rates for females were also many times higher (Barss, 1991).

In Jalisco state, Mexico, the highest drowning rates occurred among 1 to 4-year-olds, at 7.6 per 100,000 per year, followed by 15 to 24-year-old males at 5.0 per 100,000 (Celis, 1991); the rates for all ages were 4.2 for males and 1.1 for females. With the exception of toddlers, rates were very low among females. About 75 percent of toddler drownings occurred in bodies of water around the home, including 60 percent in cisterns, and the remainder in tubs, buckets, wells, and swimming pools. In victims 15 years and older, 63 percent had positive blood alcohol tests at autopsy, although the proportion above a specific limit was not specified. Many adult drownings involved lakes, rivers, or reservoirs.

Drowning rates for more developed urban areas of the tropics are lower than in rural areas; nevertheless, even there, drowning is among the leading causes of death from injury. In Singapore, a relatively wealthy urban area, the death rate from drowning was reported to be 2.1 per 100,000 per year for males and 0.4 for females, with most drownings occurring in the 15 to 24-year-old age group and related to falls into open bodies of water (Yip and Paul, 1975; Ng et al., 1978). These rates are similar to national rates in industrialized countries, but somewhat higher than would be expected in relatively low-risk urban areas.

Aboriginal toddlers are greatly overrepresented among drowning victims in Canada (Canadian Red Cross Society, 1994c, Health Canada, 1998). While aboriginals represented only about 3 percent of the Canadian population of 1 to 4-year-olds, they accounted for 22 percent of all toddler drownings in Canada during 1991–1995.

Determinants of Drowning

Personal and environmental factors are important for all drownings, and equipment factors are particularly important for boating drownings.

Personal Factors

Age and sex are important personal risk factors for drowning. Males have higher drowning rates than females at nearly all ages, with the exception of infancy.

In locations with unprotected peridomestic collections of water, young toddlers between the ages of 1 and 4 years are at highest risk, followed by older children and adult males. Children between the ages of 1 and 4 years are able to walk about and fall into unprotected bodies of water, but often lack the judgement to avoid such hazards and the physical capacity and knowledge to rescue themselves. In some communities, older children who travel longer distances from home are at greater risk (Mello-Jorge and Marques, 1985).

Adult males may be at risk because of more frequent exposure to hazards, such as travel by small boats or fording rivers, and sometimes because of ingestion of alcohol.

Certain other subgroups in a society can be at high risk for drowning. For example, in the United States, individuals from low-income families have drowning rates 3–4 times higher than persons from high-income families, although the reverse may be the case for drownings in swimming pools (Baker et al., 1992; Wintemute et al., 1987). In Australia, it was reported that children of lower socioeconomic status were less likely to know how to swim (Nixon and Pearn, 1978). Large family size (Nixon et al., 1979) and reliance on older siblings for supervision of young children (Jensen et al., 1992; Pearn et al., 1979a, 1979b) have also been noted as risk factors for drowning in developed countries; both are common in developing countries and may partially account for the observed association between socioeconomic status and drowning rates.

Epilepsy accounts for about 5 percent of all drownings and up to 45 percent of bathtub drownings in some developed countries (Canadian Red Cross Society, 1996b; Ryan and Dowling, 1993; Quan et al., 1989; Budnick and Ross, 1985; Sonnen, 1980; Pearn et al., 1978). Children 0–19 years of age with epilepsy have been found to be about 100 times more likely to drown in a bathtub and 25 times more likely to drown in a swimming pool than other children (Diekema et al., 1993).

Epilepsy is a relatively common condition that often is untreated in some developing countries. This can leave victims subject to frequent unpredictable seizures. In Cochamba, Argentina, a sample survey showed that 25 of every 1000 adults suffered from epilepsy (PAHO, 1986). Overall prevalence rates for epilepsy in sub-Saharan Africa range from 4–7 per 1000, making it the most common neurological disorder in Africa after infections of the central nervous system (Tekle-Haimanot, 1993). In rural communities in Ethiopia, 85 percent of persons with epilepsy suffered at least one seizure a month due to lack of treatment.

The high prevalence of untreated epilepsy in many developing countries, together with frequent exposure to unprotected bodies of water, suggest that epilepsy associated drownings may be a significant problem. In rural Bangladesh, it was reported that of 18 drownings of women of childbearing age, 9 were caused by falls during epileptic seizures, 6 from other falls into rivers or ponds, and 3 from falls from boats (Fauveau and Blanchet, 1989). In the Tari Basin in the highlands of Papua New Guinea, at least 7 percent (4/60) of drownings between 1971–86 were caused by epilepsy (Barss, 1991).

Alcohol consumption is associated with all types of adult drownings in developed countries and indigenous communities (Canadian Red Cross Society, 1996b; Wintemute et al., 1990; Smith and Kraus, 1988; Pleuckhahn, 1984; Davis and Smith, 1982; Corbin and Fraser, 1981), and alcohol is involved in about 20 to 80 percent of adult drownings. Data from developing countries are scarce; however, since in developing countries drownings are more often associated with activities of daily living than recreation, alcohol may be less important.

In indigenous communities in Canada, alcohol is a factor in one-half of drownings involving boat travel as part of daily life; blood levels tend to be very high, with most ranging from 150 mg% to >300 mg% (Canadian Red Cross Society, 1996b; Health Canada, 1998). Among the Greenland Inuit, it was estimated that at least one-third of drownings were alcohol related (Bjerregaard, 1992). As traditional activities decline and recreational exposures to water increase, the association of alcohol with drownings may increase.

In tropical countries with large tourist industries, tourists who swim after consuming alcohol can be a significant part of the drowning problem. A study in Barbados found that 37 percent of visitors who were victims of near drowning had evidence of alcohol intoxication documented in the medical records (Corbin and Fraser, 1981); however, no blood alcohol testing was conducted to confirm the clinical observations. Whenever possible, alcohol testing should be an integral part of drowning studies; however, samples need to be taken within 24 hours of death to avoid false positives from decomposition of the body (Wintemute et al., 1990).

Equipment Factors

Where water transport-related drownings are common, consideration should be given to the availability and use of safety equipment, such as personal flotation devices (PFDs) or life jackets, and, for large boats, life rafts. In some countries, failure to use a flotation device is strongly associated with drownings in small motorboats and canoes. In Canada, only about 10 percent of victims of boating drownings were wearing a PFD (Canadian Red Cross Society, 1994a, 1996a, 1996b, 1997). Even the most basic equipment is unavailable aboard many vessels in developing countries, and ferries and other passenger boats are often severely overcrowded.

For bodies of water in residential areas, effective barriers are needed, since a wandering toddler can drown when a caretaker's attention is diverted for just a few moments. Fences with self-closing, self-latching gates provide the best automatic protection to protect toddlers.

For snowmobile travel over ice, comfortable snowmobile suits are available that have built-in emergency flotation and hypothermia protection. Special coats and suits are also available for fishers and other boaters who work, hunt, or travel in cold conditions (Collis, 1976). Even regular personal flotation devices provide some protection against hypothermia, since the rapid swimming movements that are required to stay afloat without a PFD greatly increase conductive heat loss to the surrounding cold water. Heavy clothing, even when wet, also protects against heat loss to cold water, especially if covered with an outer waterproof layer (Keatinge, 1965).

Under conditions of reduced visibility, the high speed of modern snowmobiles, together with inadequate lighting, increases the risk of hitting a hole in the ice. Existing snowmobiles are heavy and lack a capacity for emergency flotation to keep riders up out of the water.

Small boats transporting volatile fuels, such as gasoline and propane gas, are subject to massive explosions and loss at sea. Regulations and enforcement are needed to ensure that propane cylinders are always transported on the exterior of the boat to prevent dense gases from accumulating in the bilges, and to prohibit transport of gasoline-filled drums in the passenger areas of small boats, where cigarette or cigar smoking may occur.

Environmental Factors

Residence in a rural area with unprotected peridomestic water and/or with frequent travel by water or ice is a significant risk factor for drowning.

In developed countries, drownings and near drownings among children are particularly common in man-made bodies of water near residential areas, including swimming pools and bathtubs, and to a lesser extent, ponds, ditches, and canals. Among adults, drownings occur during recreational boating or swimming in natural bodies of water such as lakes, rivers, and oceans (Pearn, 1977; Pearn et al., 1976, 1979a, 1979b; Canadian Red Cross Society, 1996a, 1996b, 1997). Wind, waves, and cold water are risk factors in boating drownings on oceans or lakes, while current is a factor in swimming drownings in rivers.

Less is known concerning the specific locations of drownings in developing countries. Unfenced ponds, various containers or cisterns for collecting and storing rain and other water, wells, and irrigation ditches are abundant in many villages, and are a significant environmental hazard for toddlers (Gordon et al., 1962; Thapa, 1984; Thapa, 1990; Celis, 1991). Some ponds are used for feeding cattle and others for raising ducks or fish; most ponds do not have protective barriers and permit many deaths from drowning.

Older children and young adults more often drown in open bodies of water such as rivers, irrigation ditches, and the sea; storm drains and canals are a hazard in some urban areas. The importance of different hazards depends on the local environment; for example, in Singapore, 45 percent of drownings were reported to occur in the sea (Yip and Paul, 1975; Ng et al., 1978).

Throughout the world, the poor are often forced to live in hazardous locations. In developing countries, the housing of poor people is often located on swampland, marshes, or flood plains with many drainage canals and open sewers that present drowning hazards. Dramatic evidence for this is the massive loss of life from heavy floods during several recent cyclones in Bangladesh.

Hypothermia is associated with many drownings in northern communities. Water temperature may also be an important contributor to drownings in mountainous areas of the tropics. Hypothermia can rapidly incapacitate even good swimmers. Hypothermia has caused fatalities after prolonged immersion even in subtropical waters (Keatinge, 1965). However, information is lacking regarding the relative importance of this factor in developing countries.

Water current may also be a factor in drownings from swimming and falls into water in developing countries. Documentation of the type of body of water in such drownings would help to establish the importance of moving water.

Organizational Aspects of Drowning Prevention

In developing countries, careful community surveys can provide baseline data on drowning and help to determine the main activities associated with drowning, together with their associated high-risk groups and determinants. Where coroners investigate most drownings, a more systematic surveillance of the circumstances of drownings could be organized collaboratively by using a standardized data abstraction form to obtain data on personal, environmental, and equipment factors from provincial coroners' reports (Canadian Red Cross Society, 1994c).

Drowning patterns differ in various regions of the world, and policies appropriate for one country or district may not be suitable for another. Until local information is available, it is difficult for governments to develop effective regulations and programs to prevent drowning. Local surveys could be completed inexpensively as a part of other studies, such as a population census. As for traffic injury data, data on drownings would be more useful if surveillance and prevention activities of different organizations involved in aquatic activities and drowning prevention were coordinated. The Ottawa Charter for Health Promotion provides a useful framework for coordinating drowning prevention activities (Canadian Red Cross Society, 1994a, 1994c, 1996a, 1996b).

As a general principle of injury prevention, "passive" protection through modification of the hazardous environment is usually more effective than "active" protection, which requires constant vigilance and action on the part of an individual. For example, studies from Australia, Hawaii, and New Zealand, where the most important environmental drowning hazard for young children is the domestic swimming pool, show that legislation mandating adequate fencing, together with self-closing, self-locking gates, can prevent most drowning deaths among toddlers (Pearn et al., 1980; Milliner et al., 1980; Langley, 1983). Such regulations are often implemented and enforced at a municipal level.

While it is obviously impossible to fence off every body of open water in a developing country, it may be feasible for municipalities to require and enforce the enclosure of wells, cisterns and tanks, small ponds and other bodies of water near residential areas to protect toddlers. Such passive protection may be more difficult to implement for adults, who tend to drown in larger natural bodies of water and in transport-related events. However, if mapping of deaths can show that drownings are particularly common at certain sites, such as

> **User-friendly and drownproofed environments protect toddlers in residential areas of villages and towns.**

Wells, cisterns, duck ponds, garbage pits, construction sites, ditches, storm drains, canals, and other similar bodies of water near residential areas where toddlers are likely to wander or play should be enclosed or covered.

This protects unattended children and other vulnerable individuals, such as intoxicated persons or those with epilepsy. Local materials can be used where resources are limited. Fencing covered with vines can be inexpensive and can even provide vine-grown food. Self-closing and self-latching gates provide automatic protection and are preferred. Closure devices should be durable.

hazardous river-crossings, construction of permanent footbridges could help to prevent deaths at such locations (Barss, 1991). Evaluations of simple interventions are needed, such as the effect on drowning rates of toddlers from enclosing village ponds and wells. However, large populations or long study periods may be needed to detect an effect, except where drowning rates are extremely high.

Overloading of boats is a common problem in developing countries, and boats often traverse hazardous reefs. Regulations must be enforced to prevent overloading, to ensure that durable, inexpensive, and comfortable personal flotation devices are routinely used, and to prohibit unsafe transport of explosive fuels. For northern aboriginal communities, sturdy fishermen's coats and suits and snowmobile suits that provide flotation and protect against hypothermia are available at reasonable cost and should be used during travel over water and ice.

If alcohol is an important local risk factor in drowning, education and legislation are needed to reduce its use and prohibit promotion and sale in association with boating and other aquatic activity and travel by snowmobile. Where epilepsy is an important factor in drownings, education of patients and their families about the risks of solitary activities near unprotected water and of the benefits of regular long-term treatment of seizures should help to protect these high-risk individuals from drownings, as well as from other hazards such as burns and falls.

While passive protection of toddlers is important, all parents need to be made aware of the special vulnerability of this age group, and that near unenclosed water, they must not leave toddlers alone or in the care of other children for even a moment. Where parental supervision cannot be assured because of other responsibilities, communities may need to consider a system of day-care in safe locations.

It was claimed that swimming instruction reduced death by drowning in East Germany (Marcusson et al., 1977). It has been suggested that swimming and water safety instruction should be targeted to high risk groups. However, Robertson (1983) suggests that more detailed studies of the value of swimming instruction are needed, since the ability to swim could potentially increase exposure to hazardous situations. Nevertheless, in villages where people wash and fish almost daily in rivers and the sea, it is difficult to imagine that water survival skills would not be an asset. In countries in northern latitudes, many professional fishermen have never learned to swim and are at high risk of drowning when they fall overboard, especially if they are not wearing a flotation device.

On balance, available information suggests that appropriate instruction of primary school children may be useful in preventing drowning from falls into water and during wading, swimming, and boating activities (Canadian Red Cross Society, 1996a). Instruction should provide practical training in the hazards of river currents and how to escape from them. Swimming instruction is not recommended for children under 3 years of age, the age group at highest risk of drowning (Committee on Accident and Poison Prevention, 1987).

Targeted efforts to train the public in basic resuscitation could be worthwhile, since survival after drowning is often possible if resuscitation is begun immediately at the time of rescue (Pearn, 1978).

Knowledge of even rudimentary resuscitation skills in most countries is largely non-existent and, where it does exist, is probably inadequate. The effectiveness of such training needs to be monitored and costs compared to those required for more permanent passive interventions, such as enclosure of hazards. Such training may best be focused on persons in high-risk environments, such as swimming pool owners or parents of toddlers in rural areas living near unprotected peridomestic bodies of water.

FALLS

Falls are a common cause of severe injuries and hospitalizations, often leave permanent disabilities, and result in many minor injuries. In some countries, falls are also a leading cause of death. While severity is seldom an issue in evaluating the health impact of drownings in developing countries and indigenous communities, it is an important consideration for falls. Severity of injuries from falls is affected by the following:

- Distance fallen;
- Nature of the surface impacted upon;
- Resistance of the victim's tissues, including bones, to damage from the energy of impact;
- Body part(s) that absorbs the energy of impact.

Importance of Falls

Falls rank third, after traffic injuries and drowning, as a cause of fatal unintentional injuries in many of the developing countries that currently provide mortality data to the World Health Organization (Table 9.2). However, in certain rural environments where traffic injuries and drownings are relatively uncommon, falls are the leading cause of mortality from unintentional injury. Among the elderly, falls are generally the main source of injury fatalities.

Falls are also the major cause of hospitalization from injury in most countries, as well as a leading cause of home and minor injuries. If good alignment of fractures is not obtained, or if rehabilitation is poor, victims can be left with permanent deformity and dysfunction of a limb. In indigenous communities in developed countries, falls are uncommon as a cause of death, but rank with motor vehicle injuries as the principal source of hospitalization for injury.

Special Circumstances in Developing Countries and Indigenous Communities

The importance and patterns of falls in any community reflect the environment, buildings and furniture, activities, and age structure of the population.

In some countries for example, building-related falls from unprotected rooftops, windows, and stairs are a common source of injury for children. In lowland areas of tropical countries where tree agriculture is widespread, falls from trees and other tree-related in-

Table 9.2 Age-specific mortality rates per 100,000 population for death by falls, selected countries

| | Sex | Deaths per 100,000 per year | | | | | | | | | year |
		<1	1–4	5–14	15–24	25–54	55–64	65–74	75+	all ages	
AFRICA											
Mauritius	M	0	0	0	0	1	0	5	0	1	1994
	F	0	2	0	0	0	0	0	0	0	
SOUTHEAST ASIA											
China, rural	M	6	5	2	4	8	12	23	61	8	1994
	F	7	4	1	1	2	5	12	56	4	
China, urban	M	2	2	1	1	3	6	21	137	6	1994
	F	1	1	1	1	1	3	16	171	6	
Sri Lanka	M	3	2	2	2	7	17	22	23	6	1986
	F	1	2	1	1	1	1	3	6	1	
Thailand	M	1	0	1	1	6	3	3	4	1	1981
	F	1	0	0	0	1	1	0	2	0	

AMERICAS

Country	Sex										Year
Ecuador	M	3	3	2	7	46	29	46	131	10	1988
	F	2	1	1	1	9	10	14	87	3	
Uruguay	M	0	0	0	1	2	3	7	85	5	1990
	F	0	2	0	0	1	1	6	77	5	
Mexico	M	3	2	1	3	7	17	24	98	6	1993
	F	1	1	1	1	1	4	10	114	3	
COMPARISON											
United States	M	1	1	0	1	2	6	12	66	5	1992
	F	0	0	0	0	1	2	6	57	5	
Sweden	M	0	0	1	1	3	8	19	132	12	1993
	F	0	0	0	0	1	1	11	116	13	
Russian Federation	M	3	2	1	5	13	19	17	27	10	1994
	F	1	2	1	2	2	4	6	22	4	

Sources: World Health Statistics Annual 1990–1992, 1995 (WHO, 1991–1993, 1996).

juries are a leading cause of death, hospitalization, and permanent disability from spinal cord injury. Victims tend to be young adult males.

Many inhabitants of rural parts of developing countries have strong bones as a result of regular weight-bearing exercise from walking (Kelsey and Hochberg, 1992); thus, the severity of injuries sustained in falls may be more a result of the distance fallen from one level to another than of poor bone strength. In developed countries, on the other hand, falls and hip fractures are epidemic among the elderly, especially women. These severe, often fatal, injuries frequently result from a relatively minor fall on the level or from a bed; thus, the severity of injury is a result of weakened bones rather than of the distance fallen.

Classification and Coding of Falls

Major categories of falls pertinent to developing countries include the following:

• Fall from tree;
• Fall from cliff;
• Fall from building, including through window or from roof;
• Fall from stairs or steps;
• Fall from furniture;
• Fall from ladder or scaffolding;
• Jump or dive into water.

Detailed codes to classify falls are available in the Tenth Revision of the International Classification of Diseases. The codes of greatest interest will vary somewhat, depending upon the age structure and activities of the local population and the environment.

Falls occur on the same level, as a trip on a path, or from one level to another, as a fall from a height. Outdoor falls often involve natural structures, such as trees and cliffs, and in northern latitudes, surfaces made slippery by ice and snow. Buildings are another major source of falls. Falls can occur from unprotected heights such as roofs, balconies, and windows. Falls in homes and other buildings often involve internal or external steps and stairs and various types of furniture. Work-related falls often are associated with specific equipment or surfaces. Injuries, other than drowning, sustained when jumping or diving into water are also classified as falls, and include head and cervical spine injuries from striking the head, as well as penetrating internal injuries from branches of sunken trees. Pointed sticks can perforate internal organs, such as intestines.

Because there is a wide range of severity of injuries resulting from falls, it is important to decide upon a definition of fall injuries and disabilities, and to develop a means of comparing the causes of different levels of severity. This may be as simple as distinguishing deaths from hospitalizations, and using the duration of hospitalization or the nature of specific injuries as basic indicators of severity and cost.

In areas where falls from trees are a frequent problem, it would be useful to document the circumstances, for example, that the fall occurred while climbing, as well as the specific activity and species of tree involved. Certain varieties of trees that attain heights exceeding a multistory building may be the source of most deaths and permanent disabilities among adult males, while shorter species may cause extremity fractures among children. Preventive interventions may differ, depending upon the age group of the population at greatest risk and the type of tree involved. Where tree-associated injuries are common, it is useful to tabulate not only falls from trees, but also related injuries from falling trees and branches. However, injuries from falling objects are classified separately by coders who use the International Classification of Diseases.

For falls that occur in the home, documentation should include the structure involved—a rooftop, window, interior stairs, external porch steps, furniture, or ladder. If there are many falls from one of these sources, a more detailed study of the precise nature of the problem may be fruitful.

In a case-control study of several indigenous communities in the United States, it was found that there were many falls associated with a particular design of house in one village (Locklear, 1991). The porch steps had a narrow depth that made people more likely to stumble and fall down the stairs if they placed a foot too far forward while descending the steps. Handrails, porch lighting, and level steps were present more often at homes of uninjured controls than of fall victims and were judged to be protective. Wider stairs appeared to protect against severe injury, by protecting people from a longer fall.

For falls at work, the specific type of equipment involved needs evaluation. Examples include unsafe ladders and scaffolds, as well as slippery or unstable work surfaces.

Data Sources for Falls

Data sources for morbidity are much more important for falls than for drownings. Hospital records are a helpful source, but only if clinical staff cooperate on an ongoing basis by recording a few pertinent details about the cause of the fall. These include how a fall occurred, such as when climbing a tree, and the type of tree (Barss et al., 1984), or the specific site of a fall in a house. When the victim of a fall dies in a health facility, the death is seldom investigated by coroners. Thus, coroners' reports are not a reliable source for assessing death rates from falls. Vital statistics may provide more complete counts, since death certificates are usually completed, at least for victims who die in a hospital. A combination of hospital records and special surveys of rural health centers can establish the approximate burden of mortality from tree falls (Barss et al., 1984—see case study in Chapter 4).

Community surveys with a retrospective recall period can document the incidence and relative importance of minor falls. A much shorter recall period must be used than for mortality interviews; a 2 month period was chosen for an Ethiopian village survey of children's injuries (Demamu, 1991). Permanent disabilities from falls can be documented as part of general community surveys on disability.

Special surveys can be helpful in documenting the circumstances of falls. If it is found from hospitalizations, mortality data, or community surveys that many falls occur in the home environment, it may be necessary to carry out a special survey of injured patients and/or of their homes to determine the specific problems that require correction, such as unprotected windows or rooftops, poorly designed steps and stairs, or hazardous furniture. If a specific hazard is identified and confirmed to be widespread in the community, then a collaborative approach to prevention for the community may be needed, as discussed below.

Examples of Mortality and Morbidity from Falls

Among females in urban China during 1989, falls were the leading cause of death from unintentional injury, and death rates from falls exceeded rates for traffic injuries and drowning (WHO, 1991; see Tables 9.2, 7.3, and 9.1).

Studies from rural hospitals in India, Sri Lanka, and Papua New Guinea have shown that in some areas, falls from trees and tree-related injuries, such as being struck by falling coconuts, are the main cause of hospital admission for trauma, as well as of deaths from head and spinal injuries (Barss et al., 1984; Gee and Sinha, 1982; Moharty et al., 1980; Krishnarajah, 1978; Sambasivan, 1977). Young boys and young adult males are at highest risk. Falls from trees are also the leading cause of spinal cord injury in some parts of Nigeria (Okonkwo, 1988; Ebong, 1978) and in certain other developing countries, including Burma (Toe, 1978). At an urban tertiary hospital in Kathmandu, falls were the leading cause of injuries treated in the casualty department, and the leading cause of admissions and deaths from injuries (Thapa, 1989). Falls accounted for 40 percent of all injuries seen in the casualty department and 46 percent of all admissions for injuries.

An international collaborative study of the incidence of nonfatal injuries in children and adolescents under 20 years of age in Brazil, Chile, Cuba, and Venezuela showed that falls were the leading cause of unintentional injury in all four countries (Bangdiwala et al., 1990b). The study was based upon institutional data from hospitals and on household interviews.

In Mexico, falls from stairways and beds were the main source of falls among children less than 10 years of age presenting to emergency departments in three pediatric hospitals (Híjar-Medina et al., 1992). The main hazards for infants were beds, and for toddlers, patios. The investigators visited homes and observed a lack of protective rails for 48 percent of staircases and 30 percent of cradles. In 44 percent of residences, there was free access to the roof.

In Ethiopia, falls were the second most common unintentional injury reported from hospitals, health centers, and health stations, and were exceeded in number only by animal bites (Larson and Dessie, 1993). Falls were the leading cause of injury among persons over 45 years of age. It was noted that in Ethiopia, many falls result in fractures and are not recorded as falls, resulting in underreporting. Falls were the most common source of hospital outpatient visits for injury among children, and ranked third as a cause of admission for injury (Tekle Wold, 1973; Tamrat, 1981). In a community-based survey in an area of Ethiopia with an 85 percent rural population, falls ranked first as a cause of injury among children of less than 15 years of age, and accounted for about 27 percent of injuries, if foreign bodies were excluded (Demamu, 1991). An injury was counted if there was persistent pain or swelling and/or restriction of activity for more than one day. The incidence of fall injuries was estimated at 128 per 1000 children per year.

In Hong Kong, not really a developing country, falls accounted for more hospital admissions than any other type of injury, with an average of 19,000 hospital discharges per year. This represented 32 percent of all trauma discharges, with an approximate rate of 416 per 100,000 population per year (Kleevens, 1982). The death rate from falls was three times the rate for motor vehicle injuries, which may be partly explained by the height of the buildings and the short network of congested roads.

Determinants of Falls

Personal Factors

Age and sex are significant personal risk factors for falls (Table 9.2). The circumstances of falls vary considerably with these and other personal factors. In many rural subsistence societies, young males are at high risk of injury from falls because of agricultural activities, and, in more developed areas, are often at high risk because of employment in construction. In São Paulo, Brazil, fatal falls of infants were mainly from beds, in 5–9 year-old children, from windows or into wells, and in 10–14 year-old children, from trees or roofs (Mello-Jorge and Marques, 1985).

The importance of alcohol has not been well-established for falls in developing countries, but where alcohol is available, it would be expected to contribute to the risk of falls among certain subgroups of adults, as it does in some developed countries such as Finland (Honkanen et al., 1983). Alcohol intoxication sometimes results in severe falls in indigenous communities, including falls on stairs.

Among the elderly of both sexes, falls are the leading cause of injury morbidity, disability, and death throughout the world. This is probably a reflection of certain risk factors that develop with age, including reductions in bone strength, vision, reaction time, alertness, and mobility. In developed countries, hip fracture has been described as an orthopedic epidemic (Wallace, 1983; Baker et al., 1992) and often results from weakened trabecular bone structure due to osteoporosis and lack of exercise (Prince et al., 1991; Waller, 1985; Cummings et al., 1985). The regular weight-bearing exercise that is a part of daily activities throughout life for most people in developing countries helps to maintain the strength of bone and to prevent hip fractures (Sattin, 1992; Wagner et al., 1992; Buchner et al., 1992; Barss, 1985c; Ford, 1989; Wickham et al., 1989; Beverly et al., 1989; Cummings et al., 1985; Zhang et al., 1992).

Equipment Factors

Tree climbers in developing countries seldom use safety equipment, such as climbing belts or helmets. In many villages, simple forked bamboo poles and other harvesting devices that could eliminate the need for climbing are unknown or unavailable. Pruning shears or saws on long poles can help to keep certain varieties of trees short enough so that fruit can be reached without climbing.

The presence or absence of protective guards or railings can affect the risk of injury from falls from windows, rooftops, stairways, wells, holes in streets, and scaffolding on construction sites.

Each tread should be about
28–30 cm deep to accommo-
date large feet. Risers should be
of uniform height, since an unexpected vertical distance between treads causes falls.

Stairs need to be designed with steps of adequate depth and width
so that the entire length of a large foot fits easily onto the step. In
the case-control study discussed above, it was found that treads av-
eraged nearly 50 cm deep in homes of uninjured controls and less
than 30 cm in homes of injured cases. Good lighting, either natural or artificial, is needed for high-risk areas such as stairs; contrast in colors can also help to highlight critical areas such as the
edges of steps. Where heavy rainfall and mold combine to make
exterior steps slippery, boat deck paint or sand on fresh paint provides a safer surface.

The height and sharp edges of furniture such as beds and coffee
tables can be risk factors, especially in homes with small children or
elderly persons. Playground equipment is an important source of pediatric injuries from falls in developed countries. Unless care is taken
to minimize the distance of a potential fall and to avoid the use of
concrete, rocks, and other hard surfaces, playgrounds can become
sources of injuries both in developing countries and indigenous
communities as new facilities are constructed (see Chapter 10).

Environmental Factors

In rural areas of many developing countries, tree agriculture is often
an important part of the rural subsistence and cash economy. In
some areas, boys climb trees not only to gather fruit, but also to obtain animal fodder (Thapa, 1990). Moderate and severe tree-related
injuries are common, as discussed above. While the height of a tree is
a critical variable, the surface beneath a tree can add to the risk of
climbing if it includes rocks, pointed sticks, or other hazards.

When coconut palms are located close to residences or paths,
falling coconuts pose a significant hazard, since a direct blow to the
head can be fatal (Barss, 1984a). For subsistence cultivators, blows
from falling objects such as trees or branches during slash-and-burn
agriculture or along forest trails can also cause fatalities or severe injuries, as can trees that fall onto village huts during storms or when
struck by lightning (Barss, 1991; Barss et al., 1984).

Falls often reflect the design of dwellings. Falls from rooftops are
common in urban and rural Nepal, because animals live on the
ground floor and people above. Children play and fly kites on flat
rooftops without any protective railings, and many boys suffer head
injuries during falls (Thapa, 1990). Falls also occur from dark steep
stairways without protective railings and from old windows with missing bars.

Poor design and maintenance of streets and drainage ditches
can be an important environmental risk factor for falls. Deep unprotected holes and ditches are often seen in pedestrian areas. Many
pose a serious hazard during the day and are potentially lethal after
dark. Such openings are sometimes a permanent feature of the land-
scape, reflecting poor urban design or management They can be a
result of poor maintenance or a failure to erect protective barriers
for pedestrians during street repairs. In some rural areas, such as villages in the highlands of Papua New Guinea, deep drainage ditches
for agriculture or defense are local hazards (Barss, 1991). For workers, construction sites with trenches or partially constructed buildings often pose significant risks for falls (Masalawala, 1975).

Implications for Prevention

The major causes of falls vary from one country to another, and from cities to rural areas. Falls can be an outdoor problem and can be related to either work or home. Environment, equipment, or host factors may predominate. Public health and clinical surveys can help to clarify local determinants and high-risk groups for falls (Barss et al., 1984).

Potential collaborators and the organizational approach for prevention are determined by local causes, together with community input and involvement. For falls related to tree agriculture, departments of agriculture, plantation owners, equipment manufacturers, tree breeders, individual farmers, and possibly occupational health workers may all need to be involved. For falls in homes and other buildings, architects, furniture designers and manufacturers, contractors, and municipal staff responsible for building codes are possible collaborators. Prevention of falls in formal working environments requires the involvement of occupational safety inspectors, plant owners and managers, engineers, and unions.

Although it obviously is impossible to prevent all injuries due to falls, measures can be taken that greatly reduce both their frequency and severity, especially among high-risk groups. New, shorter, hybrid varieties of tropical trees such as oil palm, mango, and coconut palm have been developed; some of these are more productive than taller varieties, a fact that should speed their adoption (Okonkwo, 1988). Innovative devices on long poles are being used in some areas, such as Fiji and Tahiti, to harvest fruit from tall trees. Appropriate pruning of certain types of trees, such as mango or breadfruit, in combination with simple harvesting devices, can eliminate the need for climbing. Thus, shorter trees allow crops to be harvested from ladders, by machines, or with simple hand-held implements.

Education to deter small boys from climbing the tallest trees might also help, although it would be more effective to eliminate the need to climb trees to harvest fruit or gather leaves for animal fodder. Where climbing is still necessary, harvesting of coconuts can be restricted to specialized occupational groups, as it is in some areas of south India. Climbing equipment, such as the safety belts or helmets used by telephone and electric linemen, should be evaluated for such workers.

Instruction in appropriate methods of felling trees could help to prevent some injuries. Injuries from falling coconuts may be preventable by planting trees away from dwellings and footpaths, removing coconuts in pedestrian areas when they are still green, and requiring that helmets be worn by plantation workers.

Falls into wells or from rooftops, windows, and stairs can be prevented by appropriate design modifications or barriers. In New York City, for example, windows of tall buildings were found to be a major site of fatal falls among young children. After legislation was passed to require installation of window guards by landlords, there was a large decrease in such deaths (Barlow et al., 1983). In some developing countries, the windows of houses have protective bars. These need to be maintained or installed in all areas where children could potentially sustain a severe fall. Where rooftops are used for play or other activities, protective barriers around the periphery are essential. Injuries from collapsing walls of mud houses can be pre-

> **Simple harvesting devices and barriers can prevent many falls from trees and buildings.**

Durable and inexpensive devices, such as cutters and baskets on long poles, are useful for pruning branches to maintain fruit trees at a safe height for harvesting and to replace climbing as a means of gathering the fruit of trees, such as mangoes and breadfruit. Such devices could be developed locally or introduced from other countries where they are already in use. Appropriate education of populations at risk may be useful in conjunction with technical interventions.

Shorter hybrids can sometimes be introduced as substitutes for tall varieties of species such as coconut palms, since trees can reach heights exceeding that of a ten-story building. Because some palms survive for many decades, replacement by hybrids is a long-term solution and alternative short-term measures should also be considered. There is also a problem with falls from other tall trees such as mangoes, breadfruits, and areca palms.

Where falls from rooftops and other residential locations, such as stairways or windows, are common, building codes should require protective barriers to prevent falls. Simple barriers could be developed, tested, and marketed.

vented by better design and reinforced construction. Safer furniture can be designed by rounding edges and corners and avoiding excessive heights for beds without protective rails. Substandard steps should be replaced. Creating and enforcing regulations at construction sites can ensure the appropriate use of scaffolding, ladders, safety harnesses, and other equipment, as well as stable and safe work surfaces.

The importance of weight-bearing exercise in maintaining bone strength among the elderly needs to be emphasized in cultures where regular exercise is being abandoned. For example, an increased incidence of hip fractures in Hong Kong during the past two decades is believed to have resulted from declining activity levels (Lau et al., 1990). As motorization increases, deterioration in host resistance to falls is probable in many developing countries and indigenous communities.

BURNS AND SMOKE INHALATION

Most burns are caused by open flames, hot liquids, or hot surfaces. Fatalities mainly occur in housefires or from clothing fires. Smoke inhalation, rather than burns, is often the cause of deaths in housefires.

Importance of Burns

Burns and smoke inhalation are important causes of injury mortality and morbidity in many developing countries. Burns often rank fourth as a source of mortality after traffic injuries, drownings, and falls (see Table 9.3; compare with Tables 7.3, 9.1, and 9.2). In many northern aboriginal communities in Greenland and North America, housefires are third as a cause of fatal unintentional injury, after drowning and traffic injuries (Bjerregaard, 1992; Muir, 1991). Fires have accounted for as many as 12 percent of all deaths in some communities, with a risk as much as 27 times the risk for non-aboriginals (Jarvis and Boldt, 1982).

Housefires or conflagrations and clothing fires are the most severe and lethal events, but are less frequent than scalds and other mild to moderate burns, which are leading sources of morbidity, especially in communities where open flames are widely used for cooking, heating, and lighting (Thapa, 1990; Courtright et al., 1993). Many nonfatal burns require costly and prolonged hospitalization and skin grafts with a high risk of death from infection and other complications. Burns also frequently result in disfigurement and in severe disability from complications such as scar contractures, which may need surgical correction (Learmonth, 1979; Rao, 1966). Minor burns are among the most common types of household injuries (Thapa, 1989; Demamu, 1991).

Special Circumstances in Developing Countries and Indigenous Communities

In developing countries, open flames are a common feature of many households, especially in rural areas without electrification, and include the following:

- Open hearths on floors of huts used for cooking and warmth;
- Small kerosene and naphtha stoves and lanterns;
- Candles.

Important contributors to the fire risk from these sources are the following:

- Lack of enclosure for open fires and flames;
- Floor-level location of fires and stoves (infants can crawl in, people with epilepsy can fall in, unstable pots can topple onto small children, and long, loose clothing can ignite);
- Instability of candles, small stoves, and lanterns;
- Volatile, highly flammable fuels;
- Flammable housing materials;
- Lack of exits.

An open flame in a flammable hut poses a constant threat of housefire, and many households use either an open fire, a candle, or a lantern nearly 24 hours a day. Infants can crawl into open fires on the floor of huts, and, if they sleep near the fire, their clothing can ignite. Untreated epilepsy is relatively common. A seizure can cause a victim to fall into the fire and suffer severe burns when the victim is alone, or if bystanders flee out of fear. Girls and women often wear loose flammable clothing, which is susceptible to ignition or melting.

Flammable building materials for houses and a lack of emergency exits also contribute to the risk of fatalities in housefires, especially since the smoky interior of a bush hut is often covered in creosote from years of smoke, and, like a chimney fire, burns rapidly once ignited. Volatile fuels can flash up into the face, onto hands, or onto adjacent flammable structures, particularly during lighting. If lanterns are overturned during the night and spill fuel, a flammable hut can be rapidly ignited.

If water is heated in low or unstable positions, it may tip over onto small children causing extensive burns. Less severe burns can result from some of the same sources as those in developed countries, including hot liquids such as coffee, tea, and cooking oils.

Many indigenous communities are in cold northern areas and do not always have electricity because of inaccessibility or lack of funds to pay for it. Housefires can result from candles, various types of heaters with volatile fuels, electrical wiring or appliances, smoking in bed (especially if intoxicated), or sniffing volatile solvents, such as gasoline, near a cigarette (Friesen, 1985).

In developed countries, many housefires are associated with poverty. In the United States, housefires cause over 70 percent of all deaths from burns and fires, and smoke inhalation is the main cause of death (Baker et al., 1992). Smoking and alcohol abuse, particularly in combination, have been found to be the most important factors in housefires, accounting for about one-half of all deaths (Mierley and Baker, 1983; Baker et al., 1992). Cigarettes dropped onto bedding or furniture by intoxicated individuals may smolder and later ignite the fabric. Toxic smoke can kill sleepers before they have a chance to escape, and some are too intoxicated to react. The situation may differ in other countries; the housefire mortality rate in the United States is higher than in many industrialized countries,

Table 9.3 Age-specific mortality rates per 100,000 population for death by fire, selected countries

	Sex	<1	1–4	5–14	15–24	25–54	55–64	65–74	75+	all ages	year
AFRICA											
Mauritius	M	0	0	3	11	3	0	5	0	5	1994
	F	0	2	0	6	4	3	4	32	5	
EASTERN MEDITERRANEAN											
Egypt	M	0	2	2	3	2	2	5	2	2	1987
	F	1	1	2	7	4	3	5	9	4	
SOUTHEAST ASIA											
China, rural	M	1	1	1	1	1	2	5	23	2	1994
	F	1	2	0	1	0	1	4	15	1	
China, urban	M	0	1	0	0	0	1	2	7	1	1994
	F	1	0	0	0	0	1	1	5	1	
Sri Lanka	M	0	1	0	1	2	3	4	8	1	1986
	F	2	1	1	3	3	2	3	8	2	
Thailand	M	1	1	1	1	2	2	1	5	1	1981
	F	2	1	0	0	1	0	1	4	1	

AMERICAS

											Year
Ecuador	M	7	5	1	1	5	2	3	22	2	1988
	F	9	5	1	1	2	1	2	9	1	
Uruguay	M	7	1	0	1	2	5	1	14	2	1990
	F	0	0	0	0	1	1	1	6	1	
Mexico	M	1	1	0	0	0	1	1	4	1	1993
	F	1	1	0	0	0	1	1	4	1	
COMPARISON											
United States	M	2	5	1	1	2	3	4	7	2	1992
	F	2	3	1	1	1	1	2	4	1	
Sweden	M	0	0	1	1	1	2	3	6	1	1993
	F	0	0	0	0	0	1	1	3	1	
Russian Federation	M	3	6	2	3	11	19	16	20	9	1994
	F	3	6	1	1	3	5	7	15	4	

Sources: World Health Statistics Annual 1990–1992, 1995 (WHO, 1991–1993, 1996).

possibly reflecting large pockets of poverty, inexpensive alcohol and cigarettes, hazardous heating equipment, and multi-floor apartment buildings where escape can be difficult.

Classification and Coding of Burns

Burns are classified under several major headings (WHO, 1992):

Exposure to smoke, fire, and flames;
• Contact with heat and hot substances, including hot surfaces;
• Exposure to electric current (electrical burns);
• Exposure to corrosive and caustic chemicals (chemical burns);
• Exposure to forces of nature, such as lightning or sunlight.

For developing countries, important subcategories include:

Exposure to smoke, fire, and flames:
• Uncontrolled fire in a building, such as housefire;
• Controlled fire in a building, such as open fires or fire in a stove;
• Ignition or melting of clothing, both daywear and night clothing;
• Ignition of highly flammable material, such as gasoline or kerosene;

Contact with heat and hot substances:
• Sudden blast of heat from stove;
• Hot drinks and cooking oils;
• Other hot fluids, such as water heated on fire or stove.

There are certain limitations to this classification that should be kept in mind. For example, many uncontrolled housefires originate from an open controlled fire, although these constitute two separate subcategories. Similarly, clothing fires often originate from a controlled open fire. The sequence of causality and the proximate determinants could be lost if categorical groupings are too general. Special tabulations are needed for locally important causes. A common source of housefires in many countries is smoking cigarettes in bed. The importance of this cause could also be overlooked unless there is a special subcategory under housefires for smoking. Separate codes for alcohol intoxication should also be used where appropriate.

The External Cause classification of clothing burns now includes ignition and melting. Many new synthetic fabrics cause severe burns by melting on the skin (Courtright et al., 1993). These fabrics are often widely used in developing countries because of their low cost.

Under hot substances, there is a separate category for tap water burns in ICD 10. This is of particular interest for urban or other areas with hot tap water. Small children, the elderly, and persons with neuropathies can sustain extensive burns, mainly in bathtubs.

Data Sources for Burns

For fatal burns from housefires, special surveys or demographic surveillance by lay reporting and verbal autopsy may be needed to obtain reliable data, if routine reporting is poor. Community surveys can be used to determine the incidence, relative importance, circumstances, and risk groups of mild to moderate burns that do not require hospitalization, and to ascertain the prevalence of disability from sequelae, such as burn scar contractures and disfigurement. In urban areas, more routine sources may be adequate for severe burns; however, the circumstances of burns are not always described, even in university hospitals.

Examples of Mortality and Morbidity from Burns

Mortality rates by age and sex for fires in selected countries with data are shown in Table 9.3. Rates are generally highest between 0–4 years of age and among the elderly. In certain countries, such as Egypt, Mauritius, and Sri Lanka, women of reproductive age (15–49 years) are at high risk. In a study of about 1700 deaths among married women of reproductive age in Menoufia, Egypt, it was found that burns accounted for 9 percent of all deaths in this age group (Saleh et al., 1986).

It was estimated by Gupta (1982) that in India more than 10,000 deaths occur annually from burns, and more than one million people suffer annually from moderate to severe burns. These figures from India correspond to a burn mortality rate of 1.4 per 100,000 per year, and were probably an undercount for all burn and fire deaths, because many victims of housefires never reach a hospital and their injuries go unreported.

In remote subsistence villages of the highlands of Papua New Guinea during 1971–86, mortality rates from fire and flames were several times the reported rates from other countries, about 10 per 100,000 per year for both males and females (Barss, 1991). After age adjustment to the world standard population to allow for the young population structure of Papua New Guinea, the mortality rate was about 15 per 100,000 per year. The highest rates were among those aged 55 and above, followed by young children of 0–4 years. Epilepsy was the most commonly reported personal risk factor other than age. Housefires or conflagrations were the most important cause of burn deaths, followed by falls into open fires. Open fires are maintained on the floors of huts for cooking and for warmth during cold nights in the mountainous villages. Houses are constructed of highly flammable thatched materials; moreover, for security purposes many huts have only a single exit that is barricaded at night and often not located in the sleeping room.

Most of the burn literature in developing countries is based on hospitalized cases, and misses many deaths from house fires. However, burns are a major cause of injury mortality, even among hospitalized patients. In a hospital in Zimbabwe, burns comprised 8 percent of trauma admissions, but 16 percent of trauma deaths (Auchincloss and Grave, 1976).

Burns have also been an important cause of mortality in aboriginal communities in developed countries, although the situation has been improving with changes to less flammable housing materials and safer methods of cooking, heating, and lighting. The standardized mortality ratio during 1981–82 for deaths from fire among aboriginals in the province of Manitoba, Canada was 4.3 when compared to fire deaths among the entire provincial population (Friesen, 1985).

In indigenous communities, open flames from wood stoves, candles, cigarettes, and portable heaters were the most common sources of ignition in fatal housefires, followed by electrical problems from unsafe wiring or appliances. Alcohol was an important co-factor in a majority of cases. Socioeconomic deprivation was felt to be an important underlying determinant in many deaths.

Burns are also an important cause of morbidity. In rural Nepal, burns were found to be the most common injury, after wounds of the skin, in a longitudinal survey done in 1985–86 (Thapa, 1989). In Nepal, 3 percent of the population are estimated to be disabled and 25 percent of all disabilities are caused by injuries; one-fifth of disabilities from injury are due to burns and scalds.

In Ethiopia, burns were the fourth most commonly reported unintentional injury from hospitals, health centers, and health stations, after animal bites, falls, and motor vehicle injuries (Larson and Dessie, 1993). Burns were the leading cause of injury among children under four years of age. Burns were also the leading cause of admission to pediatric hospitals for injury, and ranked third as a source of outpatient visits (Tekle Wold, 1973; Tamrat, 1981). In a rural community survey, burns were the second most common injury to children under 15 years of age, if foreign bodies were excluded (Demamu, 1991). Burns accounted for 17 percent of injuries, and 93 percent occurred inside the home. Open fires are used in a common room in the homes in this district. Using a definition of persistent pain and swelling and/or restriction of activity for one or more days, the incidence of burns was about 80 per 1000 per year among over 2000 randomly sampled children.

In three pediatric hospitals in Mexico, exposure to boiling liquids, most commonly water for bathing, accounted for the majority of emergency room visits for burns among children 0–9 years of age (Híjar-Medina et al., 1992).

Electrical burns sometimes result from improperly grounded appliances and deficiencies in wiring. In Turkey, electrical burns were responsible for 19 percent of burn center admissions (Haberal, 1986).

Determinants of Burns

Personal Factors

In some cultures, females, often both children and adults, are at higher risk of burns because of domestic activities near open flames, and because of clothing styles. In rural Nepal, females were burned more than twice as often as males, and the sex differentials were even greater for adults. This is not always the case, and males can be at higher risk because of involvement with lighting of fires, stoves, and lamps, and because of alcohol abuse. In rural Ethiopia, male children and female adults had the highest incidence of burns (Courtright et al., 1993). In some aboriginal communities in developed countries, males are at higher risk of death in housefires (Friesen, 1985).

Age is also a factor. In cold mountainous areas of Nepal, burns are common among children, since they spend much of their time clustered around open fires to keep warm (Thapa, 1990). In rural Nepal, young children and the elderly are at risk, particularly where open flames are used for cooking or heating. Toddlers are at high risk of scald burns, while older children are at risk of burns while lighting stoves and lamps (Laditan, 1987). Elderly males have substantially higher mortality rates than females in a number of developing and developed countries (Table 9.2). In developed countries, the elderly and demented are at risk of severe scalds from immersion in hot bath water (Katcher, 1981; Baker et al., 1992).

Alcohol abuse and smoking in bed are the leading causes of death from housefire in some developed countries and indigenous communities. Among Canadian Indians in the province of Alberta during 1976, fires were the most common cause of death from unintentional injury, with a death rate 27 times higher than for the remainder of the population; 90 percent of the adult victims were under the influence of alcohol (Jarvis and Boldt, 1982). Similarly, in the province of Manitoba in 1981–82, alcohol was associated with 76 percent of fatalities of Canadian Indians from fire (Friesen, 1985). Investigation of the importance of alcohol and cigarettes in housefires in developing countries is needed to clarify their relative importance.

Epilepsy is a precipitating factor in many severe burns because of the high prevalence of untreated epilepsy. The situation may be further exacerbated by traditional beliefs that epilepsy is associated with evil spirits (Tekle-Haimanot, 1993). In a survey of attitudes in rural Ethiopia, it was found that 45 percent of the people being interviewed believed that the disease was contagious if there was physical contact during an attack (Tekle-Haimanot et al., 1991); this could prevent bystanders from removing the victim from harm during a seizure. In an Ethiopian hospital, epilepsy was responsible for 29 per cent of adult burns that were severe enough to require admission (Courtright et al., 1993). In a population-based village survey, epilepsy was also the most frequently described cause of burns, along

Table 9.4 Most common causes of burns in children and adults as reported* in an Ethiopian village survey

Causes of burns	% reporting
CHILDREN	
Playing	78
Sleeping, sitting for warmth, or left alone	28
Cooking	7
Bringing fire from another house	6
Looking for child's mother	4
Naphtha lantern	3
ADULTS	
Epilepsy	44
Cooking/boiling water for coffee	44
Housefire	26
Sitting for warmth, sleeping	15
Naphtha lantern	12

Source: Courtright et al., 1993.

* Some respondents provided more than one answer.

with cooking and boiling water for coffee, and was noted by 44 percent of respondents. Table 9.4 includes causes of burns among children and adults as reported by adults in Ethiopian villages. There may be some bias towards more severe burns, since these would be more readily recalled.

In remote coastal villages in one province of Papua New Guinea, untreated epilepsy was the second most common cause of hospitalized burns, and accounted for 24 percent of cases (Barss and Wallace, 1983). Severe burns, sometimes requiring amputation of limbs, occurred when persons with epilepsy were left alone near open fires. Cerebral cysticercosis, one cause of epilepsy, presented as an epidemic of burns in West New Guinea following introduction of taeniasis (tapeworm) into the local pig populations (Subianto et al., 1978; Gadjusek, 1978). In rural Bangladesh, severe burns from falls during epileptic seizures caused 0.7 percent of all deaths to women of childbearing age (15–44 years), with a rate of about 2 per 100,000 population per year (Fauveau and Blanchet, 1989).

Although both untreated epilepsy and open fires are less common in developed countries, persons with epilepsy are at special risk (Backstein et al., 1993). Among patients under treatment for epilepsy in Leeds, England, 38 percent were reported to have been burned during a seizure, and the rates of reported burns were four times those of a similar population of diabetics (Hampton et al., 1988).

Peripheral neuropathies are a common complication of leprosy and diabetes; leprosy is the commonest cause of peripheral neuropathies in developing countries (Berhe et al., 1993). Since the ability to feel pain is lost, individuals with neuropathies are more susceptible to trauma, including burns such as scalds from hot water (Katcher, 1981; Katcher and Shapiro, 1987), from handling hot pots, and from sleeping with anesthetic feet near a fire (Backstein et al., 1993).

Personal knowledge of first-aid for burns (especially the immediate application of cool water) and proper treatment thereafter can determine the outcome of burns. Traditional remedies, some harmful and others possibly helpful, are used for burn treatment in Ethiopia, Ghana, and other countries (Courtright et al., 1993; Forjuoh et al., 1994, 1995). They include substances such as cooking oil, eggs, and soil or mud.

It is, therefore, encouraging to find that in Ethiopia, application of cool water was recommended by 80 percent of respondents, and that most villagers recommended that burn victims be taken to a health center or hospital. Although water was not always available, treatment with water was the most frequently used first-aid and had actually been applied to 46 percent of burns, while the next most common treatment was the application of egg. The use of raw egg yolk was felt not to be harmful, perhaps even useful, and was not discouraged. Potentially dangerous remedies such as application of soil or animal dung (with a risk of introducing tetanus into the wound) were recommended more frequently by persons above 40 years of age. Not many people were aware of rolling a person on the ground to extinguish a clothing fire by cutting off oxygen from the flames.

In Ghana, water was applied to 30 percent of burns, including some that subsequently received traditional remedies. Traditional treatments were used more frequently for severe burns than for minor ones.

Equipment Factors

Since the major cause of burns in many developing countries is the use of open flames in the home, the design, location, and use of heating, cooking, and lighting equipment are important considerations.

Portable kerosene and gas stoves were the cause of 63 percent of burn deaths among women of reproductive age in Menoufia, Egypt (Saleh et al., 1986). Exploding kerosene burners caused many severe burns to women in rural Bangladesh (Fauveau and Blanchet, 1989). Kerosene pressure stoves have also been identified as a major cause of burns in Singapore; clothing and other fires were caused when leaking fuel ignited or when a stove sitting on the floor was overturned (Lee, 1982; Sundarason and Kim, 1969).

Kerosene or naphtha lanterns are also a common source of severe burns, and are often kept on unstable surfaces where they can tip over and cause housefires (Courtright et al., 1993; Laditan, 1987). In an Ethiopian survey, 81 percent of lanterns were not on a stable base (Courtright et al., 1993). For similar reasons, the use of open candles and homemade bottle lamps for lighting is also hazardous.

Clothing ignition has been identified as a major cause of mortality on the Indian subcontinent, especially of women with loose flammable saris, which can easily be ignited while cooking near open flames, particularly if the stove is used on a floor where it can ignite long loose garments (Durrani, 1974). Clothing fires were also common and severe among children in Delhi, Pune, Hyderabad, and Bangalore, and their prevention was felt to be a priority (Learmonth, 1979). In Pakistan, 31 percent of hospitalized burns were a result of ignition of clothing. Similar problems have been identified in warm coastal areas of Papua New Guinea due to ignition of grass skirts; grass-skirt burns accounted for 48 percent of hospitalizations for burns from villages in one remote province (Barss and Wallace, 1983). In many areas, adults and children sleep in huts around an open fire; rolling into the fire poses a risk of clothing ignition and of house fires, while infants can crawl in.

In Ethiopia, boiling water for coffee and cooking were reported to be common causes of burns among adults in a village survey (Table 9.4). Among Nigerian children, hot liquids were the cause of two-thirds of hospitalizations for burns (Onuba, 1988).

In developed countries, hot tap water, mainly in bathtubs, is a source of severe burns in small children, the elderly, and persons with neuropathies (Baker et al., 1992; Backstein et al., 1993; Katcher and Shapiro, 1987; Katcher, 1981). The incidence of tap water burns in developing countries is unknown; nevertheless, lowering of tap water temperatures has been advocated for hotels (Forjuoh and Gyebi-Ofosu, 1993). Caution is warranted however, since there have been many deaths from Legionnaires' disease among hotel guests, as well as in hospitals and other institutions in both developed and developing countries. Sporadic community-acquired cases in homes have also occurred (Stout et al., 1992). These pneumonias have often originated from contaminated hot water systems (Barbaree et al., 1993).

Heat-tolerant aquatic pathogens such as legionellae bacteria are unable to proliferate at 60°C in biofilms in plumbing (Rogers et al., 1993; Dennis, 1993; Dennis et al., 1993), but at lower temperatures they can survive, particularly in electric water heaters (Alary and Joly, 1991). Atypical mycobacteria are another group of pathogenic bacteria that proliferate in warm water systems, and some species survive at even higher temperatures than Legionellae (Schulze-Robbecke and Buchholtz, 1992; Schulze-Robbecke et al., 1992; Vess et al., 1993). However, hot water heaters should not be maintained at temperatures above 60°C (Sörensen and Vindenes, 1993). At this temperature, a second degree burn can occur in from two to six seconds (Moritz and Henriques, 1947; Leach et al., 1943–44). At temperatures above 65°C, burning is almost instantaneous.

Fireworks, especially those held in the hand, have been identified as a significant source of burns during the festival of Divali in India (Mohan and Varghese, 1990; Mohan et al., 1984). Fireworks also cause eye injuries (Hatfield, 1970). Homemade bombs were reported to have caused 86 deaths over a 5 year period in Colombo, Sri Lanka (Saravanapavanthan, 1978).

The length of time that cigarettes smolder and the temperature at which they burn are characteristics that greatly influence the likelihood of ignition of mattresses and sofas. These characteristics can be altered by cigarette manufacturers.

Environmental Factors

The majority of deaths due to fire in developed countries result from the inhalation of toxic smoke. Many synthetics used in furniture, drapery, and building materials emit highly toxic fumes when they burn, including carbon monoxide, hydrogen cyanide, and other toxic substances (Guidotti and Clough, 1992; Haponik et al., 1988; Terrill et al., 1978). More information is needed on the incidence of death from smoke inhalation in developing countries. The use of synthetic materials in homes and hotels could pose significant new hazards, which may require legislative changes to control.

Village housing is often constructed with highly flammable materials. A flammable hut with a single exit, together with the almost continuous use of open flames for cooking, heating, and illumination, is a lethal event waiting to happen (Barss, 1991).

Where volatile petroleum-based fuels have recently been introduced for domestic use or in small industries, flash burns are a frequent and serious hazard for the domestic user, and catastrophic fatal explosions can occur with larger quantities in the workplace. Many domestic and some commercial users are completely unfamiliar with the procedures for storing and handling hazardous fuels.

Lightning strikes are a hazard for subsistence farmers in rural communities, who may be exposed in small flammable field huts during storms. The relative importance of this hazard has not been well defined in developing countries, but it is much less common than other causes of burns. Lightning strikes may be more common in mountainous areas of southern Africa with high iron content.

Consider the little mouse, how sagacious an animal it is which never entrusts its life to one hole only.
    —*Titus Maccius Plautus,*
    Truculentus *Act IV, scene iv,*
    254–184 B.C.E.

Implications for Prevention

For the prevention of severe burns and death in housefires, all open flames in homes are prime targets for intervention. Automatic protection could be achieved by enclosing them, by raising them, or by putting a barrier around them. Other interventions include providing a more stable surface, using less hazardous fuels, or switching to a totally different alternative source of heat and light. Untreated epilepsy and hazardous clothing provide two examples of factors that can be dealt with directly and separately, the first by treatment and the second by substitution of safer fabrics or reduction of thin, flowing garments. An alternative strategy for dealing simultaneously with both problems would be to eliminate the usual source of ignition. Either or both of these approaches might be most feasible in a particular situation. To prevent burns from hot liquids, cooking surfaces should be stable and inaccessible to small children.

Clothing burns and housefires can best be controlled by addressing the heat source. Safer stoves should have an immediate impact on the health of women and children by preventing acute burns. Their long-term impact would prevent permanent disabilities and disfigurement from burns, scars, and contractures.

In the Indian subcontinent, high burn death rates among females result from the use of small portable stoves on uneven surfaces where they can overturn, or on the floor where long skirts can catch fire, and where refueling and maintenance are difficult. However, in Bali, where similar kerosene stoves were used on a firm raised surface, only one of 1,214 deaths among women of reproductive age was associated with a cooking stove.

Stove designs that keep heat and flames away from clothing and out of reach of children could help reduce risks associated with cooking. Where petroleum fuels are used, the manufacture of kerosene pressure stoves should be discouraged. They can be replaced by improved designs such as multiple wick stoves, which are safe and efficient.

Where wood, charcoal, dung, or other similar fuels are used for heating and cooking, a change to enclosed stoves made of metal or other materials can improve safety and save on valuable fuel by increasing efficiency. If smoke was channeled directly outside, there could be positive effects on common acute and chronic respiratory illnesses that are exacerbated or caused by smoke (Lancet editorial, 1992d).

Simple enclosed stoves can be constructed inexpensively from local materials. A study in rural Nepal, where burns are the second most common source of injury, showed that a program to introduce low-cost, enclosed, wood-burning stoves known as chulos led to a substantial and significant decrease in the number of burns (Thapa, 1989). It was estimated that 90 percent of hospital admissions for burns of African children could be prevented by measures such as barriers around fires, although data were not provided to substantiate this claim (Auchincloss and Grave, 1976). Where housefires from unstable candles and bottle lamps are a problem, simple stabilizing holders can be made easily and inexpensively. A safe, stable holder is also needed for lanterns. Where feasible, the replacement of kerosene lanterns and other hazardous lamps by electrical lighting or other safer alternatives would help to reduce burns from this source.

Modifications to designs and materials of housing, including regulations to mandate designs that facilitate rapid exit from sleeping quarters, could also help to prevent deaths in housefires. Other interventions used in developed countries to prevent deaths in con-

National policy and simple technical improvements should provide automatic protection of women and children from burns.

Policy initiatives are needed in developing countries to provide safer alternatives to open flames for heating, cooking, and lighting. Where clothing ignition is an important factor, safer materials and/or styles for womens' and childrens' clothing need to be developed. Another consideration in many developing countries is the high prevalence of untreated epilepsy.

Enclosure of flames could prevent many of the most severe burns among persons with seizure disorders or other problems of the central nervous system. An additional consideration is that smoke from open fires is an important source of indoor air pollution and may be associated with acute respiratory infections in children (Lancet, 1992d).

flagrations have included sprinkler systems and smoke detectors (Baker et al., 1992). Smoke detectors can be installed inexpensively in new housing, even in developing countries. For existing homes with smoky interiors, smoke detectors would be best introduced in conjunction with other measures such as enclosed stoves; users will disconnect them if there are many false alarms. Periodic inspections are needed, and batteries may have to be supplied in poor rural areas. Sprinkler systems are especially important in hotels and apartment buildings where it is impossible to exit quickly; they are required in new family homes in some areas of the United States.

Clothing characteristics influence the likelihood of ignition. Flammability is a factor of both fabric and design, including looseness and length. The flammability of fabrics is related to the chemical nature of the fiber or fiber blend; fabric structure, including tightness, thickness, type of surface, or nap; finishing treatment; and the type of garment (Pakkala, 1980). Other factors that affect the severity of clothing burns include ease of ignition of the fabric, ease of flame spread, tendency to shrink and melt, and rate of heat transfer from the fabric to the skin.

Clothing ignition used to be a major cause of burns in girls in the United States (Baker et al., 1992). In 1968, 40 girls and 11 boys aged 5–9 died following clothing ignition, while in 1986 there were no deaths at all in this age group and only three deaths of younger children. The marked improvement was attributed to decreased flammability of fabrics, flammability standards for children's sleepwear, a change from loose, frilly dresses to more close-fitting clothes for girls, and better treatment. However, a change to safer methods of heating may also have contributed to this improvement.

The application of existing knowledge to developing countries, particularly to standards for fabrics and designs for children's or women's clothing, could significantly reduce clothing ignition injuries. Cotton is a common fiber in clothing in developing countries and is quite flammable. The experimental addition of a borax rinse following washing has been shown to reduce the flammability of materials in common use (Durrani and Raza, 1975). However, cheap new synthetic fibers that melt can also cause severe burns.

Better treatment of epilepsy can reduce the incidence of seizures and thus prevent some of the more serious burns among affected individuals (Buchanan, 1972). Persons with epilepsy and their families need to be advised of the danger of leaving a person at risk of seizures alone near an open fire or other hazards. More general education about the nature of the disease is also needed in many countries. The development of effective barriers around open fires or the substitution of enclosed stoves could help to prevent many burns, from seizures even where medications are not always available or are not used.

Most cigarette ignitions of upholstered furniture in the United States could have been prevented at no cost by simple modifications, such as a reduction in the porosity of cigarette paper, lower density of tobacco, smaller circumference of cigarettes, and elimination of chemical additives that make cigarettes burn more rapidly. While less desirable than smoking cessation, such changes could save many lives and much property, since cigarettes with low-porosity paper tend to self extinguish when dropped. The tobacco industry has opposed this change, perhaps because such cigarettes would burn more slowly and decrease total consumption (Ruegg et al., 1987). In indigenous communities where smoking rates are high, this change could be quite helpful in fire prevention. In developing countries, data are needed on the role of cigarettes in housefires to establish the relevance of such interventions.

The sale and use of fireworks needs to be strictly regulated, and in many developed countries fireworks are no longer sold to the general public. In the United States, states that do not restrict the sale of fireworks have fireworks-related injury rates seven times the rates in states that do (Berger et al., 1985; Harris et al., 1983).

The immediate application of cool water to burns in order to lower skin temperature and reduce the severity of the burn is a simple measure that can be used when water is available. It was reported that among 68 burn victims who applied cool water immediately after a burn, only one required a skin graft, compared with 4 of 36 who did not (Mathews and Radakrishnan, 1987). The use of cool water to treat burns from fireworks has been promoted successfully in India (Mohan and Varghese, 1990). Knowledge about first-aid is appealing to many people and may be more acceptable and easier to teach in the short-term than more fundamental changes to their environment and equipment. First-aid offers a means of capturing peoples' interest; they can simultaneously be provided with information about primary and secondary prevention.

chapter 10

Unintentional Injuries: Poisonings, Bites, and Other Injuries

This chapter considers acute poisonings, wounds and envenoma-tions from land and marine animals and insects, cutting and penetrating wounds, eye injuries, and various other injuries.

POISONING

Acute poisonings are classified with injuries as external causes of death or illness. Chronic poisonings by substances such as lead are also an important public health problem in developing and developed countries (Guthrie, 1988). Chronic diseases, including cancers, caused by drugs such as tobacco/nicotine and alcohol are the leading cause of premature death among adults in many countries. However, in spite of their obvious importance, it is beyond the scope of this publication to consider such chronic poisonings. This section will discuss the major groups of agents of acute unintentional poisonings. Agents that are frequently used for suicide are noted, but this topic is discussed in greater detail in a later chapter.

Importance of Poisoning

As a source of unintentional injuries, poisonings rank after traffic injuries, drownings, falls, and burns, and in some areas, animal bites. In Ethiopia during 1990–91, poisoning ranked sixth after the above causes in frequency of reports from hospitals, health centers, and health stations (Larson and Dessie, 1993). However, among young children, poisoning often ranks higher as a cause of hospital admission for injury. In many indigenous communities in North America, deaths and brain damage among adolescents from abusive inhalation of solvents such as gasoline are a major concern.

The relative importance of different specific poisons will depend upon the data source that is used for reporting, since the agents that cause the most deaths and hospitalizations are not necessarily the most commonly ingested. The latter may result in a greater service load with more outpatient visits or calls for advice but with less morbidity and mortality.

Special Circumstances in Developing Countries and Indigenous Communities

Although there are few studies of deaths by poisoning in developing countries, there appear to be marked differences between developed and developing countries in the causes and age distributions of victims of poisonings. In developing countries, there tends to be greater involvement of children in fatal poisonings.

Many poisonings result from chemical products or byproducts that have been recently introduced into the culture and that become widespread before people are knowledgeable of the hazards. Kerosene is widely used for small stoves and lanterns, and pesticides are widespread in rural agricultural communities. These substances are often sold in unlabeled bottles, and even if there are labels, they may be in a foreign language or unintelligible to illiterate subsistence farmers. Similarly, many people are unaware of the lethality of carbon monoxide from heaters and small generators.

Inhabitants of developing countries are also exposed to toxins and poisons in food plants, ornamental plants, and seafood. If commercial seed grain is eaten in time of famine, poisoning results from added chemicals.

Pesticides are widely used in developing countries for agriculture and for control of insect vectors of diseases such as malaria. Some pesticides cause acute paralysis that can be fatal, and their use requires appropriate equipment and handling. In Sri Lanka, there were over 1,000 deaths reported from pesticide poisoning in 1978, compared to only 572 deaths from polio, diphtheria, tetanus, and whooping cough combined, while no deaths were reported from malaria (Jeyaratam et al., 1982). More recently, pesticide poisoning was reported to be the main cause of death among young adults of both sexes aged 15–24 years; however, most of these deaths were suicides (Berger, 1988).

Pharmaceuticals and drugs are increasingly widespread, and potentially toxic drugs are available in some countries without a prescription. In many rural cultures, methods of suicide, such as hanging, are being abandoned in favor of poisoning with drugs or new chemical products.

A study in South Africa of all hospital outpatient and inpatient visits for poisonings found marked differences between blacks and whites in the patterns of poisonings (Joubert, 1982). Poisonings among whites showed a typical developed country pattern, with a bimodal age distribution among children and adults, a predominance in females (especially in adults), a high incidence of poisoning by drugs, and more intentional than unintentional poisonings. Blacks, on the other hand, showed the pattern of poisoning typical in most developing countries, with the majority of cases occurring in children, a slight excess in males, and the vast majority (87 percent) being unintentional. The major causes in hospital patients differed from those in fatalities (Table 10.1).

In developed countries, unintentional fatal poisonings often involve illegal drugs such as cocaine and heroin, and the victims are

Table 10.1 Causes of poisonings among South African blacks, including deaths and hospital outpatient and inpatient cases

Cause of poisoning	% of hospital cases	% of deaths
Kerosene	56	10
Drugs	10	2
Carbon monoxide	8	29
Household products	6	0
Organophosphate insecticides	4	18
Corrosives	0	9
Metals	0	9
Herbal medicines	*	16
Other/unknown	16	7
Total	100	100

Source: Joubert, 1982.

*Hospital cases of poisonings from herbal medicine included in other/unknown category.

usually adults (Baker et al., 1992). Death rates from poisoning are several times higher among the poorest quintile of the population compared to the richest; the poor/rich difference was found to be about five times for men and three times for women in Canada (Wilkins et al., 1989). There are also many suicides and suicide attempts from overdoses of prescription drugs. Young children are frequent victims of non-fatal poisonings from various substances in the household. Children are often poisoned by medications, but smaller containers and childproof containers have helped to reduce fatalities. Ingestion of corrosive alkalis in the form of household cleaning products causes esophageal burns and is a frequent source of hospital admission in some countries.

Classification and Coding of Poisonings

Poisonings can be grouped into three broad categories, including:

- Poisonings from pharmaceutical agents/drugs;
- Poisonings from chemicals and toxic gases;
- Poisonings from naturally occurring plants and toxins.

These major groupings include a number of subcategories in the Tenth Revision of the International Classification of Diseases (WHO, 1992). Medications involve many subcategories. For non-medications, some of the most important for developing countries include:

- Poisoning by organic solvents and their vapors, especially petroleum derivatives like kerosene;
- Poisoning by pesticides, including insecticides and herbicides;
- Poisoning by alcohols, including methanol and ethanol;
- Poisoning by corrosives and caustics, particularly alkalis;
- Poisoning by gases and vapors, including carbon monoxide;

• Poisoning from toxin-containing natural substances ingested as food, including plants such as mushrooms and cassava, and fish and shellfish.

Like injuries, poisonings are classified using one group of codes to describe the external cause of injury and a second set to describe the nature of injury. For poisonings the Nature of Injury codes describe more precisely the specific agent involved than the External Cause codes. The Nature of Injury or Product codes for poisonings are more similar to their corresponding External Cause codes than for other types of injuries.

In all poisonings, intent will affect classification. Because many suicides involve poisoning and since it is often difficult to distinguish unintentional from intentional poisonings, there are special categories for poisonings where the intent is unknown. Intentional poisonings are coded under suicides, and occasionally as homicides.

While ingestion of corrosives and caustics can cause burns of the mouth, throat, and esophagus and are classified as poisonings, skin burns can also result from these chemicals. The latter are coded separately under rubrics for burns and may be overlooked, unless they are verified under the appropriate code.

The classification of poisonings from medications is somewhat more complex. In the case of poisoning with pharmaceuticals, it is necessary to distinguish unintentional iatrogenic poisoning as a result of treatment errors, such as an incorrect dose, the wrong medication, or misuse of a drug, from adverse side-effects related to properties of the medication or the host, such as an allergic reaction. Adverse side-effects are classified separately under adverse effects of treatment.

Multiple substances, such as alcohol and drugs, may have been ingested, and the relative importance of different substances must be taken into account in assigning causality. This can pose considerable problems in classifying deaths of drug addicts or suicides, and poisonings from pharmaceuticals.

Data Sources for Acute Poisonings

The public health burden of mortality and severe morbidity from poisonings can be assessed by counting deaths and hospitalizations from different categories of agents, while the clinical burden of poisonings can be measured by data from outpatient visits, and, where there is a poison control center, by calls for advice. It is important to consider different sources of information, since otherwise prevention campaigns run the danger of emphasizing nuisance poisonings, while overlooking and failing to take action on the most dangerous poisons. Poison control centers often are not informed of fatal poisonings.

Specific Poisons

Pharmaceuticals

The difference between a therapeutic dose and a toxic or fatal dose is small for some medications, and the potential for acute poisoning is high with self-medication or inappropriate prescribing by health practitioners. With rural development and increased availability of many drugs, it is believed that poisoning from drugs has increased, although there is a lack of detailed information.

Several studies have identified the problem of inadvertent poisoning through use of prescribed medications. In Afghanistan, the most common unintentional poisoning was overdosage by excessive medication (Choudhry et al., 1987). The inappropriate use of drugs was an important problem; 17 percent of drug poisonings were due to the antipsychotic drug chlorpromazine, which for some reason was used to control vomiting in children.

Chloroquine, an antimalarial drug, is also a significant cause of fatal poisoning in some areas. Poisonings by ingestion are confined largely to adult suicides, with few childhood deaths, probably because of its intense bitter taste. In a study of 33 chloroquine deaths in Papua New Guinea, the youngest case reported was aged 16 years (Sengupta et al., 1986). However, when given to children by injection, dosage errors have resulted in fatalities.

Patterns of poisoning from drugs differ from many developed countries, where most unintentional poisonings involve adult addicts. In the United States, adults account for 99 percent of the 13,000 deaths from poisoning that occur each year, including suicide by poisoning (Baker et al., 1992).

Petroleum Products

Kerosene ingestion is one of the most common causes of poisoning among children in many developing countries (Thapa, 1990). In India and various parts of Africa, kerosene was found to be the most common agent of poisoning among children under the age of 5 years (Baldachin and Malmed, 1964; Bwibo, 1969; Gaind et al., 1977; Banerjee and Bhattachariya, 1978). In a pediatric hospital in Tanzania, poisonings were the leading cause of admissions for injuries, and kerosene was the most common agent of such poisonings (Kimati, 1977).

In India, it has been recommended that kerosene be made unpalatable by bittering agents, and perhaps also dyed blue to distinguish it from water (Mohan, 1986a). Otherwise, a thirsty child may drink kerosene that has been stored in containers such as soft-drink or beer bottles, mistaking it for soda or water; kerosene poisonings have been reported to be most frequent during the hottest months of the year (Baldachin and Malmud, 1964). In Korea, to prevent the use of soft drink bottles for kerosene, it can be sold only in distinctive green containers.

Toxic Products of Combustion

Unintentional carbon monoxide poisoning is a problem in virtually all regions of the world. Since carbon monoxide is a colorless, odorless gas, tragedies can occur when people use heaters in enclosed rooms or try to stay warm in vehicles. Fatalities have also occurred from gasoline generators when villagers slept in a room with the engine running.

Carbon monoxide is the most frequent specific agent implicated in deaths from poisoning in developed countries such as the United States, and, excluding smoke inhalation in housefires, motor vehicle exhaust is the leading source of carbon monoxide poisoning (Baker et al., 1992). In some developing countries, however, sources of poisoning by carbon monoxide differ. In Seoul, Korea, the use of coal or charcoal to heat poorly ventilated homes resulted in 252 deaths in one year, which was more than three times the number of reported deaths from communicable diseases and more than all deaths from motor vehicle injuries (Lee et al., 1971). Many deaths still occur because of leaks in heating systems that circulate hot air laden with carbon monoxide under floors.

In Singapore, 30 percent of suicides were due to victims putting their heads into gas ovens (Chao, 1971), while occupational poisonings were responsible for most other deaths from carbon monoxide (Seah and Chao, 1975). Suicides and unintentional poisonings by stove gas have now been eliminated in many countries; this was achieved by replacing coal gas, which has high carbon monoxide levels, with other gases such as natural gas or propane (Seiden, 1977; Kreitman and Platt, 1984). The change was made for profit rather than prevention (Lester and Abe, 1992). A similar fortuitous improvement in suicides from carbon monoxide has been observed with the introduction of the catalytic converter to reduce air pollution from automobiles (Clarke and Lester, 1987).

Alcohols

Acute methanol poisoning can result in blindness or death. Methylated spirits are widely available in rural communities, where they are sold for purposes such as preheating of kerosene stoves and lanterns.

Contaminated liquor has been responsible for large numbers of deaths. In India, more than 200 persons died in New Delhi after drinking liquor mixed with methanol during the Hindu festival of Deepawali during November 1991 (Lingam, 1992). The following month about 30 persons died from the same cause in Rajkot in the state of Gujarat. At a New Year's celebration in Bombay, 90 poisonings with 60 fatalities resulted from the consumption of contaminated liquor. Contaminants in traditional alcoholic beverages are also a problem in Tanzania (Nikander et al., 1991).

Large "outbreaks" of methanol poisoning have followed social gatherings where methanol is served as cheap alcohol (Naraqi, 1979). In the Middle East, 25 cases of acute methanol poisoning occurred following the introduction of a new methanol-containing eau de cologne (Hammoudeh and Snounou, 1988). Fatal acute poisoning from uncontaminated ethanol also occurs in countries where concentrated spirits are consumed rapidly for their intoxicating effect. Some deaths occur from aspiration of vomitus.

Pesticides

Poisoning from pesticides, including insecticides, herbicides, rodenticides, and fungicides, is a major problem in many developing countries, with rates far exceeding those in developed countries (Jeyaratam et al., 1982, 1987; Berger, 1988; WHO, 1984a, 1986, 1986a; Mowbrey, 1986). The World Health Organization estimated that there were over 10,000 deaths worldwide from unintentional and occupational pesticide poisonings during the 1970s, but a more recent study of excess mortality in the Philippines alone suggests that there may be an excess mortality of "many tens of thousands" from pesticide use (Loevinsohn, 1987). People have been poisoned by occupational exposures during mixing and handling, by exposure of villagers during spray operations, by consumption of contaminated food or grain, and by ingestion of improperly stored liquid formulations (Igbedioh, 1991).

While most pesticide poisonings are due to suicides and to occupational exposures, unintentional poisonings, especially from the organophosphate insecticides, are also a serious problem among subsistence cultivators and their families. Occupational poisonings from pesticides are discussed in more detail in Chapter 11.

Organophosphates have replaced organochlorines such as DDT. Organophosphates are less toxic to the environment since they do not bioaccumulate; however, acute toxicity is high and their use demands better equipment and much more skilled handling.

Nonfatal poisonings often go unrecognized. A study in Nicaragua showed that during peak agricultural activities up to 40 percent of the workers at risk had significantly depressed serum cholinesterase activity, an indicator of organophosphate poisoning (Cole et al., 1988). In the same study, rates of pesticide poisoning requiring medical attention were 75 per 100,000 population per year; in rural areas the rate was 165 per 100,000. The mortality rate was 1.2 per 100,000 per year.

The herbicide paraquat has been recognized as particularly hazardous; ingestion of a small amount (>15 ml) is almost uniformly fatal (Crome, 1986). About 1300 deaths per year, many of them suicides, were reported from paraquat poisoning each year in Japan (Crome, 1986; WHO, 1984a). In Papua New Guinea, there have been a number of deaths among children who have ingested paraquat stored in soft drink bottles and subsequent to the use of paraquat for the treatment of head lice (Bull, 1982; Davies et al., 1982; Binns, 1976).

The total number of deaths from paraquat in developing countries is unknown; however, the toll is believed to be considerable because of poor handling procedures and the many illiterate users who are unable to read warning labels. Regulations that mandate better labeling, addition of an emetic and stenchant (a bad-smelling additive), and restricted availability of the concentrated form of the chemical, were said to have "lessened the chances" of paraquat poisoning in Papua New Guinea (Mowbrey, 1986); however, no data were provided to support this assertion.

Another pesticide that has been reported to be a major means of suicide in India is the insecticide aluminum phosphide (Joshi, 1991). A single tablet that costs about ten cents is said to be potent enough to kill 10 people. This agent has often been used by poverty-stricken farmers and their families and also by young women. In a hospital in Rohtak, near New Delhi, 418 patients with poisoning from aluminum phosphide were admitted during a 7 year period, with 286 deaths. Suicide by this method was reported to exceed other forms of poisoning in Haryana state, a farming region surrounding New Delhi. Aluminum phosphide was supposed to be sold only to government granaries, agriculture departments, and approved pest controllers, but was frequently sold to the public by unauthorized retailers.

There have also been a number of reports of mass poisonings

following the use of grain contaminated by pesticides and other chemicals such as mercury (W.J. Hayes, 1980; WHO, 1976). A study from India also suggested a correlation between the intensity of pesticide use and the prevalence of permanent disabilities such as blindness and limb deformities (Mohan, 1987a).

Plants

Poisonings from various plants occur in endemic and epidemic forms in many developing countries. Such plants include those used for food and for other purposes such as herbal medicines.

Several epidemics of food poisoning from acute and chronic cyanide toxicity have been documented in Africa as a result of improper preparation of cassava. This root crop is widely used as a food source, especially during times of famine when epidemics of poisoning can occur. In some cases, this has left victims disabled by paralysis from nerve damage (Ministry of Health, Mozambique, 1984).

A spastic paraparesis results from damage by cyanide to upper motor neurons. The toxic effects of cyanide are exacerbated by the low sulfur content of a diet based almost entirely on cassava. The paralysis is permanent and in Africa is known as *konzo*. *Konzo* has been described from Mozambique, Tanzania, and Zaire (Tylleskär et al., 1992).

In order to remove cyanogens from cassava flour, it must be soaked in water for about three days. Storage of flour also reduces toxicity by gradual hydrolysis of cyanohydrins and volatilization of hydrogen cyanide. Cases of *konzo* appeared in Bandundu, Zaire, after construction of a new road. Cassava became an important cash crop and soaking time was often reduced from three days to one. Outbreaks of *konzo* also occur when rapid population growth and declining agricultural yields result in the use of high-yielding bitter cassava as a staple food. The use of traditional processing methods or simple adjustments to new methods can prevent cyanide poisoning from cassava (Tylleskär et al., 1992)

Plants that contain pyrrolizidine alkaloids occur throughout the world and have resulted in many deaths from acute hepatotoxicity (WHO, 1988b). Chronic disability and death also occur as a result of hepatic venous occlusion. Outbreaks have resulted when cereal grains such as wheat and millet were contaminated with fragments of alkaloid-containing plants. Among the many outbreaks was one in Afghanistan where 8,000 persons were afflicted with veno-occlusive disease, with many deaths. Outbreaks are most likely to occur in areas where there are food shortages and during droughts when certain weeds infest grain crops.

The other main source of alkaloid poisonings has been herbal medicines such as infusions; however, cases may occur sporadically after treatments and the cause may not be recognized. Many cases have been documented, but because of poor reporting, no rates are available.

Where wild mushrooms are collected as a food source, mushroom poisoning can result. For example, in a population of about 30,000 villagers in remote villages in the highlands of Papua New Guinea during 1971–86, 15 deaths from poisoning were reported by community surveillance (Barss, 1991). Of these poisonings, 9 had resulted from ingestion of poisonous mushrooms, 3 from acute ethanol intoxication, 1 from ingestion of cassava, and 1 from carbon monoxide.

Although chronic poisonings are somewhat beyond the usual scope of injury control, subacute poisoning from heavy ingestion of grass peas can occur after as little as one month and deserves at least a brief mention. Lathyrism is a crippling motor paralysis caused by a neurotoxic amino acid in these legumes. It is endemic in India, Bangladesh, and Ethiopia, affecting many productive young villagers. Among peasants in some Ethiopian villages with soil unsuitable for other crops, the annual incidence is 0.6 percent and the prevalence is as high as 3 percent (Haimanot et al., 1993). As for cassava, soaking and discarding excess water after boiling reduces toxicity. Other preventive measures include the development of varieties that contain less of the neurotoxic amino acid as well as the supply of alternative foods during famines.

Marine Biotoxins

Another source of poisonings in coastal areas is the consumption of seafood containing biotoxins. Paralytic poisoning results from saxitoxin in shellfish and tetrodotoxin in puffer fish, while ciguatera is caused by ciguatoxin (WHO, 1984b).

It was reported by the World Health Organization that as of 1971, about 1600 cases of paralytic shellfish poisoning had been reported, mainly from developed countries. The pattern changed during the last two decades, with more cases being reported from developing countries. For example, 201 cases were reported from Malaysia in 1977, with 4 deaths from clams; 171 cases were reported from Venezuela, with 10 deaths from mussels. It is probable that many cases go unreported in rural areas, but as surveillance improves, there may be an apparent increase in the number of cases.

The incidence of ciguatera poisoning from consumption of ciguatoxic fish ranges from 1–50 cases per 10,000 population in different islands of Micronesia and Polynesia, and has been estimated to be as high as 300 per 10,000 on the Virgin Islands. It has been suggested that there may be an association between the observed increases in ciguatera poisoning and the following: French nuclear testing in Polynesian atolls, development projects that disrupt the marine environment, and dietary and cultural changes due to urbanization (ND Lewis, 1986).

Other Poisons

The incidence of poisoning from toxic cooking oils in developing countries is unknown, but the possibility should be kept in mind in view of the 800 deaths and 20,000 poisonings reported from denatured rapeseed oil in Spain in 1991 (WHO, 1992a).

Implications for Prevention

In planning strategies to control poisoning in a developing country, information is needed about the most important local causes of poisoning, since the situation may differ substantially in different locations. A consideration of factors involved in some of the poisonings discussed above may be helpful.

In developed countries, there has been a marked decline in poisoning deaths among young children in recent decades. This is attributed in large part to childproof packaging of medications, decreased use of kerosene for heating (as it is replaced by electricity), and the development of regional poison control centers that provide rapid advice by telephone (Baker et al., 1992).

Similar decreases in acute poisoning have not occurred in developing countries. There should be immediate application of already existing preventive strategies, such as proper storage and labeling for toxic substances and medications. Childproof containers are needed not only for medications, as in developed countries, but also for household supplies of kerosene, insecticides, herbicides, and caustics. Hazardous products should be stored out of sight and reach of children. Special consideration should be given to modifying the taste and color of kerosene, as well as its containers and storage practices.

Legislation is needed to restrict the sale of especially hazardous substances, such as paraquat, to persons with adequate training. Restrictions are needed on the sale of methanol, and the public should be educated regarding its highly toxic effects. Physicians must be better informed and more restricted in prescribing certain toxic medications. Other innovative solutions may be required as more local data become available regarding specific agents and risk factors for poisonings.

Prevention of solvent poisoning among adolescents poses a greater challenge, since gasoline is ubiquitous. However, parents must know and identify all solvents and keep them in locked storage. At the same time, the underlying community and family disturbances and external pressures that are at the root of solvent abuse must be addressed.

Integrated pest management using biological and cultural measures has been successfully developed in Cuba (Igbedioh, 1991). This is a highly desirable method of primary prevention of injuries, since the need to purchase, store, and use large quantities of toxic pesticides is reduced. However, in many cases, pesticides were still necessary; this was addressed through regulations governing storage and worker exposure to pesticides. A training program in safe handling of pesticides for vendors and in integrated pest management for farmers has been developed in Sri Lanka (Cormier, 1993). Further program development is needed to address the use of agricultural pesticides for suicide.

The identification of toxic food plants by multidisciplinary research is needed. Where such plants are an important food source, the development of simple processing methods that reduce toxicity to acceptable levels is feasible, as demonstrated in Africa for cassava (Tylleskär et al., 1992). It may be possible to prevent some poisonings from plants by educating the public about the toxic effects of cassava, mushrooms, other plants, and certain herbal medicines. Simple field tests are now available to test for pyrrolizidine alkaloids in plant materials; more careful screening of herbal medicines is also needed.

In developed countries, regional or provincial poison control centers accessible by telephone to public and health professionals have allowed for a concentration of clinical and toxicological expertise regarding acute poisonings. In countries where telephones are

> **Restricted sales, packaging, and labeling of toxic chemicals help to prevent lethal poisonings.**

Extremely toxic herbicides, such as paraquat, or insecticides, such as the organophosphates, should never be sold to illiterate farmers in unlabeled soft-drink bottles. Locally intelligible visual labels should be required for all toxic chemicals, including those imported from other countries. Where toxic substances are essential to the local economy, they should, whenever feasible, be sold to the public only in diluted forms and/or packaged in small amounts to reduce the likelihood of death from ingestion.

Other common sources of poisonings include cheap intoxicating alcohols and solvents, carbon monoxide gas, toxic medications, and plants. Medications and hazardous household products, such as caustic alkalies, should be sold only in childproof containers.

widely available, such centers can help to ensure the most efficient use of limited resources and can actually save money by providing advice directly to the public, thereby eliminating unnecessary visits to hospital emergency departments or health providers (Sanfaçon and Blais, 1991; Mathieu-Nolf and Furon, 1990; Buzik and Hindmarsh, 1987). In low-income countries with more limited telephone access for most of the public, such centers could be operated on a national basis to provide specialized advice to health providers rather than directly to the public.

BITES, WOUNDS, AND ENVENOMATIONS FROM LAND AND MARINE ANIMALS AND INSECTS

Animal bites can cause severe physical damage, internal injuries, infection, and rabies. Many snakes, arthropods, and certain marine species injure by envenomation with local effects such as severe pain, tissue necrosis, and infection, or systemic effects such as paralysis or hemorrhage (Nishioka et al., 1993b; Nishioka & Silveira, 1992a, 1992b; Auerbach, 1991; Barss, 1984b).

The types of injuries seen in an area are often predictable based on the prevailing environment and activities and customs of the people. In a survey of rural health centers in the Ivory Coast, where the incidence of animal bites was 11 per 1,000 population per year, dog bites predominated in the north of the country, and snake bites in the south (LeBras et al., 1982).

Importance of Bites and Envenomations

Injuries from animals are an important public health problem in many developing countries. However, the burden of mortality and morbidity from this source is not well documented and the relative importance of injuries from animals is therefore unknown in many countries. This is probably because, with the possible exception of dog bites, such injuries tend to occur in rural areas where reporting is poor.

Nevertheless, in Ethiopia, where packs of wild dogs roam the country, animal bites were the most frequent unintentional injury reported through routine Ministry of Health data from hospitals, health centers, and health stations during 1990–91 (Larson and Dessie, 1993). The ages most affected were 5–44 years, and about 60 percent of victims were males. However, in a rural community study of injuries in Ethiopian children 0–14 years of age, animal and insect bites accounted for only about 6 percent of injuries (Demamu, 1991). People may seek medical attention more often for animal bites than for other injuries, particularly if rabies is feared in the area.

In some rural areas, animals such as cattle, water buffalo, pigs, and camels cause severe injuries, while needlefish, stingrays, and crocodiles are hazards in coastal zones. Envenomation from bites can cause death or disability. Bites and stings from arthropods, including insects and arachnids, can initiate skin infections and ulcers, as well as cause envenomation. Severe infection or tetanus can complicate open wounds.

Special Circumstances in Developing Countries and Indigenous Communities

Dogs often run loose in developing countries and many indigenous communities. Resources are often lacking for impoundment and sterilization or destruction of stray dogs, and many owners do not take responsibility for restraining their animals. In China, the government took a stand against private ownership of dogs, and legislation was firmly enforced by destruction of animals (Wong, 1994a). While this approach may appear draconian to westerners, the alternatives are also unpalatable. In densely populated urban neighborhoods, dogs can create problems of injury and fear, infection, poor hygiene, and intolerable incessant rounds of barking and wailing throughout the night.

Rabies vaccine is expensive and often unavailable for many dog owners, and sometimes even for human victims of bites. The modern diploid cell vaccines that are used in developed countries are unavailable in most developing countries because of cost. As a result, neural tissue vaccines, which cost about 30–100 times less, are used, with an incidence of neurological complications ranging from about 0.8 to 8.0 per 1000 (Petricciani, 1993). Because fear of reactions to the injections and the high number required (up to 24), many people who are bitten by potentially rabid animals avoid being vaccinated.

Rural agriculture and fishing expose people to various animal and marine bites and envenomations and can attract venomous snakes. Rats can be a plague in houses (Cummins, 1988) and in leprosy wards in hospitals, where they sometimes consume the anesthetic toes of sleeping patients. Biting insects cause innumerable tiny wounds that frequently become infected, while stinging insects cause envenomations individually or in swarms, either of which can be fatal.

Children are sometimes placed in charge of herds of large animals. Travel on bush trails for gardening or other purposes can lead to encounters with animals or snakes, especially after dark or in long grass.

In developed countries, dogs are generally kept enclosed by regulation. When they are in the streets, they must be restrained on a leash. Immunization for rabies is mandatory and many health departments have special programs for rabies control that deal with dogs and human bites, and often employ veterinarians. There are more resources for enforcement, and unrestrained dogs are impounded and can be destroyed.

Classification of Bites and Envenomations

The two principal ICD 10 categories with pertinent subcategories for classification of bites and envenomations include:

Physical injuries:

- Bitten by dog;
- Bitten by rat;
- Bitten or struck by other mammals, such as cattle, pigs (feral and domestic), camels, water buffalo, and others;
- Bitten by non-venomous insects or other arthropods;
- Contact with marine animals such as needlefish, sharks, and others;
- Bitten or struck by crocodiles or alligators.

Injury Prevention

Envenomations:

- Venomous snakes and lizards;
- Hornets, wasps, and bees;
- Centipedes and venomous millipedes;
- Scorpions;
- Spiders;
- Venomous marine animals and plants such as stingrays, stonefish, fire corals, and jellyfish, among others.

Data Sources for Bites and Envenomations

Brief questionnaire surveys of senior staff at a broad sample of rural health centers and/or hospitals can provide an inexpensive estimate of the relative impact and circumstances of different bites and envenomations.

With the exception of particularly common injuries, such as dog bites, where emergency room records could be useful, reviews of hospital records to retrieve data on severe injuries can require several years of data review and is laborious. Surgeons sometimes record brief histories of severe injuries from animals and other sources in operating theater logs of surgical procedures.

In urban areas with rabies immunization and response programs, records may be maintained of animal bites, and these could provide estimates for the minimum incidence of bites, particularly from dogs.

In Thailand, the distribution and varieties of venomous snakes responsible for bites was mapped by a national study that involved collecting and identifying the dead snakes brought with victims to district and provincial hospitals (Viravan et al., 1992). The species were correlated with the patients' symptoms and signs, such as neurotoxicity with paralysis, incoagulable blood, and local necrosis. Of 1,631 snakes collected at 80 hospitals in 67 provinces, 1,145 were venomous. Species identification is important in Thailand, where antivenin is monovalent.

Specific Bites and Envenomations

Dog Bites

Cave canem (Beware of the dog).

—Latin proverb

Dog bites and rabies are a common threat in many rural villages in developing countries. Dogs are also an important cause of morbidity in many northern aboriginal communities, and fatalities have been reported among the Greenland Inuit and Alaskans (Dalton et al., 1988; Bjerregaard, 1992). Children are the most frequent victims and sometimes are bitten on the head. Complications such as infection and prolonged psychological stress are common.

The attack rate from dogs among Alaskan aboriginals during 1979 was reported to be 680 per 100,000 population per year, but in Barrow, where there was a special reporting system for dog bites, the rate was 1,490 per 100,000 per year during 1982–86. These rates were substantially higher than for most areas of the United States. The proximity of houses appeared to be a factor in bites. Dog bites were most frequent during summer months, perhaps because people were outside more often and wearing less heavy clothing.

The widespread custom of keeping dogs as pets, and the presence of large numbers of uncontrolled stray dogs in poor countries and northern communities appear to be the most important sources of injuries from animals in many countries (Thapa, 1990). In an urban tertiary hospital in Kathmandu, Nepal, animal and insect bites were the fifth most common injury (6 percent of all injuries) seen at the casualty department during a 1 month survey in 1987; 69 percent (63/91) of these were dog bites (Thapa, 1989). In Nigeria, one hospital reported that over 1 percent of casualty department attendances were for dog bites (Kale, 1977).

Rabies

Although wounds from dog bites can result in many problems if they become infected, the most serious potential complication of dog bites is rabies (Warrell and Warrell, 1988). Rabies, a fatal disease caused by a virus that affects the nervous system, is widespread among dog populations in developing countries because of a lack of resources for vaccines, ignorance, and large populations of wild stray dogs.

Rabies is endemic in dogs in much of the developing world. Adequate immunization of dogs and post-exposure immunization and treatment of dog bite victims in rural, and even urban, areas is a tremendous administrative and economic burden and is essentially impossible for many developing countries.

Both rural and urban areas are affected; however, in many developing countries rabies is sustained by urban dog-to-dog transmission and appears to be a growing problem in crowded urban slums where there is close contact between a reservoir of plentiful stray dogs and the human population. However, in developed countries rabies tends to be maintained in wildlife reservoirs (Acha and Arambulo, 1985)

It is reported that of the total estimated and reported human deaths from rabies, 99.9 percent were in the tropics, but only 89.4 percent of post-exposure treatments were given to persons in the tropics (Acha and Arambulo, 1985). Of the total known animal rabies cases in the world, 47 percent occurred in the tropics, where 76 percent involved dogs in urban areas (Figure 10.1). Although 53 percent of reported cases of rabies in animals occurred in Europe and North America, only 0.01 percent of human cases occurred there, while Asia, with 17 percent of reported animal cases, had 98 percent of human cases.

Mortality and Morbidity from Rabies

The greatest human rabies problem today is in the Indian subcontinent (Steele, 1988). There were 25,000 reported human cases in India in 1985, but the actual total was estimated to be 50,000 cases. Rabies was responsible for 1 of every 2000 admissions in a survey of 41 university hospitals. Each year, 700,000 persons had to undergo a series of anti-rabies immunizations at tremendous public expense (Petricciani, 1993; Sehgal, 1992); 96 percent were due to dog bites. About 75 percent of victims were males, and 40 percent of all cases were children less than 14 years of age. Dog bites caused 98 percent of human rabies cases. More than one-third of victims never received any immunization or treatment, and the remainder had received either ineffective modes of treatment or incomplete regimens.

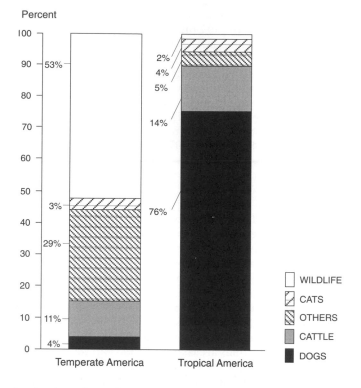

Figure 10.1

Proportion of rabies cases in animals in temperate and tropical americas
Source: *Rabies in the Tropics.* E. Kuweert et al. (eds.) Acha PN, Arambulo PV. Rabies in the tropics—history and current status. p. 349, Fig. 7. Copyright 1985, Springer-Verlag. Reprinted with permission.

In the Americas, the countries of Brazil, Colombia, Ecuador, El Salvador, Mexico, and Peru together accounted for 84 percent of all reported cases of rabies in the region (PAHO, 1986). In Brazil, there was a range of 87 to 190 reported human cases of rabies per year from 1970–84, while in Mexico there were 55 to 83 cases per year. Children 1–4 years of age accounted for 11 percent of cases, and children from 5–14 years for 47 percent. In Latin America, 90 percent of human rabies cases resulted from dog bites.

Epidemics of bovine and human rabies caused by vampire bats occur in several countries in the Americas, from northern Mexico to southern Argentina (Lopez et al., 1992). Between 1989–90, 177 human cases of bat-associated rabies were reported in the Americas, including 27 in Brazil (PAHO, 1991). Attacks of humans by bats have been associated with environmental changes or reductions in other species, such as pigs and cattle; bats then attack people as an alternative food source (McCarthy, 1989).

An outbreak of human rabies was caused by the bites of vampire bats in 1990 in the Amazonian rain forest in Peru. The population affected were Aguarunas Indians living in remote villages, and most bites were to the head. The 29 deaths among 636 residents represented a loss of 5 percent of the local population. Deaths were most common among children 5–14 years of age. Recommended preventive measures included the use of soap and water to vigorously cleanse bat bites, together with physical barriers to prevent bat bites, including bat-proofing of houses and use of mosquito nets to keep bats out.

Attacks by vampire bats have also been reported from a Brazilian village (Batista-da-Costa et al., 1993). Villagers were bitten while asleep, mainly on the toes. It was believed that bats began to reside near humans after changes in their natural habitat. Another explanation was that the use of pyrethrins to control an insect pest of cattle may have repelled the bats from the animals, inducing them to seek an alternative food source.

In a WHO survey that attempted to document the incidence of rabies in 30 developing countries, India had the largest number of reported human cases, with 20,000 in 1979, followed by Ethiopia with 412; the highest incidence of cases was in India with 29 cases per million population, followed by Ethiopia with 13 (Bogel and Motschwiller, 1986). The lowest reported incidence among the 30 countries was for South Africa, with 0.1 cases per million population in 1979. In Ethiopia, 98 percent of over 60,000 persons who required anti-rabies treatment had been bitten by dogs, mainly in towns (Kloos and Zein, 1993; Makonnen, 1982).

Such differences among countries may reflect the efficacy of programs for control of rabies in animals and elimination of stray dogs, the thoroughness of wound treatment after animal bites, the availability and use of effective rabies vaccine and globulin, and variability in the completeness of reporting.

Injuries from Other Animals

Injuries from other animals are less general in their distribution, but are important in many areas. Bites and the injuries inflicted by animals are relatively common agricultural injuries in India (Qadeer and Mohan, 1988). The literature includes reports of goring by cattle in India (Tanga and Kawathekar, 1973), by water buffalo in Kampuchea (Tournier-Lasserve et al., 1982), and by feral and domestic pigs in Melanesia (Barss and Ennis, 1988) and Brazil (Nishioka et al., 1994), but no rates are available.

Some breeds of cattle that are common in Africa, India, and elsewhere have long pointed horns that can inflict deep penetrating injuries of viscera or limbs. In rural areas, many of the injured are cattle attendants. Animals may step on a foot or toes, or may suddenly run, causing the securing rope or chain to tighten around hands and fingers.

Many injuries from pigs in Melanesia occur during hunting of feral pigs or attempts to capture or move domestic pigs (Barss and Ennis, 1988). In Brazil, injuries from pigs are related to capture, transport, and immobilization for slaughter (Nishioka et al., 1994).

In desert areas of Africa and India where camels are used for domestic and agricultural purposes, they are reported to cause severe penetrating wounds and compound fractures from bites with their large teeth. Camels can also cause severe internal injuries and injuries of the limbs by kicking, trampling, or lifting and throwing persons. In Bikaner, Rajasthan, India, 153 patients injured by camels were admitted to the orthopedic wards of a single hospital during the 4 year period 1976–79; all of the injuries occurred during the rutting season, when male camels can become violent and difficult to handle (Saxena et al., 1982). Nine cases were described from Sokoto, Nigeria; it was recommended that camels should be handled only by experienced personnel (Tahzib, 1984).

A snake lurks in the grass.
—*Virgil*, **Eclogues**, *III,*
70–19 B.C.E.

Snakebites

Snakebite is often overlooked as an important cause of death in many countries, and has been described by one authority as "the most neglected area of tropical medicine" (Warrell, 1987, 1990). This is attributed to the fact that the majority of bites occur in rural areas remote from hospitals and are, therefore, never reported in national statistics.

It has been estimated that almost 10,000 deaths from snakebite occur annually in the savanna regions of Nigeria, and about 23,000 in all of West Africa. In northern Nigeria over one percent of all deaths were estimated to be due to snake bites (Pugh and Theakston, 1980). Among the Waorani Indians in Ecuador, almost 5 percent of all deaths were attributed to snake bites (Theakston et al., 1981). About 20,000 snake bites per year were reported to the Brazilian Ministry of Health, and in southern Brazil the incidence was about 24 per 100,000 per year (Nishioka and Silveira, 1992b; Silveira and Nishioka, 1992a, 1992b). The true number of cases was believed to be higher. The case fatality rate ranged from 0.6 to 0.9 percent of victims. Snakebite is also reported to be an important cause of death in Burma and other countries of southeast Asia (Warrell, 1990).

In rural areas of many developing countries, such as in rice-growing areas, farmers are frequently bitten on the feet when walking home from their fields in the dark, although certain species are also reported to enter huts and bite people while they sleep (Warrell, 1990). In Brazil, the male to female ratio of victims was 5:1 and was attributed to occupational exposure (Silveira and Nishioka, 1992b). A 5 year-old Brazilian child who was bitten in the eye by a viper while asleep required enucleation of her eye (Brandão et al., 1993).

In rural Bangladesh, snakebite was the fourth most common cause of death from unintentional injury among women of child-bearing age (15–44 years) between 1976–86, and accounted for 20 percent of all unintentional injury deaths and 0.9 percent of all deaths in this group, with a death rate of 2 per 100,000 per year (Fauveau and Blanchet, 1989). Gardening, fetching water and firewood, and going into the bush to defecate, especially at night, were activities commonly associated with bites in Bangladeshi villages. Unfortunately, antivenins were unavailable at rural health centers.

Human disturbances of the natural environment often create favorable conditions for snakes in close proximity to humans. In agricultural regions of central Brazil, constructions of hydroelectric dams have created lakes, which are surrounded by rodents and armadillo burrows. This habitat provides water, food, and shelter for venomous snakes (Nishioka and Silveira, 1992a).

Antivenin can be highly effective in reducing mortality from snakebite. In Thailand, the Thai Red Cross Society has been producing antivenins since the 1920s. The number of reported fatalities from snakebite declined from over 200 per year in the 1940s to less than 20 per year in the 1980s, even though there were at least several hundred venomous bites per year (Viravan et al., 1992).

It is important that victims of snakebite be transported rapidly to a health facility where antivenin can be administered immediately, if signs and symptoms of envenomation develop. However, since antivenins occasionally cause severe or fatal anaphylactic reactions, they should not be used for non-venomous bites if there is no clinical evidence of envenomation. If the snake is available and is clearly a non-venomous species, this may also be helpful. In a hospital in São Paulo, Brazil, about 40 percent of snake bites involved non-venomous species (Silveira and Nishioka, 1992b), while 18 percent of victims admitted to hospital in Uberlandia had been bitten by non-venomous snakes.

Delays in communications, transport, and administration of antivenin greatly increase the risk of complications and death. In Brazil, the risk of renal failure from rhabdomyolysis and of tissue abscesses from venom of South American rattlesnakes and lance-headed vipers was significantly increased with delays in treatment, and also with increasing age of the victims over 40 years old (Silveira and Nishioka, 1992b; Nishioka and Silveira, 1992a).

Many rural inhabitants still use tourniquets following snakebite. Prolonged constriction has resulted in limb loss. It is much safer to immobilize the bitten limb and apply a firm but non-constrictive pressure dressing with a cloth pad and elastic bandage, if available, (Auerbach, 1991).

Marine Injuries

Although sharks are often thought to be a hazard in developing countries, injuries are rare. Injuries inflicted by needlefish (Barss, 1982, 1985a) and stingrays (Barss, 1984a) are a problem in some areas and can result in death, visceral injury, gangrene, and severe disability.

Most villagers attacked by crocodiles disappear without a trace and their deaths are never reported. While many species of alligators and crocodiles are relatively harmless to humans, two species of crocodile are particularly ferocious and often attack humans (Pooley et al., 1989). The Nile crocodile, widely distributed throughout Africa, weighs up to 1000 kilograms and reaches 6.5 meters in length. Indopacific crocodiles grow to be 7 meters long. In a village in Irian Jaya, 62 villagers were reported to have been killed by a single rogue crocodile. If these crocodiles have successfully taken humans from a particular location, they return repeatedly and lie in wait hoping for another meal. In Papua New Guinea, villagers have been dragged away after dark by salt-water crocodiles while sleeping under huts near a beach or while defecating at a riverside. Fishing among mangrove roots, swimming, and paddling small canoes can also be hazardous in certain locations.

Many fish, molluscs, jellyfish, and other marine creatures have venoms for protection or for immobilizing prey (Auerbach, 1991). These venoms can seriously injure and occasionally kill humans. Stingrays and stonefish are a source of many of these injuries.

Stingrays have venom in the tail barb that causes severe tissue necrosis (Barss, 1984b). Most injuries occur when a stingray is stepped on by a wader, and involve the lower limb. Some cases are severe enough to necessitate amputation, particularly if surgical debridement is delayed. Thoracic wounds involving the heart or lungs have caused myocardial rupture or pneumothorax. Stonefish have venom in small sacs on barbs; venom is injected into the foot by the pressure of the foot on the sacs.

Neurotoxic envenomations from other species are relatively

It has been related that dogs drink at the river Nile running along, that they may not be seized by the crocodiles.
—Phaedrus, **Fables,** *Bk I, Fable 25, 8 C.E.*

rare, but can be fatal. Cone shells inject a venom to paralyze fish as prey; this can cause respiratory paralysis in humans who pick up these beautiful shells in their hand. The venom of sea snakes and the blue ringed octopus can also cause respiratory paralysis.

My father hath chastised you with whips, but I will chastise you with scorpions.
—Old Testament, 1 Kings, 12:11

Insects and Arachnids

Bites and stings from arthropods, including insects and arachnids, are well recognized as entry points for many tropical diseases such as malaria. The importance of tiny wounds from insects as foci for initiation of various skin infections such as cellulitis, tropical ulcers, pyodermas and other more severe infections has been suggested (Manson-Bahr and Bell, 1987), but better documentation of their relative importance would be useful.

Scorpion stings are said to be more important than snakebite in large areas of the world, including Mexico, Trinidad, North Africa, and parts of Brazil. A 1979 study in southern Libya reported 900 scorpion stings and an incidence of at least 7 deaths per 100,000 population per year (Warrell, 1987). The deaths were mainly of small children under the age of 2. In Mexico, there are between one and two thousand deaths from scorpion sting per year, with an incidence of mortality ranging from 3 to 84 per 100,000 per year in various states (Warrell, 1987). In Brazil, about 3800 scorpion stings are reported each year (Nishioka et al., 1993a; Nishioka et al., 1992). The toxic effects of wasp and other hymenoptera stings are moderately well documented (Barss, 1989), but the incidence of envenomations or fatal allergic reactions from these and other arthropods is unknown.

Spiders are another source of bites and envenomations. In Brazil, 1863 cases were reported in 1988, but this number is believed to be low, since there were 680 cases at one hospital in São Paulo that year (Ribeiro et al., 1990). In São Paulo, 515 wolf spider bites were reported in a single epidemiological study. While some spider bites result in tissue necrosis from local envenomation, most wolf spider bites were relatively minor injuries of the hands and feet. Many were previously misdiagnosed as due to the more toxic brown recluse spider.

Implications for Prevention

Many developing countries need assistance in developing effective public health programs to deal with dog bites and prevention of rabies. Legislation, enforcement, and availability and promotion of neutering programs are needed to control excessive numbers of domestic and stray dogs. Unclaimed strays should be destroyed. Legislation and enforcement are also necessary to ensure immunization of all dogs. Assistance with purchase, storage, and possibly manufacture of modern rabies vaccine and immune globulin is needed so that these products can be made available to governments at affordable prices. While modern veterinary vaccines produced in cell lines are widely used for animals in developing countries, humans have been condemned to receive the far more hazardous neural vaccines (Petricciani, 1993). Modern vaccines can apparently be produced at very low cost. Their availability to developing countries would spare hundreds of thousands of individuals the need to undergo a prolonged course of hazardous immunization with obsolete products.

It has been suggested that in many populations the most cost-effective approach may be to concentrate on human post-exposure vaccination with or without passive immunization, but that in some situations elimination of the reservoir by canine vaccination may be considered (Bogel and Motschwiller, 1986; Cifuentes, 1988; Belotto, 1988; Wandeler et al., 1988). In Chile, house-to-house canine vaccination is carried out by special teams. In many cities and states of Brazil, one-day mass vaccination campaigns, using army, police, and health workers, have virtually eliminated rabies. In China, dogs have been largely eliminated by special government teams.

To effectively implement programs, educational campaigns directed at the general public are necessary. In many communities, simple epidemiologic studies are needed to define the extent of the problem, so that public support for programs can be generated. In some countries, religious beliefs hinder the elimination of stray dogs.

Information about the true incidence of serious injuries due to animals such as cattle and pigs, on the age and sex groups of victims, and other details may help in prevention. Blunting or capping of horns, using safer breeds, and avoiding use of young boys as herders could help to prevent injuries from cattle; however, such measures need to be evaluated. The more widespread use of suitable footwear could help to reduce the severity of toe injuries from cattle; however, more comfortable shoes for tropical conditions need to be designed. Melanesian pig hunters who carry only one spear or use an inadequate number of dogs appear to be at increased risk of severe injury from pig goring (Barss and Ennis, 1988), while in Brazil and elsewhere, safer methods for capturing and immobilizing pigs for transport may be needed.

Since proximity of snake populations to people is often increased by human modification of the environment, ecologic studies of the conditions under which snake bites occur are indicated. This could help to determine ways in which food storage and the local habitat could be altered to discourage snakes from residing near homes and to reduce their numbers. Improved rodent-proof storage facilities, for example, may help to control both rodents and snakes, while also reducing food wastage. Keeping the edges of paths clear in grassy areas and using lights when walking at night might also reduce the incidence of snakebite. Appropriate footwear could also help; it is said that the use of rubber boots by fish farmers in Thailand has reduced the incidence of cobra bites (Warrell, 1990). Adequate supplies of effective antivenins at rural health centers, staff trained to use them, and a rural public educated to seek help would prevent many deaths; however, the costs may be prohibitive for many countries. Rapid transport of snake bite victims to hospital before signs of envenomation develop should improve the outcome of treatment.

A better understanding of the ecology and biology of various marine creatures may prevent some injuries. Surveillance and careful study of the circumstances of specific types of injuries can be helpful in developing preventive interventions. Prompt recognition of the potentially serious nature of certain injuries, such as those resulting from needlefish and stingrays, together with resuscitation and rapid transfer for basic surgical treatment, may help to reduce mortality and disability. Shark attacks at large public swimming beaches near tropical cities have been greatly reduced by the use of hanging nets. The vibration of the nets attracts sharks which become entangled and suffocate. The training of lifeguards in resuscitation and hemostasis has saved a number of persons attacked by sharks in South Africa (J.A.M.White, 1975). In Australia, areas that pose a significant risk for attack by salt-water crocodiles are posted with warning signs. It is important that simple methods of first-aid be more widely publicized, since rural populations are often unfamiliar with even the most basic measures. For example, the use of plenty of soap and water to clean and irrigate dog bites reduces the risk of infection and rabies, but even this simple first-aid is rare in some countries. Periodic prophylactic immunization against tetanus is also an important preventive measure for all types of wounds, since fatalities can result from tiny wounds that go untreated. Washing small wounds and insect bites with plenty of water and covering them to keep flies off helps prevent infection.

Basic first-aid can be quite effective in the early management of many marine envenomations. Soaking an injured extremity in hot water is simple and effective for envenomations from stingrays, stonefish, and other venomous fish, since the heat destroys the venom (Auerbach, 1991). Vinegar is the best first-aid for jellyfish and coral stings, since the mild acid neutralizes the venom-containing nematocysts. A limb bitten or stung by a cone shell, blue-ringed octopus, or sea snake should be immobilized and a pressure bandage applied (not a tourniquet) to slow the spread of venom while the patient is transported; patients may require respiratory support if neurotoxic paralysis develops.

SKIN WOUNDS, PENETRATING WOUNDS AND INJURIES FROM CUTTING TOOLS

Superficial skin wounds, cutting and piercing wounds, and injuries from cutting tools and small machines are a major source of morbidity and disability in developing countries, and much greater attention is needed to both research and prevention. While the injuries in preceding sections have been organized by external cause, this topic indicates the nature of injury. These injuries are considered by both nature and external cause, since classification by external cause is poorly developed. Crushing injuries are much less common, but become more prominent as loading equipment and powered machinery are introduced.

Importance of Cutting and Piercing Wounds

In developing countries, wounds of the skin are generally the most common cause of morbidity from injuries, and are among the leading causes of morbidity from all diseases and injuries. When treatment is inadequate or delayed, severe morbidity, permanent disability, or death frequently result. Death can occur from hemorrhage, septicemia, or tetanus or from malignant transformation of chronic ulcers, giving rise to squamous cell carcinoma.

Data are limited on such injuries since their external cause is seldom specified and coded in official reporting. In addition, many minor skin wounds become infected and treatment is sought only when the wound is already infected; the case is then frequently reported as an infection rather than as an injury.

Special Circumstances in Developing Countries and Indigenous Communities

Cutting tools such as knives, axes, and machetes are common possessions in most tropical villages. The machete, also known as the panga or bush knife, is inexpensive and ubiquitous. While the great utility of this simple device is undeniable, severe and disabling injuries result from its use both as a multipurpose tool and as an offensive weapon.

Laccrations from machetes are frequently deep and may sever multiple tendons, nerves, vessels and even bone, especially in injuries to the palm of the hand. Such wounds often receive inadequate surgical treatment or none at all, leaving victims permanently disabled. Other modes of injury include running and falling onto unsheathed knives; such impalements can result in deep thoracic and abdominal wounds. When the machete is used as a digging tool, the hand can slip down onto the blade since there is usually no safety guard between handle and blade. Other tools, such as long grass knives, can also result in severe injuries, such as lacerations of the achilles tendon, if users work barefoot with no protection for the ankles.

Small children are often left alone playing with sharp pointed knives, spears, or sticks. Penetrating wounds of the eye or the hand may result in blindness or other disability.

The development of powered machinery for use on small farms in countries such as India has increased the potential for severe hand injury. Many machines have no protective guards.

Although the serious damage from dramatic injuries caused by tools and machinery is obvious, smaller wounds occur much more frequently and may cause surprisingly severe complications. These wounds include punctures from insect bites, as well as small cuts, punctures, and abrasions from grass, sticks, bushes, stones, and glass. Since many people walk barefoot, injuries of the feet and lower legs are common. Foreign bodies such as pieces of wood or dirt are often implanted in penetrating wounds. Unless the wound is opened, debrided, and irrigated, such foreign bodies can cause severe acute wound infections, or chronic disability by festering for months or even years.

In areas where flies, tropical heat, dirt, and sweat are common, small wounds can rapidly become septic or develop into large tropical ulcers (Manson-Bahr and Bell, 1987). Sepsis can be life threatening, while more indolent infections of soft tissues can cause permanent damage of important structures such as tendons; destruction or scarring of such vital structures in the hand can cause permanent disability. Even small skin wounds can result in tetanus, if the affected individual has not been immunized.

If tropical ulcers are neglected, they may become chronic and fester for many years. Malignant skin cancers eventually develop in many chronic tropical ulcers. Such cancers frequently require amputation of a leg and sometimes cause death by metastatic spread (Foster and Webb, 1988).

Classification and Coding

The classification of cutting and piercing wounds by external cause is less well developed than for most other categories of injury, probably because, although they are frequent causes of morbidity, the International Classification of Diseases was initially developed to classify mortality. Thus, the classifications of leading causes of mortality are more highly organized.

There is a need to analyze all cutting, piercing, and crushing wounds in developing countries and to organize a practical classification system for external causes. In addition, skin infections need to be reviewed to determine the distribution of underlying causes, including the relative importance of different types of injuries. Similar work is needed for disabilities from these wounds.

The Nomesco classification systems, developed for coding hospitalizations in Europe and the Arctic, provide much greater detail than the ICD (Nordic Medico-Statistical Committee, 1990, 1993), although they are not adapted for tropical developing countries. However, the mechanism of injury, the implement involved, the environment, and the sector and type of activity appear to be useful general categories in the Nomesco classifications. Thus, an injury can be classified as follows:

Mechanism of injury:

- Cutting;
- Piercing;
- Crushing.

Equipment:

- Cutting hand tool, such as machete, small knife, axe, or grass knife;
- Powered tool such as a fodder cutter, sugar cane crusher, or electric saw;
- Pointed object such as a stick, spear, or pointed knife;
- Bites and stings;
- Lifting equipment such as loaders for logs and boxes, and other machines that can crush.

Environment:

- Home;
- Garden;
- Workplace;
- Other.

Activity:

- Daily living, such as pierced by branch while walking through bush, cut with knife while preparing meal, cut with machete while trimming hedge, injury while playing with pointed object;
- Subsistence agriculture;
- Remunerated employment by specific sector, such as cutting sugar cane on a plantation, construction, logging.

Data Sources for Cutting, Piercing, and Crushing Wounds

Until better classification systems for cutting, piercing, and crushing injuries are developed, standard data sources for mortality and morbidity are not very useful. Potential sources of data may include special surveys of communities, emergency rooms, hospitalizations, and operating room logs. Surveys will need to be done prospectively and data collection and classification tailored to the leading external causes in the location and population being studied.

Examples of Morbidity

In an 18-month household survey in rural Nepal, the most common injury was a wound to the skin surface such wounds accounted for 67 percent of all injuries, deep cuts added another 7 percent, and puncture wounds, 3 percent (Thapa, 1989). Thus, in this rural population, various types of skin wounds accounted for over three-quarters of all injuries. Wounds to the skin surface were also the most common injuries to workers in all occupations, with an average of 1.5 injuries per laborer and 0.8 per skilled laborer during the 18-month study period. The rates were high in both sexes, with only a slight excess in males.

At the Mulago teaching hospital in Kampala, Uganda, 56 percent (48/68) of soft tissue injuries resulted from assault, and more than half were inflicted with a machete (DeSouza, 1968). In northern Indian villages, injuries from hand tools were found to be the most frequent cause of minor agricultural injuries. The majority of serious injuries resulted from mechanized equipment such as fodder cutting machines, wheat threshers, tractors, and sugar cane crushing units (Mohan et al., 1989; Mohan and Qadeer, 1988; Patel et al, 1989; Qadeer and Mohan, 1988; Varghese and Mohan, 1990a; Gordon et al., 1962).

In Ethiopia, infections of the skin and subcutaneous tissues were the second most common cause of outpatient visits at government health facilities, after respiratory infections, and accounted for 4 percent of the total (Kloos and Zein, 1993). Although a precise classification of the underlying cause was not available, tropical ulcer, infestation by sand fleas (*Tunga penetrans*), and trauma were much more frequently associated with such infections in rural areas than in towns.

Implications for Prevention

Simple first-aid in the home, such as early cleaning and covering of wounds, could do much to prevent complications from developing in minor skin wounds. Unfortunately, it is still all too common in many tropical villages to see uncovered wounds swarming with flies. Low levels of personal hygiene and environmental sanitation, and the increased risk of wounds in rural areas need to be addressed by basic education about hygiene, sanitation, and first aid (Kloos and Zein, 1993). Screening homes against insects could help reduce exposure to flies, and may be needed if enclosed stoves are introduced to control burns, since the smoke from open fires helps to control flies and associated diseases such as trachoma (Alemayehu and Cherinet, 1993; Sahlu and Larson, 1992).

Many chronic tropical ulcers can be closed by simple skin grafts carried out under local anesthesia. Adequate tetanus immunization can prevent deaths that may otherwise occur in persons with minor wounds or chronic ulcers.

Redesign of the machete to provide a simple guard to prevent the hand from slipping onto the blade could prevent some injuries, as could the use of a sheath when carrying such knives. The installation of safety guards on machinery or other design changes can be highly effective in preventing injury. Simple guards that are easy to use have been developed for some of the agricultural machines that are used in villages in India (Patel et al., 1989; Qadeer and Mohan, 1988, 1989; Varghese and Mohan, 1990a).

Instructing villagers in the potential hazards of cutting tools and in safe handling procedures may prevent some injuries, although the effectiveness of such educational efforts has not been evaluated in developing countries. Even in developed countries, education is probably most effective in occupational settings where there is a more structured environment (Waller, 1985; Robertson, 1983).

Further research is needed to develop and evaluate suitable methods of prevention for developing countries. Since data are so scarce, population-based descriptive studies of disability from cutting tools and other cutting, piercing, and crushing injuries would be useful to determine the magnitude of the problem, and could be carried out collaboratively with surgical staff. Many axes sold in developed countries now carry labels that warn users to wear eye protection; such labels cost very little but their efficacy needs to be evaluated.

EYE INJURIES

The eye is particularly vulnerable to injury and an infected eye wound often leads to loss of the eye. As in the preceding section on skin wounds, the heading for this topic denotes the nature of the injury, rather than a specific external cause.

I have only one eye, I have a right to be blind sometimes . . . I really do not see the signal.
    —*Horatio Nelson, At the battle of Copenhagen, 1801,* in **Life of Nelson**

Importance of Eye Injuries

A clear distinction must be made between binocular blindness that renders a person functionally blind, and monocular blindness, which is much less debilitating. Fortunately, most eye injuries affect only one eye (Schwab, 1990). In a rural survey in Ethiopia, the prevalence of monocular blindness was double that of binocular (Alemayehu and Cherinet, 1993). Injuries were the leading cause of monocular blindness and accounted for 32 percent of the total, while injuries accounted for only 2 percent of binocular blindness.

In developed countries, eye injuries are also an important cause of blindness and range from 4 percent of cases in Japan to 35 percent in Finland (Niiranen, 1978). The extent to which this represents differences in reporting or in risk factors is unknown.

Special Circumstances in Developing Countries

Domestic, subsistence, and occupational activities are common sources of penetrating eye injuries. Severe complications from delays in obtaining expert treatment is common to most such injuries, particularly in rural villages.

Common sources of eye injury are debris from chopping firewood, thorns, sharp objects such as knives, needles, and arrows, metal fragments from grinding activities, and chemical irritants or corrosives used in occupational settings. Chopping wood is an everyday activity in many villages; it is also the most important cause of severe eye injury in many developing countries. In Malawi, 25 percent of eye injuries occurred during wood chopping (Ilsar et al., 1982). Sharp sticks can fly up into the eye, sometimes as a result of improper positioning of the sticks, or perhaps because of a blunt or inappropriate tool.

When treatment is delayed, even minor injuries can result in permanent blindness because of extensive infection. A study in Nigeria found that only 20 percent of patients with eye injuries at a hospital had been seen within one week following the injury (Olurin, 1971); many patients tried traditional remedies first, and sought medical advice only when the traditional treatments failed to resolve their symptoms. In another study, it was found that more than 80 percent of eye injuries had occurred in rural areas where treatment was usually unavailable (Adala, 1983). Foreign bodies or objects that cause penetrating wounds are often heavily contaminated, and flies will swarm around any wound, including the eyes.

In Ethiopia, there is a widespread belief that blindness is associated with evil spirits or sent as a punishment by God (Alemayehu and Cherinet, 1993). This fatalistic belief leads to delays in seeking treatment for eye injuries.

Classification of Eye Injuries

There is no specific classification for external causes of eye injuries in the ICD. Therefore, in surveys it is necessary to organize a classification based upon local priorities. Some of the leading causes of eye injuries include:

- Foreign bodies either from natural sources, such as wind-blown dust, or from occupational hazards, such as metal or stone chips from grinding or pounding;
- Penetrating and cutting wounds from pointed tools such as knives and spears and from sticks;
- Blunt trauma from fights.

Small foreign bodies are often embedded relatively superficially in the cornea, but infection, ulceration, and scarring can occur if they are not promptly removed. Perforating wounds can lead to internal infection and/or hemorrhage with loss of the entire eye. Blunt trauma can result in internal hemorrhage of the eye with potential loss of vision.

Subcategories for classification can also be organized on the basis of determinants such as activities and personal, equipment, and environmental factors.

In classifying eye injuries, estimates of severity are essential. Examples include the following:

- Bilateral or unilateral blindness;
- Total loss of light perception in an eye or partial loss of visual acuity;
- Simple indicators of functional visual acuity such as whether a person can read, recognize others, and see hazards at a distance; or actual visual acuity measured with standard tests for non-literate populations.

Examples of Morbidity and Mortality from Eye Injuries

Disability from Eye Injuries

While data on the prevalence of blindness due to injury are not available for most developing countries, the large number of clinical articles on eye injuries suggests that they are a significant problem. Among the few developing countries for which data are available, the proportion of blindness attributable to injury varies substantially.

In some countries, most blindness is due to conditions of older age, such as cataract or glaucoma, or to infectious disease such as trachoma or onchocerciasis. However, among cases of preventable blindness, excluding degenerative and congenital causes, injuries and infection tend to be most important. Injuries often affect the young and can cause lifelong disability.

In a national survey of the handicapped in China in 1987, only 2 percent of visual disabilities were attributed to blindness (WHO, 1991). Although injury was less common than degenerative conditions as a cause of visual disability, visual disability due to injury tended to affect children and young adults, and would result in a much longer duration of disability than conditions of older persons, such as cataract and glaucoma.

In less developed, more rural societies, injuries appear to be more common as a cause of visual disability. In a 1981 survey of disability in Zimbabwe, unintentional injuries accounted for 29 percent of visual impairments and war for another 7 percent (WHO, 1991). These cases included both near-total visual impairment of both eyes and profound visual impairment of one eye. Domestic injuries were the most common cause of both types of visual impairment, accounting for 47 percent of binocular and 67 percent of monocular impairment. Agricultural activities caused 21 percent and 9 percent respectively, traffic injuries 14 percent and 3 percent, and assault 7 percent and 12 percent. About 80 percent of persons who were visually impaired as a result of war were civilians.

In India, a 1981 national survey of the handicapped showed that 9 percent of cases with a known cause of total visual impairment of both eyes with no light perception were due to injuries in urban populations and 7 percent in rural residents (WHO, 1991). Of near-total visual impairment of both eyes with light perception, 6 percent of cases with known causes in both urban and rural areas were a result of injuries. In about one-half of all cases of visual impairment, however, no cause was specified.

A 1981 population census in Sri Lanka identified 9,331 blind persons with total visual impairment of both eyes (WHO, 1991), which represents a prevalence of about 60 per 100,000 population. Among both urban and rural males, 9 percent of cases with a specified cause were due to unintentional injuries and 1 percent to violence. Among urban females, 3 percent of cases were due to unintentional injuries and none to violence, while among rural females, 4 percent of cases were due to unintentional injuries and 0.1 percent to violence. In about 11–15 percent of all cases of visual impairment, no cause was specified.

Eye injuries with visual impairment accounted for about 16 percent of patients at an eye hospital in Ethiopia (Alemayehu and Cherinet, 1993). About 7 percent of cases of optic atrophy were attributed to trauma, and frequently affected children, along with phthisis bulbi and corneal scarring. Childrens' eye injuries resulted from falls, injury by another child, and bombs. Adult males were blinded more often than females, due to occupational eye injuries.

Implications for Prevention

Improvement in the early treatment of eye injuries is needed but is unlikely to be available in many remote villages where the risks are greatest. It is also unclear whether vision could be saved by available treatment in the more severe injuries that result in loss of vision. However, since foreign bodies embedded on the surface of the cornea are a relatively common injury in many settings, rural health workers could be trained to recognize and manage many of these injuries to prevent corneal ulceration and scarring. Since prompt access to expert treatment will often remain the exception rather than the rule, primary prevention of eye injuries is very important for developing countries and also for isolated indigenous communities. Nevertheless, education of the public is needed, not only in prevention but also in prompt treatment. If fatalistic beliefs about eye injuries lead to avoidable delays in seeking treatment, then measures may need to be taken to address such beliefs.

Primary prevention for eye injuries includes eye protection such as glasses or goggles for hazardous activities such as chopping wood and chipping stone and appropriate eye shields on machinery likely to cause eye injuries. Labels on hazardous tools, such as axes, should warn the user that safety glasses are needed. Safety glasses could be supplied with hazardous tools, or at least made available at cost with the tool. When feasible, guards are usually more effective than goggles, particularly where high temperature and humidity make the latter uncomfortable or subject to fogging.

When metals and tools to work them are newly introduced and unfamiliar, appropriate devices to afford eye protection should be introduced simultaneously. While passive automatic protection is to be preferred, education in schools and the community on the safe use of common tools as well as of hot and caustic substances is essential.

OTHER INJURIES

Abortion

Wounds or sepsis sustained during induced abortion were reported to be the leading cause of death from injury among women of childbearing age in rural Bangladesh, and accounted for 5.5 percent of all deaths in this 15–44 year age group, with a mortality rate of 15 per 100,000 per year (Fauveau and Blanchet, 1989). The root of a creeper plant was inserted into the cervix in 46 percent of cases, while a traditional or allopathic medication was used in another 46 percent. Unmarried teenagers were at highest risk. Profound cultural changes and better family planning services are needed to address this tragic problem.

Sports Injuries

The extent and nature of the sports injury problem in developing countries is unknown, but the potential for injury is expected to be significant where resources for supervision and protective equipment are limited. For example, in Papua New Guinea, rugby players are sometimes picked up and "speared" head first onto the field; this can result in spinal cord injuries of the neck, quadriplegia, and death. Spearing was also common in American football in the United States, but the incidence of quadriplegia was reduced dramatically by changes in football rules that outlawed the practice. Sports injuries are an important problem in developed countries; however, appropriate epidemiologic research and interventions have helped to minimize their impact (Baker et al., 1992). If certain practices or equipment can be shown to be linked with specific types of injuries, then changes in regulations or equipment will help to prevent the associated injuries. Schools, universities, community groups, and other responsible organizations should consult the available literature on sports injuries to consider potential hazards of their own specific sports activities and to aid in developing local surveys.

Playground Injuries

While playgrounds can prevent pedestrian injuries by giving children a play location away from busy streets, they must be carefully planned to avoid introducing a new source of injuries into the community. The surface beneath the equipment should be free of rocks and sharp objects and be soft enough to cushion the impact of a fall. Hard surfaces such as concrete or bricks should be avoided. Packed earth, although better than rocks, offers little impact attenuation. Wood chips, fine "pea gravel," and sand offer good energy absorption (U.S. Consumer Product Safety Commission, 1990; Lewis et al., 1993), but only wood chips offer good protection in freezing conditions.

Equipment should be evaluated for excessive height and spaces that could result in entrapment of the head or other body parts (Chalmers et al., 1996; Bowers, 1989). Standards for equipment and surfaces have been developed in a number of countries and are useful for municipalities that are planning new playgrounds or improving existing ones.

Foreign Bodies

Foreign bodies can be classified into three main groups, as follows:

- Foreign bodies ingested, inhaled, or inserted into natural orifices of the body;
- Foreign bodies on the surface of or in the eye;
- Foreign bodies in skin or subcutaneous tissues as a result of penetrating wounds.

Only the first is considered here, since the others were discussed above. In developed countries, asphyxiation as a result of choking on food is common among both small children and the elderly. Peanuts and many seeds are small enough to pass into the trachea and bronchi; if immediate death does not result from aspiration, victims require anesthesia and bronchoscopic removal. Children are also at risk from asphyxiation by small toys, pacifiers, and plastic bags (Baker et al., 1992). The extent of the problem in developing countries is unknown, but could be significant, particularly in communities where children are exposed to the following:

- Small round food items, such as peanuts;
- Small round objects, such as seeds used as toys or in "pea shooters" (Barss, 1985b);
- Poorly constructed toys and those with small parts;
- Small infant pacifiers;
- Plastic bags used without an appreciation of their potential hazard.

Where a problem has been identified, the public must be educated concerning the hazards of small round objects and plastic bags to children, and there must be in place appropriate regulations preventing the sale of hazardous toys and other items, such as undersized pacifiers or those made in several pieces that can separate.

In an Ethiopian community survey of rural children 0–15 years, the incidence of a child requiring treatment at a health facility for removal of a foreign body was about 50 per 1000 children per year (Demamu, 1991). These foreign bodies included items such as seeds, which children placed in their ears. Objects composed of natural materials or plant fiber can absorb moisture and swell, making them difficult to remove.

Asphyxiation with Intoxication

In cultures where it is common to consume alcoholic drinks rapidly to achieve intoxication, aspiration of vomitus may be an important mechanism of death by asphyxiation; however, more information is needed about the relative importance of this factor.

Sudden Infant Death Syndrome

Sudden infant death syndrome has been associated with asphyxiation in the prone sleeping position and hyperthermia from excessive wrapping with clothes and blankets (Dwyer and Ponsonby, 1992).

The condition is more prevalent among low socioeconomic groups and aboriginals (Irwin et al., 1992; Rhoades et al., 1992). Sudden infant death syndrome accounted for 40 percent of postneonatal infant deaths among United States aboriginals. The importance of sudden infant death syndrome and the significance of various causative factors need to be clarified in developing countries, since mothers sometimes transport their babies inside cloth bags and tend to wrap their infants in many layers of warm clothes, even when ambient temperatures are high. People may also have been erroneously instructed that the prone position is preferable for sleep.

chapter 11

Occupational Injuries

Injuries at work represent a substantial proportion of all injuries. The tremendous variety of occupations and working environments in many countries provides a challenge for the surveillance and prevention of occupational injuries. In other countries or regions, most occupational injuries occur during subsistence activities, but few are ever reported or investigated. Although the study of occupational injuries can be a somewhat complex and specialized undertaking, the general principles of surveillance of mortality and morbidity, as discussed in the introductory chapters, also apply to occupational injuries. The specific occupation, tasks and activities, working environment, equipment, and personal factors must be considered when implementing injury surveillance and prevention.

A substantial portion of adult life is spent in the working environment, and yet, until recently, relatively little emphasis has been given to the health effects of the workplace. In developed countries, occupational injuries and diseases are now recognized as a significant public health problem. Although often inadequate, some measures are now being taken to address such injuries. In most developing countries, the situation for workers is less favorable for a variety of reasons.

SPECIAL CIRCUMSTANCES IN DEVELOPING COUNTRIES AND INDIGENOUS COMMUNITIES

Many occupational injuries result from hazards associated with a task, working environment, equipment, or activities. However, other occupational injuries arise from hazards in the general environment and society. For example, in the United States, as the physical safety of worksites and machines has improved, motor vehicle injuries and homicide have become increasingly prominent as leading causes of death from injury on the job (Baker et al., 1992; Weeks, 1991; Kraus, 1991; Robertson, 1991).

In many developing countries the situation differs, since the working environment is often less controlled, with many hazardous exposures due to old or poorly shielded machinery, toxic exposures, and other features of the working environment. Poverty often forces people to accept dangerous jobs, while fear of unemployment may prevent them from protesting against specific hazards in their working environment.

Many agricultural workers in developing countries are subsistence cultivators. Occupational injuries of subsistence cultivators have rarely been studied in a systematic manner, but are considered here, together with injuries from other traditional and newly introduced occupations.

The magnitude of the problem of occupational injury is relatively unknown in developing countries; however, most of the labor force is employed in workplaces with minimal or non-existent safety standards. Factory regulations enacted several decades ago in colonial times are sometimes all that is available to provide for workers' safety, even in complex modern industries such as pesticide or other chemical factories. For example, it was noted in Pakistan as recently as 1989 that the only occupational safety and health regulations dated back to the British Raj (Nathani, 1989). However, regulations for factories have been introduced in many developing countries during the past two decades.

For many people in developing countries, any job, no matter how hazardous, is seen as preferable to the alternative of unemployment (Vilanilam, 1980). For workers, "today's wage is more important than tomorrow's health" (Dhara, 1989). This is particularly disturbing when modern principles of industrial hygiene and safety engineering can do much to prevent injuries. In the absence of a well-educated and unionized work force to demand such preventive measures, government intervention is essential to regulate and enforce the protection of workers by employers.

In indigenous communities, many jobs involve subsistence activities, such as fishing, hunting, and trapping. This includes frequent exposure to travel over water or ice by small boat, canoe, snowmobile, or on foot. It also includes the use of firearms, the use of fire and stoves in flammable tents, extremes of weather, and isolation. In remote areas, paid employment in construction and other occupations may be less well supervised and regulated than in more accessible communities.

REPORTING OF OCCUPATIONAL INJURIES

Any injury at work, however humble the occupation, should be considered preventable and worthy of attention by public health policymakers. However, generally only the injuries that occur in large industrial settings are counted as occupational injuries by reporting systems.

The types of injuries that must be reported often vary from one jurisdiction to another. A practical and objective method of classifying the severity of occupational injuries is needed to determine which injuries must be reported and investigated. Both the circumstances of the incident (external cause) that resulted in the injury, as well as the nature and severity of the injury, should be recorded and reported. Data should be grouped by occupation and by the type of industry. For example, welders may be employed in several different types of industry, but share common hazardous exposures such as flash burns of the eyes.

Some of the categories that have been used for classifying the severity of occupational injuries include the following:

- Fatalities;
- Hospitalizations;
- Incidents that cause more than a specified number of lost workdays for an individual, including temporary and permanent disability (lost time may be expressed as the lost-workday incidence rate per 100 full-time workers per year);
- Injuries that affect more than a specified maximum number of workers;
- Injuries that require medical treatment or first-aid, but do not result in lost workdays;
- Near-misses that nearly result in a fatality or severe injury;
- Damages to materials and equipment, since they could reflect potential hazards for workers.

These approaches are general, but do provide an overall estimate of the extent of the injury problem. Another method of measuring occupational injury severity is to calculate the median number of lost workdays for groups of workers who suffer similar disabilities from specific types of occupational injuries (Bureau of Labor Statistics, 1993). This can help to identify types of injuries that cause prolonged disability, such as back injuries. In occupations where repetitive motions are required to perform the same task many times per hour, repetitive strain disorders of tendons and nerves can become epidemic and must be reported and carefully monitored.

In most countries where employers are required to report occupational injuries to the government, small workplaces (often those with fewer than ten employees) are completely excluded from the reporting requirement. Many workers on job sites are self-employed and management maintains no records for them. Some managers attempt to hide injuries, or reduce the severity or lost time, to maintain a good safety record for their department, and to protect their own reputation and employment history. Thus, even in developed countries, it is often difficult to get an accurate estimate of the number of workers affected by occupational hazards (Kraus, 1985). Where they exist, reporting requirements in developing countries are even more incomplete or are limited to certain groups of the workforce. Reporting of agricultural injuries is rare (Larson and Dessie, 1993).

Examples of Reporting for Occupational Injuries by Country

In some Latin American countries, occupational injury data are available for workers who are enrolled in social security plans, but coverage is often incomplete (PAHO, 1984). On the basis of the available data, it has been estimated that about ten million occupational injuries, with 50,000 deaths, occur each year in the Americas (PAHO, 1981).

In India, it has been estimated that each year one to two million workers are disabled or seriously injured and 100,000 are killed (Mohan, 1984). However, Indian government labor statistics in 1981 reported only 1,028 fatal and 345,000 nonfatal occupational injuries in factories, mines, and ports (Dhara, 1989).

In India, only factories, mines, or ports, which employ about 15 percent of the work force, were required to report disabling injuries. Powered workplaces with ten or less workers and unpowered workplaces with 20 or less workers were excluded from reporting requirements. Reported deaths in factories increased from 474 in 1961 to 742 in 1981, with a corresponding increase in the death rate from 9 to 16 deaths per 100,000 workers per year. In mines, the number of deaths decreased from 344 to 254, while the reported rate fell from 77 per 100,000 to 34. The number of reported deaths in ports increased from 12 to 32 (Dhara, 1989). As a comparison, in the United States in 1978, there were said to be 9 deaths per 100,000 factory workers (Mohan, 1984).

Even in industries where reporting of injuries is required, serious under-reporting often occurs (Dhara, 1989). Four million construction workers and 150 million agricultural workers in India are said to be completely uncovered by any safety regulations.

In the meantime, there has been astounding growth in certain industrial sectors. The increase in production of a few of the leading industrial products in India from 1970 to 1981 gives some idea of the rapidity of change: tractors 4,040 percent, mining machinery 1,400 percent, propylene 1,200 percent, industrial boilers 940 percent, paper 890 percent, chemical machinery 560 percent, fertilizer 340 percent, powered two-wheelers 340 percent, and diesel engines 340 percent.

In Pakistan, according to figures from the Labor Inspectorate, there was an average annual rate of fatal occupational injuries of 24 per 100,000 workers, of serious injuries 120, and of minor injuries 700. These data are based only upon injuries among permanent factory workers and are believed to be affected by severe underreporting (Nathani, 1989). Casual workers, who are often given the most hazardous jobs, are not covered, nor are workers in high-risk industries such as mining and construction. Occupational illnesses apparently are not reported at all.

In Brazil, the National Institute of Social Security estimated the occupational injury mortality rate to be 31 per 100,000 workers in 1970 and 18 in 1982 (Ferreira and Mendes, 1981; PAHO, 1984). In the smelting and foundry industries of Mexico, reported rates of fatal and nonfatal injuries were 2,600 per 100,000 workers, double the rate of all factories combined (Cuellar, 1980).

For non-industrial workers, the available information tends to be mainly qualitative rather than quantitative. An exception may be China, where the work force is relatively stable and where record keeping and surveillance are facilitated by organized health services (Christiani and Xue-qi, 1988). Some of the successes in China are discussed below under pesticide poisoning.

TYPES OF OCCUPATIONAL INJURIES

Workers are subject to a variety of occupational exposures to physical and chemical hazards. Skin wounds are common and can lead to prolonged disability if appropriate treatment is delayed. These in-

The seaman's story is of tempest, the plowman's of his team of bulls; the soldier tells his wounds, the shepherd his tale of sheep.

    —Sextus Propertius,
Elegies *II, i, 54 B.C.E.– 2 C.E.*

clude cutting wounds from hand and power tools and machines, as well as piercing wounds from other hazards.

Burns tend to be the second most common occupational injury to the skin in developed countries (Hipp and Taylor, 1988). In South Korea, a survey found that burns, mostly "major" ones, constituted 8 percent of reported occupational injuries (Eun, et al., 1984). In rural Nepal, it was found that wounds of the skin surface were the most common injury in all occupations; burns were the second most common injury and affected mainly women working in the home (Thapa, 1989).

Permanent disability from amputations and crushing are common during the use of poorly designed machinery. Blows from falling objects, crushing or suffocation by collapsing trenches or structures, and falls from scaffolds are common in some industries. Hearing loss is a frequent problem wherever power tools or machinery are used.

Eye injuries and blindness or permanent loss of binocular vision are another problem. In the United States, about one-fourth of all eye injuries were occupational (Verma, 1991), but 20 years earlier in Singapore, 51 percent of all eye injuries were reported to be occupational (Loh and Ramanathan, 1968). Foreign bodies are the most common source of industrial eye injury. Other types of occupational eye injuries include penetrating wounds, blunt trauma, and welding flash burns (Verma, 1991). Eye injuries frequently result from failure of employers to provide appropriately shielded machines or personal protective devices such as eye goggles, especially for activities such as pounding, chipping or grinding metal or stone.

In factories, workers are often exposed to chemical hazards of poisoning by vapors and dust inhalation, and explosive hazards from dusts or combustibles. China has considerable heavy industry and major current occupational health problems include poisoning by industrial chemicals and heavy metals, as well as physical hazards such as noise and vibration (Christiani and Xue-qi, 1988). Pesticide poisoning is also a serious problem in China.

In agriculture, poisoning by pesticides is a common hazard. The World Health Organization has estimated that there are about 3 million severe acute cases of pesticide poisoning annually worldwide, with about 2 million of these related to suicide attempts; about 220,000 deaths per year were attributed to acute pesticide poisoning (Levy and Widess, 1991). Fifty million persons are estimated to be at high risk of pesticide poisoning by virtue of heavy exposure, while another 500 million are subject to less intensive exposure, but may also be at considerable risk due to lack of knowledge and experience in handling pesticides.

Where rapidly repeated motions are required, as in meat-packing plants and many other industries, such as garment assembly, that require rapid piecework, crippling repetitive-motion damage to nerves and tendons frequently occurs (Punnet, 1991a, 1991b, 1991c; Bureau of Labor Statistics, 1993). Carpal tunnel syndrome of the wrist is a common example of a peripheral nerve entrapment syndrome that can be bilateral and completely disabling. Tendinitis and nerve entrapments, as well as many back injuries (Himmelstein, 1991), often result from damage from cumulative trauma rather than a single acute injury.

In some occupations, motor vehicle injuries are the leading fatal injury hazard (Weeks, 1991; Robertson, 1991). In high-crime areas, clerks and shopkeepers are at significant risk of assaults and homicide after dark (Kraus, 1991).

INJURIES BY TYPE OF OCCUPATION

Injuries are discussed by major sectors, including agriculture, fishing, resource extraction, construction, and production.

Agriculture

Subsistence agriculture is widespread and is still the most common occupation in many countries, although in Latin American nations the percentage of the workforce employed in agriculture has decreased. Nevertheless, the total workforce in Latin America is now doubling every 25 years, so the number of workers in all sectors who require protection is also rapidly increasing (Michaels and Mendes, 1988).

Although a large proportion of the labor force of developing countries is involved in agricultural activities, most injuries are not reported. In one industrialized country, the United States, death rates in agriculture have not declined as much as death rates in other high-risk occupations. Agriculture is now the most dangerous industry; in 1993, the mortality rate for agricultural workers was 35 per 100,000 workers per year, while in construction it was 22 and in mining 33 (National Safety Council, 1994).

Injuries from farm equipment in India are described in the section on penetrating injury. Women were the most common victims of fodder machines. Children were injured when playing with unshielded machines that were left unattended. Rural Indian workers frequently sustained prolonged disability lasting from weeks to many months. Disability was frequently a result of failure to obtain skilled professional treatment of wounds, amputations, crush injuries, and fractures, and to the use of ineffective or harmful first-aid techniques such as the application of oils, pastes, and tight splints.

A high rate of injuries to the left hand has been noted when sugarcane is harvested under a piece-work system using machetes (Suchman and Munoz, 1967). This system of compensation encourages workers to labor excessively fast and long, which may increase productivity in the short term but often has adverse long-term effects in the form of acute injuries and repetitive motion disorders, such as tendinitis and peripheral nerve entrapments.

The use of pesticides has increased greatly with changes in agricultural practices. Many of the most hazardous pesticides are used in developing countries. It has been reported that about one-third of pesticide exports from the United States to Latin America are products that are prohibited from use in the United States because of their extreme toxicity (Michaels and Mendes, 1988).

Most agricultural exposures to toxic pesticides occur via the skin, and the heaviest exposures are reported to be on the hands. Persons at high risk include individuals who produce, mix, and apply pesticides for farms and plantations or who are involved in control of pests in buildings (Levy and Widess, 1991). Field workers who carry out tasks such as harvesting fruit and vegetables are at risk when they enter contaminated fields, unaware of the toxic properties and safe handling practices for the chemicals to which they are exposed. Household contacts, including children, are exposed to pesticides on clothing, in food and drink, and from improperly-stored pesticides. Ready accessibility to pesticides often leads to high suicide rates, and in many villages in India, pesticides are the preferred means of suicide (Mohan, 1993).

It has been estimated that over 40 percent of Central American workers are now migrant farm laborers. Many of the workers who are most heavily exposed to toxic pesticides are illiterate migrants. A study of Central American cotton workers found that three-fourths were unable to understand pesticide warnings or instructions, and that protective clothing was seldom available. Exposure occurs not only in the workplace, but also by contamination of the workers' drinking and washing water and during spraying operations near on-site temporary housing.

Among Ecuadorean farm workers who regularly used toxic pesticides, knowledge about symptoms and treatment of pesticide poisoning was limited (Grieshop and Winter, 1989). Safety equipment was unavailable for most workers. The majority of farmers believed that it was unnecessary to use safety equipment, and about one-half felt that it was too uncomfortable. Many farmers were unaware of the hazard of skin contact with pesticides.

In Sri Lanka, a survey reported that 17 percent of all pesticide poisonings were occupational; it was estimated that about 5 per 1,000 agricultural workers in the country were hospitalized each year for such poisonings (Jeyaratam et al., 1982), with a total of about 1,000 deaths per year from occupational and other unintentional pesticide poisonings. This led to the development and implementation of a special curriculum and training program on pesticides for vendors and on integrated pest management for farmers (Cormier, 1993).

More than 80 percent of China's population work in the countryside where pesticide poisoning is a serious occupational hazard (Christiani and Xue-qi, 1988). When certain organophosphate insecticides were introduced to the rural counties of Shanghai, acute poisonings occurred at rates as high as 130 cases per ton of pesticide. However, a control program was implemented, and within three years the rate was reported to be less than two cases per ton. In one Shanghai district from 1981 to 1983, the number of persons occupationally exposed to pesticides increased by 159 percent to 326 million and the amount of pesticide applied increased by 206 percent to 10,086 tons. However, during this period the cumulative incidence of pesticide poisoning reportedly dropped from 7.1 percent to 0.2 percent, with a corresponding drop in mortality from 4.4 to 0.1 deaths per 100,000 workers per year.

Such successes attest to the potential efficacy of control programs in organized socialist societies, even where most of the population are low-income rural workers. The controls that were implemented included training programs, use of full-body personal protective equipment, and substitution of less toxic insecticides.

In the United States, migrant seasonal farm workers are frequently minorities or immigrants and are heavily exposed to pesticides. The most severe exposures occur during the mixing of concentrated pesticides. Such exposures can be prevented by engineering controls, including the use of a closed system to transfer the pesticide to the mixing tank; this eliminates direct contact by the workers with the chemicals (Coye and Fenske, 1988). Appropriate training for workers is also important.

The most effective method of protection against acute poisoning for field workers is reported to be the use of appropriate reentry intervals, so that pesticides are substantially degraded by the time the workers enter the fields. Personal protective equipment may also be needed, especially suitable gloves. However, the use of inappropriate materials or damaged gloves can increase exposure if chemicals become concentrated inside the gloves. It is undesirable to base the prevention of acute pesticide poisonings solely upon constant vigilance by workers and the use of hot and uncomfortable personal protective equipment. Substitution of less toxic pesticides, as they become available, is also important and provides more automatic protection of workers. Integrated cultural and biological pest management to reduce dependency upon chemical pesticides is another desirable option (Igbedioh, 1991).

Fishing

Another important subsistence activity in coastal areas is fishing. Subsistence fishers, working from small open boats or canoes, face a number of hazards, such as wounds and envenomations from needlefish, stingrays, and other marine fauna as described in Chapter 10.

The mortality rate from injuries among commercial fishers is very high in developed countries; drownings account for most of the deaths (Schilling, 1971; Reilly, 1987a, 1987b). Drowning rates among subsistence fishers in developing countries have not been reported, but are probably high. Garments that contain flotation and protect workers from hypothermia in extremely cold water should be more widely used, especially in northern indigenous communities.

Resource Extraction

Resource extraction, such as logging and mining, has a history of high rates of serious and fatal injury, although in well-run unionized mines there have been highly significant decreases in fatalities in recent years. Loggers are exposed to skin wounds, falling objects, noise, and vibration from trees and chain saws. Many loggers sustain permanent disability from injuries to the head, spine, or extremities (Holman et al., 1987). Machinery operators are exposed to falling trees, overturning tractors, and severe noise and vibration. Miners are exposed to crushing injuries, noise, and explosions.

In China, tree fellers have a rate of injury about 30 times greater than processors (Qi-chun and Fend-chong, 1989). The two leading sources of injury were being struck by objects and vehicle-related injuries, such as injuries sustained from rollovers. Severe vibration and noise in tree harvesting machines apparently cause the rapid onset of fatigue in workers, increasing the risk of injuries.

The use of safer chain saws to protect against injuries has been recommended. To be effective, such saws must have well-maintained anti-vibration and anti-noise devices, as well as automatic brakes and other safety equipment. Other interventions include cabs on harvesting machines to protect the operators against rollovers and falling objects, as well as engineering changes to reduce vibration and noise, thereby preventing driver fatigue. In Nigeria, many chain saws had no automatic brakes or chain covers and anti-vibration devices were often broken (Udo, 1989). A survey of tree fellers showed that only 37 percent used safety helmets, 23 percent work boots, 6 percent gloves, and 6 percent hearing protection. Fellers often worked long hours with very little food. Because of inadequate protection of the hands and feet, injuries to the upper and lower limbs were frequent and accounted for two-thirds of all injuries. One-third of injuries resulted from chain saws and another one-third from being struck by objects; 61 percent of all injuries occurred during tree felling.

Coal mining is one of the highest-risk occupations throughout the world (Bennett and Passmere, 1984). Most mining injuries described from developing countries resulted from explosions, roof cave-ins, and flying debris (Laxminarayan and Dhanbad, 1968; Asogwa, 1980b, 1988).

Construction

The construction industry is another source of many injuries and fatalities; however, reporting systems do not tend to provide surveillance for workers in this sector. Construction workers are exposed to the hazards of falls from inadequate scaffolding, to blows from falling objects, and to crushing by collapse of trenches and buildings.

In Tanzania, cave-ins of inadequately reinforced trenches and collapse of concrete structures have been reported (Machumu, 1989). Among road construction workers in Nigeria, motor vehicles were the leading cause (48 percent) of occupational injuries (Jinadu, 1980). Quarrying rocks for construction can be hazardous because of explosions of blasting powder (Urasoda, 1968).

Production

Many factories in developing countries contain hazardous machinery and/or toxic chemicals. Workers in small factories and also in some larger ones are exposed to physical injury, including noise and vibration from unprotected machines, poisoning by inhalation of solvents and other chemicals, and explosions caused by static electricity in the presence of vapors or dust.

There is some evidence that the risk of injury varies with the size of a factory or work site (J.A. Waller, 1985). Small plants represent a particular problem with respect to monitoring. It has been reported that middle-sized plants often have higher rates of injury than large ones (Bureau of Labor Statistics, 1993).

Over 90 percent of industries in the Americas have less than 100 employees (Mendes, 1982). The risk of injuries in these industries is reported to be four times greater than in larger ones. Such businesses are engaged in all types of industrial activities and employ from 48 to 95 percent of the labor force in various countries (WHO, 1976). Rates of injury are high because the working environment tends to be relatively unstructured and unregulated. This allows for minimal investment in safety measures, and safety regulations that do exist are difficult to enforce. It is reported that engineering controls of toxic exposures are almost unknown in smaller Latin American factories and are grossly inadequate in most other workplaces (Michaels and Mendes, 1988).

In India, employment in small industries is increasing rapidly and accounts for almost 50 percent of industrial production and 25 percent of exports. In 1985, about nine million persons were employed in such small industries, including foundries, engineering, ceramics, bangle shops, and lead battery reconditioning plants (Parikh et al., 1989). Working conditions were generally poor, no records of occupational injuries were kept, and most workers had no access to medical facilities. Many industrial injuries resulted from unsafe or defective machinery, including unshielded hazards, as well as from inadequate training of workers.

Hand and finger injuries are generally the most common type of industrial injury (Leung and Ng, 1982); one study showed that such injuries represented between 34 and 43 percent of industrial injuries (Vaidhya et al., 1982). Lack of safeguards on conveyer belts and machines have been reported to cause many injuries (Gupta et al., 1982). In Brazil, a survey of 290 press machines in ten plants found that none of the machines had safety devices to prevent amputations or fatal injuries (Carmo et al., 1989).

Among industrial workers in Addis Ababa, Ethiopia, the overall injury rate was 200 per 1,000 person years of exposure, and 75 percent of injuries involved the extremities. The leading source of injuries was heavy machinery, and only 13 percent of workers wore any type of protective equipment (Fulle, 1993). Injuries were most common at the beginning and end of the work week in this study, and also in another study of port workers who had a similar rate of injury (Demissie, 1993). In a textile factory near Addis Ababa, the injury rate was somewhat lower at 80 per 1,000 person years; falls and being struck by falling objects accounted for 63 percent of all injuries (Elias, 1991).

In most developed countries, noise-induced hearing loss is the most common permanent disability resulting from chronic occupational injury. Cumulative hearing loss from injury by sound pressure has been shown to be a serious problem in older cotton and silk mills in China where noise levels were estimated at 95 to 110 decibels. Similar noise problems are found in textile mills and shipyards (Christiani and Xue-qi, 1988). Noise injury has been reduced in some Chinese textile plants by substitution of plastic spindles for metal, by the use of quiet energy-efficient motors, and by enclosure of machines.

In Nigeria, many new, highly toxic, and unidentified chemicals have been pouring into the country (Onyoyo, 1989). Chemicals are handled by many different agencies, and there has been no control over the flow of such products. Many chemicals are inadequately labeled, and management and workers frequently know nothing about their hazards. It has, therefore, been recommended that legislation be developed to control the importation, manufacture, storage, transport, use, and disposal of chemicals.

Explosions are a hazard in certain plants and mines. They occur when uncontrolled static or other sparks ignite unsafe accumulations of dusts or vapors. Even metal dust can lead to such explosions. Dust control and shielded ignition sources can prevent most explosions, while appropriate pressure release vents in buildings can minimize the effects of any explosions that do occur (Jar et al., 1989).

Severe explosions, sometimes involving a chain reaction, have been triggered by static electricity in factories that produce fireworks and explosives, in the fuel depots of machinery factories, and in the holds of certain ships (Fang, 1989; Shun, 1989; Xin, 1989). The risk of such explosions is high when workers with plastic shoes and clothing made of synthetic fabrics work in an ungrounded, crowded, and cluttered environment. Explosions have also resulted when volatile fuels, such as crude oil, were improperly stored near sources of ignition in tanks that had been designed to store less-volatile fuels, such as fuel oil.

IMPLICATIONS FOR PREVENTION

The introduction of new industries from developed countries continues and results in the importation of new and often unfamiliar technology (Conway, 1984; Fernando, 1970). Potential injury hazards should be anticipated and met with appropriate safety regulations and enforcement. Policy-making and regulatory bodies of developing countries, company management, and workers must be involved in developing and implementing safety measures and controls.

Well-organized programs to monitor and prevent occupational injuries should include the following:

- Routine reporting of injuries by severity as discussed earlier in this Chapter;
- A systematic approach to investigating and recording the circumstances of injury-causing incidents and near misses, including established criteria for determining which incidents must be investigated;
- Regular review of physical environment, and correction of hazards by engineering controls and other measures;
- Regular review of work procedures and safety/protection practices;
- Information and training targeted to improving dangerous procedures and deficient practices.

Occupational injury surveillance should be organized so that systematically recorded data include the specific occupation/task and hazardous activities, as well as environmental, equipment, and personal risk factors. Data collection must be kept simple and sustainable. Information about the circumstances of specific types of injuries should be tabulated on a regular basis. A legal requirement for surveillance, with severe penalties for non-compliance, helps to ensure that companies in high-risk industries maintain appropriate records. In Brazil, it was found that when workers and unions were actively involved in epidemiologic inspection and surveillance, improvements were more likely to be made by management (Carmo et al., 1989).

Workers in small enterprises are usually unprotected by any oc-

> **Special studies are needed to monitor and control injuries in small farms and worksites; unions have been helpful in larger workplaces.**

Special surveys can assess injury hazards and means of control for vulnerable workers in poorly-monitored small-sector industries, home industries, and agriculture. The level at which agricultural workers are exposed to hazardous pesticides and machines must be assessed for large commercial farms and smaller family farms, and improvements recommended to policymakers as indicated.

Trade unions should be encouraged to include worker safety clauses in their negotiated agreements (World Bank, 1989). Unions and their members should be encouraged to be actively involved with their managers in epidemiologic surveillance, hazard identification, and control of occupational injuries (Carmo et al., 1989). Safer worksites have been found to improve worker morale and productivity.

cupational injury surveillance, and it may be more difficult to actively involve them in prevention. In Latin America, there is reported to be a serious shortage of programs for the training of health and safety technicians. Such technicians are needed to serve as inspectors for governments and as safety officers and industrial hygienists for industry (Michaels and Mendes, 1988).

Unfortunately, even transnational companies that routinely employ industrial hygienists to control hazards in their plants in developed countries frequently fail to do so in similar plants that they operate in developing countries (Michaels and Mendes, 1988). Company management is expected to be interested in injury prevention, if only because of the potential economic benefits from reduced disability and deaths among their workforce. However, until compensation costs and litigation or government penalties become sufficiently high to force management to take effective action to protect workers, the active involvement of workers is needed to bring about substantial improvements.

In agriculture and small industries, owners often try to keep their expenditures on safety to a minimum to remain competitive with larger businesses. Legislation and enforcement are essential to ensure that workers are paid for the time required to learn how to handle hazardous materials and machinery safely, and are not simply thrown into dangerous situations. They must also be provided with data sheets about hazardous chemicals and with protective equipment that is practical for local climatic conditions.

In spite of such obvious problems, strategies already exist for the control of occupational injuries in some developing countries. In China, where occupational health is an integrated part of many of the rural epidemic prevention stations, the government has proposed seven strategies to control occupational hazards. These include the following (Christiani and Xue-qi, 1988):

- Setting occupational health standards;
- Engineering controls;
- Personal protective equipment and hygiene;
- Worker education;
- Preventive diagnosis;
- Professional training;
- Worker's compensation.

Nevertheless, these strategies remain to be implemented in many parts of China and other countries. A major problem in China and other developing countries is the exportation by companies in developed countries of their hazardous operations. In the developing countries, the companies may not be required to comply with the more stringent safety regulations that protect workers for the same companies in developed countries.

Although occupational injury death rates have been reported to be about five times as high in Brazil as in North America and Western Europe, there have been substantial improvements in industrial safety in São Paulo since the 1970s (World Bank, 1989). These improvements were attributed to gradual familiarization of workers with the industrial environment and to three specific interventions. The most important intervention in São Paulo is believed to have been the organization of independent trade unions in the 1970s. As a result, worker safety clauses are now written into collective agreements, and unions monitor the work of safety professionals. Second, every plant with 50 or more workers is required to have a specialized service of occupational safety and health. These services are staffed by occupational health professionals trained by the Ministry of Labor's Foundation of Occupational Safety and Health. Third, appropriate legislation has been passed to prevent occupational injuries and diseases in plants with 50 or more workers.

In Pakistan, Nathani (1989) outlined several improvements to address the alarming situation that he described there. His recommendations, relevant to the situations in a number of other developing countries, include the following:

- Updating occupational safety and health rules and regulations;
- Establishing training for inspectors and safety professionals for industry;
- Creating a body such as a National Safety Council to monitor injuries in the workplace and to engage in activities to increase safety awareness among employers and workers;
- Developing an effective inspectorate;
- Organizing safety consulting services.

In addressing the problem of death and disability from occupational injuries, high priority must be given to permanently engineering hazards out of the workplace to provide long-term protection for as many workers as possible. This can be implemented according to the well-known and respected "hierarchy of controls" (Office of Technology Assessment, 1985). In such a hierarchy, strong emphasis is given to permanently eliminating the most serious hazards in order to provide continuous automatic protection for workers at all times, so they are protected even if inexperienced or momentarily fatigued.

The concept of passive protection of workers was established at least 150 years ago by Villerme (1840) in his classic study of the terrible working and living conditions of workers in cotton, wool, and silk mills in France. It is, therefore, entirely unacceptable for present-day governments and plant managers to claim ignorance of such principles. While Villerme clearly recognized the critical importance of plant owners and managers in protecting workers from machinery, he did place some of the blame for injuries on child workers who failed to take "safety measures", which is unfortunate, since elsewhere in the document he describes exhausted malnourished children as young as seven-years-old falling asleep at their work. Work often consisted of 12 to 15 hour shifts, alternating night and day for seven days a week, with fatigue exacerbated by long walks into cities to get to and from work.

> . . . the rather frequent accidents that occur during the work day. These are normally injuries to hands or fingers that are caught in machines or gears. Sometimes bones are broken, limbs are severed, or even death can occur. These accidents are always the fault of the manufacturer who has neglected to isolate or surround the dangerous parts of machines with a casing or screen, or of the workers themselves, especially children,

who neglect to take safety measures. I do not know how frequent they are, but I believe that the very serious ones are not very numerous and generally result from oversight on the part of the victims. Most of these could be prevented by use of the screens that I mentioned above. Some manufacturers have already made this expense, however, others, and these are the majority, have not taken this safety measure. Legislation should be passed to make this compulsory.

—Louis R Villerme,
Tableau de l'État Physique et Moral des Ouvriers Employés dans les Manufactures de Coton, de Laine et de Soie,
Vol 2, 1840.

As noted by Villerme, implementation by engineers, hygienists, and managers should be based upon locally appropriate regulations. Such regulations must be developed and enforced by a body of trained personnel. Thus, the training of suitable staff and the development of effective legislation are priorities for governments that are concerned with the safety and well-being of their work force.

For occupations that require the handling of dangerous chemicals, such as pesticides, workers must be guaranteed access to copies of material safety data sheets from suppliers or makers of the chemicals. Data sheets must be in the local language and fully explained to workers and their supervisors before starting work with the chemicals. The European Union has acquired extensive expertise in the development of standardized warning risk symbols for different groups of hazardous chemicals and in preparing uniform risk phrasing for written materials to facilitate translation into the multiple languages of the union countries. This expertise and the written material should be of great practical interest to developing countries.

Work practices and procedures and protective equipment must also be reviewed with each new worker. The feasibility of substituting less hazardous substances should be reconsidered periodically.

For occupations that involve repeated movements, the workplace and the process must be adapted to the task and the worker (List, 1994). Taller and shorter workers may have different needs. In addition to improved equipment and processes, changing daily routines and switching tasks with other workers at regular intervals are helpful in avoiding strain. Changes such as these can pay off, since healthy workers produce higher quality products, and lost time can be cut to a tenth or less. Safety audits, records of lost time, and quality of work can provide objective measures of progress.

chapter 12

Injuries from Disasters

Injuries from disasters have a major adverse impact in certain areas of the world; human activities contribute to or greatly exacerbate the effects of many disasters. The impact of disasters on human populations is much more severe in countries with environmental degradation, poorly constructed buildings, adverse climatic conditions, and large poverty-stricken populations (Noji, 1997). The effects of a disaster are also much more serious in countries that lack the skilled personnel, organization, communications, transport, and other resources to manage the disaster rapidly and effectively.

DEFINITIONS AND TYPES OF DISASTERS

Disasters have been defined as "any disruption of the human ecology that exceeds the capacity of the community to function normally" (Lechat, 1990a). An event that is a disaster in one community may not be so in another, since disaster occurs only when a community is unable to absorb the impact of a physical event upon its people.

Other definitions for disasters reflect the particular perspective of different organizations. The Pan American Health Organization has defined a disaster or major emergency as "a natural or man-made occurrence that produces a massive disruption in the normal delivery of health services, and that poses such a great and immediate threat to public health that the affected country requires external assistance to respond to the situation" (PAHO, 1990). The World Bank defines a disaster as "an extraordinary event of limited duration, such as war or civil disturbance, or a natural disaster that seriously dislocates a country's economy" (World Bank, 1989).

Each disaster usually captures world-wide attention and causes widespread devastation. Viewed over a span of time, natural disasters are not a major cause of injury mortality in most developing countries, but do cause considerable losses in certain individual countries. Nevertheless, disasters occur more often and have a proportionately greater impact on poor countries than on rich ones. Development

It wont be long now it wont be long man is making deserts of the earth it wont be long now before man will have it used up so that nothing but ants and centipedes and scorpions can find a living on it.
—*Archy (the cockroach)*,
what the ants are saying in:
Archy does his part,
D.R.P. Marquis, 1935

With man, most of his misfortunes are occasioned by man.

—*Pliny the Elder,* **Natural History,** *23–79* C.E.

projects sometimes increase susceptibility to disasters and can result in severe economic and human losses when a disaster does occur (Anderson, 1991).

Disasters result from natural and technological sources; however, the human impact of natural disasters is often greatly exacerbated by technical factors, such as the design and construction of housing (Kreimer and Munasinghe, 1991). Natural disasters include earthquakes, floods, cyclones, typhoons, hurricanes, volcanic eruptions, droughts, desertification, wildfires, and infestations of grasshoppers and locusts. The most common disasters today are droughts and flooding, and both appear to be increasing. Environmental degradation because of overpopulation has been a critical factor in some countries, while in others, disasters have resulted from short-sighted destruction of the natural environment for farming or other uses.

Many disasters are acute events, while others, such as drought, are chronic. Nevertheless, even though many disasters occur suddenly, they are often precipitated or exacerbated by long-term predisposing factors in the manmade infrastructure or by anthropogenic damage to the natural environment. Many disasters have a long-term impact on populations that persists for a generation or much longer (Stackhouse, 1994), and some disasters are significant determinants of political violence (Homer-Dixon, 1993).

CLASSIFICATION AND REPORTING OF INJURIES FROM DISASTERS

The most basic classification involves coding the type of disaster. Individual deaths or morbidity from technological disasters may be coded as due to a specific toxic chemical, explosion, or radiation. For natural disasters, the following categories are provided for in the ICD-10 (WHO, 1992) under the heading natural forces of nature:

- Earthquake;
- Volcanic eruption;
- Avalanche, landslide, and other earth movements;
- Cataclysmic storm, such as a cyclone, hurricane, tornado, tidal wave from storm, torrential rain, or blizzard;
- Flood, as a direct or remote effect of storm, or from melting ice or snow;
- Other and unspecified forces of nature.

Accurate reporting of injuries by type and severity provides documentation of the impact of a disaster. Comparison between the circumstances of the injured and the non-injured at the time of the disaster can provide important insights into determinants of injury and protection from injury.

The immediate needs of disaster relief lead to a natural preoccupation with relieving such needs. This should not preclude epidemiologic study of injuries and their circumstances for the purposes of planning prevention of future disasters; however, classifications of injury severity and determinants should be relatively simple so that they are workable in the context of the post-disaster situation.

The classification of injury severity should be adapted to the type of disaster. For example, for disasters that result mainly in deaths, classification into dead and alive may be all that is needed. For disasters that cause both deaths and severe injuries, classification into three categories may be used, with the non-injured group actually including minor injuries ignored for the purposes of expediency. For technological disasters that result in many permanent disabilities from injuries, such as toxic brain damage, it may be necessary to include permanent disability as another category of injury severity.

A count of the death certificates issued in a village immediately following a disaster and a simple census count of survivors can provide fatality rates. Counts of a random sample or all of the injured from hospitals and/or clinics should provide an estimate of the number of severe injuries. For technological disaster, all exposed survivors must be counted and registered for long-term follow up, since it is otherwise impossible to separate those who were exposed from unexposed persons who may attempt to obtain a share of any financial compensation.

Similarly, the circumstances for comparison between the injured and non-injured must be adapted to the type of disaster and based upon hypotheses as to the most pertinent personal, equipment, and environmental factors. However, the natural curiosity of investigators must be restrained, and only the most important determinants investigated. When it is unclear from a review of previous disasters which circumstances should be included in a post-disaster study, a post-disaster field pretest on a small group of victims and survivors may help to assess the final variables that should be retained for the complete survey and acceptability of survivor interviews.

In a study of the impact of housing design on the risk of injury in a Guatemalan earthquake, injuries were classified as either fatal or severe (Glass et al., 1977). Severe injuries were defined as all those that required hospitalization or outpatient care with extended follow-up of more than two weeks duration. The risk of fatal and severe injuries was then compared between residents of adobe and non-adobe houses. In addition, injury risk was compared within the same types of houses for different age and sex groups and for various types and sizes of rooms.

The researchers were able to show that adobe houses were lethal for small children and the elderly, and that houses made of wood, cornstalks, or concrete were protective. Thus both house (equipment) factors and host (personal) factors were important in survival. While only the type of housing was a modifiable determinant of injury, in assessing this factor, it was important to control for other determinants of injury, such as host resistance to injury related to age and sex.

By also counting deaths from other disaster-related causes, it was possible to assess the relative importance of housing-related injuries and other causes of mortality and morbidity from the disaster. All deaths during the disaster period occurred from injuries related to housing collapse, with not a single death from infectious disease, lack of food, landslides, or other problems. It was also found that a better emergency response for the injured could have prevented no more than 7 percent of the deaths.

For disasters, such as floods, that result mainly in fatalities, it may be adequate to simply count the number of fatalities and survivors and use this as a basis for comparison between areas with different circumstances, for example, islands with and without protective equipment, such as cyclone shelters (Siddique and Eusof, 1987).

INJURY PATTERN BY TYPE OF DISASTER

Injury patterns depend upon the type of disaster and the part of the world affected. Earthquakes are one of the most dramatic sources of deaths and injuries from disasters, and vulnerability may be increasing as populations become concentrated in crowded urban areas with poorly constructed multistory housing. Droughts and floods may, however, be the disasters with the greatest potential for future morbidity and mortality, mediated by starvation and drowning. The threat of deaths from droughts and floods is increasing as ecological damage mounts, in part from population pressures on fragile tropical soils. Deforestation can lead to rapid run-off of rain and consequent flooding, while poor land management can cause landslides (Lechat, 1990a).

Earthquakes cause many deaths and large numbers of severe injuries requiring extensive care. Multiple fractures are a common pattern of injuries after earthquakes (PAHO, 1990). Earlier studies of large earthquakes found a ratio of injuries to deaths of approximately 3:1 (PAHO, 1981), and suggested that the number of deaths may be a useful guide to predict the number of injured persons requiring treatment (Lechat, 1979; DeBruycker et al., 1985). However, a more comprehensive analysis found that this ratio only applied to a limited number of earthquakes (Alexander, 1985). In the recent earthquake in Armenia, an estimated 25,000 people were killed and 31,000 injured (UNDRO, 1989). Thus, there were almost as many dead as injured. This was attributed to inadequate construction of buildings (EQE, 1989). It could be that large buildings constructed of heavy materials with inadequate reinforcement lead to higher ratios of fatalities to injured.

It has been estimated that about 75 percent of fatalities from earthquakes result from collapse of buildings (Coburn et al., 1989). The majority of deaths occur in masonry buildings constructed from materials such as adobe, rubble stone, rammed earth, or unreinforced brick or concrete.

High winds cause few deaths and moderate numbers of severe injuries. Tidal waves and flash floods cause many deaths and few injuries, whereas other floods generally result in relatively few deaths or injuries (PAHO, 1981). Certain areas, such as the Bangladesh delta, have been subject to regular massive floods after cyclones, resulting in high fatality rates (Siddique and Eusof, 1987).

In addition to injuries, another effect of many natural disasters that has significant public health implications is the widespread disruption of reticulated systems of water and sewage supplies (PAHO, 1990).

Technological disasters such as the massive release of poisonous gas from a pesticide plant at Bhopal, India, the explosion of a butane plant in Mexico, and the explosion of the nuclear reactor at Chernobyl, USSR, are becoming increasingly common (Lechat, 1990b;

Gregg, 1989; Bertazzi, 1989; Mohan, 1987b; PAHO, 1986). The worst of these, such as Bhopal, can cause thousands of deaths and hundreds of thousands of injuries, including permanent disabilities (Stackhouse, 1994).

EXAMPLES OF MORTALITY AND MORBIDITY

Most of the deaths, casualties, and damage from disasters occur in the poorer countries of the world (Lechat, 1990a). The true burden of nonfatal injuries from disasters is often difficult to determine, in part because there is no consistent definition for an injury in most published data.

The greatest numbers of fatalities from earthquakes during this century have occurred in developing countries. The two earthquakes with the largest number of fatalities in the past half-century were the Tangshan, China, earthquake of 1976, which resulted in 242,469 fatalities, and the 1970 earthquake of Ankash, Peru, which caused 66,794 deaths (Coburn et al., 1989). Almost half of the total number of earthquake deaths in the world have occurred in China, and about 80 percent of all deaths from earthquakes have occurred in China, Japan, Iran, Peru, Turkey, the former USSR, Chile, and Pakistan.

Floods cause more damage than any other natural disaster and account for about 40 percent of the total damage from all disasters (French and Holt, 1989). The Hwang Ho, or Yellow River, in China is the most flood-prone river in the world. There have been at least three major floods in the past 100 years, including one in 1969, with estimated losses in each flood ranging from several hundred thousand to 900,000 lives.

The Pan American Health Organization compiles records of all disasters in the Americas, and Table 12.1 provides a summary of some of these disasters. This gives an overview of the impact of various types of disasters in the region (PAHO, 1986, 1990). In the Americas from 1970–90, nearly 150,000 persons died from natural disasters, about 500,000 were injured, millions of people were affected, and economic losses of many billions of dollars were sustained (PAHO, 1990). Two major sources of injuries during this period were the 1985 volcanic eruption in Colombia with 23,080 deaths and 4,420 injuries, and the 1985 Mexico City earthquake with 10,000 deaths and 30,000 injuries.

The Asian Disaster Preparedness Center (1990) has summarized information about disasters in Asia between 1964–86. During this period, the largest numbers of deaths resulted from earthquakes and cyclones/typhoons/storms (Table 12.2). In contrast, the largest numbers of persons were affected by drought and floods. Earthquakes and floods caused the greatest economic losses. Earthquakes, floods, and wind storms often leave a majority of affected persons homeless.

Nur (1990) has compiled from multiple sources a list of the effects of recorded disasters in African countries from 1980–89 (Table 12.3). In comparing the data for Asia and Africa in tables 12.2 and 12.3, it is evident that in Africa the numbers of deaths and persons affected are much smaller for acute disasters, such as earthquakes and cyclones, than for long-term disasters, such as drought and famine.

Table 12.1 Most important disasters in Latin America and the Caribbean, 1980–88

Year	Type of Disaster	Countries Affected	No. of Deaths	No. of Injuries	Number Affected
1980	Hurricane Allen	St. Vincent			20,000
		Saint Lucia	17	1,000	70,000
		Jamaica	9		10,000
		Haiti	220		835,000
		Argentina	31		36,000
1982	Earthquake	El Salvador	8	96	5,000
	Hurricane Albert	Cuba	40		105,000
	Flood	Nicaragua	71		52,000
		El Salvador	600		600,000
		Honduras	200		52,000
	Volcanic eruption	Mexico	100		60,000
1983	Earthquake	Colombia	102	228	150,000
	Flood (el nino)	Ecuador	300		950,000
		Peru	233		830,000
		Bolivia	40		700,000
	Hurricane Tico	Mexico	135		10,000

Year	Event	Country			
1984	Flood	Colombia	152		192,000
	Gas explosion	Mexico City	400	5,000	700,000
1985	Earthquakes	Argentina	7	230	38,000
		Chile	177	2,500	170,000
		Mexico	10,000	30,000	60,000
	Volcanic eruptions	Colombia	23,080	4,420	200,000
	Hurricane Kate	Cuba	2	41	476,000
	Floods	Brazil	200		60,000
		Argentina	15		100,000
1986	Earthquake	El Salvador	1,100		500,000
1988	Hurricane Gilbert	Jamaica	45		500,000
		Mexico	250		200,000
	Hurricane Joan	Nicaragua	116		185,000

Adapted from Pan American Health Organization, Health Conditions in the Americas, 1986, 1990.

Injury Prevention

Table 12.2 Effects of major Asian disasters 1964–86

Type of disaster	Deaths	Persons affected	Losses in U.S.$
Earthquakes	677,000	3,250,000	1,438,000
Cyclones/typhoons /storms	409,000	74,323,000	4,539,000
Floods	65,000	359,588,000	9,582,000
Droughts	9,000	533,744,000	481,000

Source: Asian Disaster Preparedness Center, 1990.

The volcanic release of massive quantities of carbon dioxide gas asphyxiated more than 1,700 persons near Lake Nyos in the Cameroons (Lechat, 1990b; Kling et al., 1987; Palca, 1987). Another disastrous source of enormous loss of life in many African countries has been widespread civil unrest and population movements due to ethnocentricity and civil unrest.

In the explosion of the pesticide plant at Bhopal, India, methyl isocyanate gas caused over 4,000 deaths, and immediate medical attention was required by between 50,000 to 200,000 persons. While there were about 3,000 immediate deaths, 1,700 deaths were expected from late effects (Stackhouse, 1994; Gregg, 1989; Bertazzi, 1989; Mohan, 1987b). In Mexico, the explosion of five million liters of butane gas resulted in 400 deaths, 1,000 people unaccounted for, and 5,000 injured (PAHO, 1986). Nuclear mishaps, such as the 1986 Chernobyl explosion in the former USSR, can result in massive acute casualties, as well as delayed effects in areas adjacent to the facility, and widespread contamination of populations in other countries (Lechat, 1990b).

For technological disasters that result in many permanent disabilities and delayed deaths, if the initial registration and follow-up of exposed victims are inadequate, immense suffering can result from delayed compensation. Ten years after the Bhopal disaster, only 1 percent of the 615,000 death and injury claims had been settled and only $3 million of the $470 million compensation settlement with Union Carbide had reached the victims (Stackhouse, 1994). Delays were attributed to poor communication between the excessive numbers of doctors and the different hospitals involved with the victims, as well as failure of the government to release funds to victims. However, many victims have been denied compensation because of a lack of documentation proving their status as victims. Bhopal represents a tragic example of the importance of organizing and provid-

Table 12.3 Effects of major African disasters 1980–89

Type of disaster	Deaths	Persons affected
Earthquakes	2,700	479,000
Cyclones/typhoons/storms	1,700	
Floods	900	4,875,000
Droughts	303,800	60,174,170

Source: Nur, 1990.

ing sufficient resources for a meticulous and complete registration of all exposed victims in the immediate post-disaster period and a coordinated follow-up to document and promptly compensate permanent disabilities.

For disasters such as the Bhopal chemical plant explosion, the public health impact and costs of permanent disability among the survivors can greatly exceed the impact and cost of immediate deaths. While the explosion of the Bhopal chemical plant killed about 4,000 people in 1984, estimates of the number of survivors with long-term damage ten years later ranged from 200,000 to 500,000 (Stackhouse, 1994). The total number of persons affected is even greater, since many brain-damaged parents with memory loss are unable to provide for their children.

ORGANIZATIONAL ASPECTS OF DISASTER PREVENTION

In an analysis of the costs and benefits of responses to natural disasters, it was concluded that for developing countries, as for developed countries, prevention is economically and politically preferable to recovery, and can be justified on the basis of cost-effectiveness (Anderson, 1991). In Bhopal, for example, the lack of basic industrial safety measures (Lillibridge, 1997) resulted in far more costly human damage.

As part of the International Decade for Natural Disaster Reduction proclaimed by the General Assembly of the United Nations in 1987 and initiated in 1990, it was recommended that special attention be given to assisting developing countries with assessment of the potential for damage from disasters, and in establishment of early warning systems and disaster-resistant structures (Lechat, 1990a; Merani, 1991). The objective of the Decade is to reduce, through concerted international action, the loss of life, property damage, and social and economic disruption caused by natural disasters, especially in developing countries.

An integrated approach to all types of disasters has been proposed to help avoid previous fatalistic attitudes that limited action to the provision of relief after disasters had already occurred (Lechat, 1990a). This integrated approach includes the following five phases:

1. Anticipative phase: planning, preparedness, and prevention;
2. Alarm phase: appropriate warning;
3. Rescue phase: the local affected population should be prepared in advance for this role so that they will be actively involved when a disaster occurs;
4. Relief phase: emergency post-disaster assistance;
5. Rehabilitation phase: this should be closely related to the process of general development.

The emphasis has shifted from post-disaster improvisation to pre-disaster planning and preparedness. In order to plan for prevention and even to make long-term provision for permanently disabled survivors, the relief phase needs to include an injury surveillance and research component that should be preplanned whenever possible, and be activated immediately once a disaster is known to have occurred. Careful documentation is necessary, not only to

Advance planning minimizes injuries from disasters.

Advance planning for disasters at a national level includes setting up a national committee and a national plan for disaster prevention. Specific activities include developing profiles of the most probable types of disasters for the country, mapping hazards and the vulnerability of warning systems and methods for rapidly publicizing warnings, training of emergency teams, and education of the public in the areas at risk.

Since many disasters result from hazardous man-made structures and environmental degradation, long-term prevention also includes safe building codes and measures to protect and repair the environment.

prevent future disasters, but also to ensure that, where appropriate, disaster victims are registered and promptly compensated to avoid long-term problems such as those suffered by Bhopal residents, as noted above.

While body counts may be available for many natural disasters, few epidemiologic studies have been conducted to determine risk factors for injury (Logue et al., 1981). The value of good epidemiologic information was demonstrated by a study of the 1985 cyclone in Bangladesh (Siddique and Eusof, 1987). On one island with no cyclone shelters, the study group lost 40 percent of its family members, while at a similar island with eight shelters, only 3 percent of the study group lost family members. Similar studies of earthquakes and tornadoes have led to useful suggestions for preventing loss of life from disasters (Glass et al., 1977; Glass et al., 1980). Disaster planning and preparedness can reduce the overall impact of disasters, but often basic planning is not done, even in countries at high risk (PAHO, 1986).

The adobe construction that was such a crucial factor in the Guatemala earthquake was not traditional to the indigenous inhabitants of the affected village, but had been copied from the houses of wealthy Spanish inhabitants of Guatemala city. In a previous earthquake prior to the introduction of these houses, there had been no deaths in the village. The research documented the lethal impact of housing "development" on the inhabitants and the fact that the risk of earthquake injury had gone from minimal to maximal in the space of 40 years.

Examples of the types of epidemiologic studies needed include research to determine risk factors for death following building collapse, injury patterns in relation to building design, factors responsible for survival, the most appropriate means of rescue and emergency preparedness, and other factors that could help in planning appropriate interventions either to prevent injury in a natural disaster or to mitigate its effects. The low fatality rates in recent disasters in the United States, including hurricanes Gilbert and Hugo in 1988 and 1989 and the California earthquake in 1989, were in part the result of the application of previous research findings (Lechat, 1990a, 1990b).

Architectural and anthropological studies should be carried out prior to disasters to determine the best type of housing to rapidly replace houses that are lost in a disaster. This will vary for different countries, regions, and ethnic groups. While architects and epidemiologists should be able to assess the resistance of structures to locally-important disasters, advance surveys of inhabitants of high-risk areas by anthropologists can determine the cultural acceptability and practicability of proposed designs. This could help to avoid situations where crisis planning and political considerations lead to immense pressure for rapid construction of foreign and inappropriate house designs in the wake of a disaster.

The 1993 earthquake in India flattened more than 32,000 homes in 57 villages, damaged as many as two million more, and killed about 20,000 people, all in less than a minute (Stackhouse, 1993). The sudden lack of housing together with offers of foreign assistance resulted in immense political pressure to construct thousands of Japanese concrete igloos and American suburban bungalows, although the designs were alien to the local culture and lifestyle. In the 1982 Yemen earthquake, foreigners built homes that were so inappropriate to local needs that they are now used as cattle sheds.

At Tonji University in Shanghai, studies of strategic systems planning for the prevention and relief of disasters have already begun. Four major research groups have been organized, including urban earthquake engineering, wind engineering, disaster prevention in engineering structures, and urban traffic safety (Rongfang et al., 1989).

New technology will increasingly be used for disaster surveillance, both to predict the spread and extent of certain disasters and to provide advance warning to the general public. Satellite imaging has been particularly effective in mapping the effects of floods, and can be used to obtain advance warning for affected populations (Morgan, 1989; Hassan and Luscombe, 1991; Carter et al., 1989). Satellite communications have also facilitated the development of remarkable networks for global communication.

In both "natural" and technological disasters, many deaths result from man-made changes in the environment and habitat. For example, earthquakes themselves seldom kill; collapsing buildings do the damage. It has been reported that in an intensity IX earthquake, a person living in an adobe or weak masonry building is 20,000 times more likely to be killed than someone living in a reinforced concrete frame building that has been properly designed for a minimum seismic load of UBC2 (Coburn et al., 1989).

Such engineering problems should be amenable to intervention if technical knowledge and funds can be made available; however, the costs can be considerable. It has been estimated that an increase of investments in preventive engineering of somewhere between 10 and 1,000 times in the buildings in the worst seismic areas would cause the problem of fatalities from earthquakes to disappear (Coburn et al., 1989). However, earthquake-safe housing in rural villages need not always be more costly than hazardous structures, since, as noted above in the Guatemala study, simple traditional houses were much safer than the newer introduced designs. Reduced insurance premiums and taxes for disaster-resistant housing have been suggested as market incentives to promote safer building construction (Natsios, 1991).

Other strategies of low to moderate cost proposed for reduction of deaths from earthquakes have included the restriction of building construction on the most unsafe land, better forecasting of earthquakes to allow evacuation of buildings before collapse occurs, and effective rescue. Creative solutions are urgently needed to avoid further massive losses of life, since many of the highest-risk areas have limited resources and high population densities.

Simple multipurpose buildings that can function as cyclone shelters have been effective in preventing loss of life in the Bangladesh delta, and should be built in other flood-prone areas. Other obvious preventive strategies, such as not rebuilding in areas subject to frequent disasters such as floods, are often not observed because of land shortages and the fact that the land in flood-prone deltas is often the most fertile.

Injury prevention in disasters can be considered at a local micro-level and at a national or international macro-level. For prevention at the micro-level of injuries in the household or workplace, the United Nations (1975) has prepared a manual of low-cost construction resistant to earthquakes and hurricanes. UNESCO has published a similar manual for the protection of new and existing educational buildings, such as schools, against earthquakes (Arya, 1978). The United Nations Centre for Human Settlements (Habitat) has provided (1989) practical examples of disaster-resistant housing and reconstruction programs in various countries.

With respect to injury prevention by planning at a macro-level, Siegel and Witham (1991) have outlined the importance of integrating disaster prevention into general development planning and Ciborowski (1978) has discussed urban and town planning as a mechanism for prevention of injuries in disasters. Pantelic (1991) has emphasized the importance of careful planning during reconstruction so as to reduce the risks of future disasters. Clark (1991) has detailed the importance of planning for coastal settlements and the hazards of disrupting natural environmental barriers such as fringing reefs, mangroves, and sand dunes. Nkwi (1990) provides a detailed account of the problems and long term strategies in attempting to resettle populations at risk after the Lake Nyos gas explosion in West Africa. Nur (1991) has outlined a detailed action plan for disaster preparedness in Africa.

Unfortunately, in many countries national disaster preparedness programs are established on an ad hoc basis with limited staff and funding or not at all (PAHO, 1990). The larger problems of overpopulation, environmental degradation, and settlements on marginal unsafe habitats are even more challenging to deal with. Exceptional multisectoral, political, and international cooperation and leadership are needed. Failure to act leads not only to local impact, but also to long-term political violence that can affect neighboring countries (Homer-Dixon et al., 1993). In some situations, a point of no return has been reached and irreversible environmental degradation of renewable resources is now an independent variable, rather than a dependent one.

chapter 13

Intentional Injuries: Homicide, Suicide, and Other Violence

INTENTIONAL INJURIES

Intentional or violent injuries are injuries purposely inflicted by an aggressor or self-inflicted by the victim. Such injuries include homicide and nonfatal assaults, as well as suicide and attempted suicide. Definitions of violence usually include the use of physical force with the intent of causing injury or death, but violence may also occur from other behaviors intended to cause pain, damage, or destruction of a person, such as neglect of children, adolescents, and the elderly, or oneself (Jeanneret and Sand, 1993; Rosenberg and Mercy, 1992; D.O. Lewis, 1991).

It has been stated that throughout history, the two leading causes of premature death have been infectious diseases and violence (Foege, 1986). While the control of many infectious diseases has been achieved, the prevention of violence is less well understood. In addition, the control of violence, as for many other injuries, tends to require multisectoral interventions. While the study of violence has often been left to criminologists, sociologists, and psychologists, the techniques of epidemiological and demographic analysis can provide another dimension for policymakers in choosing and evaluating interventions.

Importance of Intentional Injuries

Deaths by violence are a leading cause of loss of young adult lives in many countries. In the Americas, deaths by violence exceed the number of deaths for any other cause in the age group 5–24 years (PAHO, 1986). In certain countries such as El Salvador, homicide and assaults have been reported to be the leading cause of death (Lundgren and Lang, 1989). In some cities supposedly not at war, homicide has displaced motor vehicles as the leading cause of death from injury. Even the family home is no longer a safe haven, if it ever was, and has been declared as one of the most violent environments on earth (Krugman, 1993).

Although the 1990s were proclaimed to herald a new world or-

I pray that love may never come to me with murderous intent, in rhythms measureless and wild. Not fire nor stars have stronger bolts than those of Aphrodite sent by the hand of Eros, Zeus's child.

> —*Euripides*, **Hippolytus**, *l. 525, 428 B.C.E.*

Manufacturers of armaments that maim and kill civilians after hostilities have ceased should be legally responsible for costs.

Weapons of war that are particularly harmful to children and other civilians and that continue to maim after hostilities have ceased, such as land mines, must be banned.

Severely affected countries and international bodies may need to undertake class action suits or other legal action in order to recover from manufacturers the costs of treatment and rehabilitation of surviving victims and support of surviving families, the expenses of detecting and removing armaments that remain after military conflicts, and loss of productive farmland.

Epidemiologic and cost studies of deaths and disabilities from land mine injuries by country are essential in legal action by governments and individuals against manufacturers. Teams of epidemiologists and economists will conduct such studies.

der, there were about 30 armed conflicts in progress during the first few years of the decade (Last, 1993; Zwi and Ugalde, 1993). All wars in the 1970s and 1980s were fought in developing countries, with direct or indirect participation by many developed countries. The majority of victims of war are civilians, especially children, women, and the elderly. With weapons such as land mines, new injuries continue to occur long after the war has ended, and from that point onwards, all of the victims are civilians.

Suicide rates have increased markedly among young adults around the world in recent decades, and are also high among the elderly. Suicide is now among the leading causes of preventable loss of life in many countries. Since the meaning of suicide is often culture-specific, there are important differences among countries and regions in the population groups at greatest risk. For example, although males tend to be at greatest risk of suicide in many developed countries (Diekstra and Gulbinat, 1993), young women are the principal victims of suicide in the rural villages of some developing countries (WHO, 1991; Barss, 1991; Li and Baker, 1991).

Violence as a Public Health and Community Problem

In the past, the prevention of violent deaths was ignored by most health professionals because they tended to consider violence as largely unpreventable. Such attitudes are gradually changing, and the control of violence is now considered a leading public health priority (PAHO, 1990; Rosenberg and Fenley, 1991). However, since violence is a complex problem, it is unlikely to be resolved by interventions from a single sector, such as health. Nevertheless, public health workers can help to draw attention to the problem of violence by documenting and publicizing rates of different types of violence and their consequences. Epidemiologic analyses can be used to identify groups at high risk of violence, and major determinants of injury. Unfortunately, health professionals themselves are sometimes the targets of violence, as recently seen in El Salvador, Nicaragua, Guatemala, and Mozambique (Zwi and Ugalde, 1991; Garfield, 1989; Lundgren and Lang, 1989), and attempts to document violence may entail considerable risk.

Research has shown that certain social and environmental conditions are conducive to high rates of violence. Such conditions include the following:

- Large social class gradients, as seen in many developing countries and the United States;
- Male dominance;
- Racial, cultural, and religious ethnocentrism;
- Rapid population growth, with large numbers of unemployed young males in cities (Cohen, 1989);
- Freely-available concealable firearms, as seen in certain developing countries and in the United States;
- Widespread use of alcohol and other addictive drugs.

Attempts to control violence by repressive measures, such as law enforcement and imprisonment of large proportions of the population, while simultaneously ignoring the root causes described above, are reminiscent of previous unsuccessful efforts to control immunizable diseases using only hospitals and curative medicine. The best "vaccine" for violence may be profound social, political, and economic changes to empower and increase the well-being of disenfranchised groups in the community. However, more immediately achievable interventions also must be pursued, such as controlling lethal agents by banning concealable weapons, outlawing armaments such as land mines that take a major toll on civilians, and tightening controls over lethal pesticides that are used for suicide.

Classification of Violence

The standard classification of violent deaths in the International Classification of Diseases (WHO, 1992) includes the following major categories:

- Various types of assaults, including homicide;
- Operations of war;
- Legal intervention;
- Intentional self-harm;
- Injury event of undetermined intent.

These major categories are subtended by detailed subcategories that define the weapon or agent used to cause the death or injury. A major limitation of the standard WHO subcategories is that, while they describe the method of killing in considerable detail, the underlying cause of the violence is often ignored. Thus, there are no codes to describe collective state violence against the people, even though this is a major cause of death in many countries.

The use of codes varies among countries, with some countries making excessive use of categories such as "other violence" or undetermined intent (Jeanneret and Sand, 1993). Some homicides and suicides are misclassified as various types of "accidents", such as burns, falls, or drownings. Misreporting of homicides of women is particularly common in countries where dowry murders are widespread (Heise, 1993). The definitions and classification of various types of assaults and self-harm are discussed below in the sections for these topics.

Public reporting of intentional injuries does not always occur, even when data exist. Misclassification is a common subterfuge in countries with high levels of collective violence by government against the population. In other cases, as in the Gulf war of 1991, data are available but are withheld for political reasons (Zwi and Ugalde, 1993).

HOMICIDE AND ASSAULT

Homicide and assaults may involve individual violence between two or more persons or collective violence between citizens and authorities (Jeanneret and Sand, 1993).

Most data from developing countries pertain to fatal assaults, and even homicides are poorly documented in many countries. Nevertheless, there is increasing interest in identifying and preventing nonfatal domestic violence. A number of surveys of violence against women have documented the prevalence of assaults in the home (Heise, 1993; Belsey, 1993). The underlying determinants of such assaults are incompletely understood and poorly addressed throughout the world, since domestic violence is widespread in both developed and developing countries, as well as in indigenous communities in developed countries. Political violence is also an important category, but the study of these phenomena, including state terrorism and police violence, is not without risk in many countries (Zwi and Ugalde, 1991).

In view of its frequency as a cause of fatal and nonfatal injury, relatively little is known or has been done to prevent homicide and other assaultive injury. Effective long-term solutions that deal with the underlying causes of violence are often unpalatable to powerful groups with strong incentives to maintain the status quo. Such groups include the ruling elite, wealthy minorities, and foreign powers with extensive business and strategic interests. Preventing violence in the home requires major changes in societal norms, as well as other determinants, such as aggressive marketing of alcoholic beverages.

Classification and Reporting of Homicide and Assault

The standard WHO classification of homicides and nonfatal assaults includes the three major categories noted above—assault, legal intervention, and operations of war (WHO, 1992). The subclassification of assaults and war injuries focuses upon different types of weapons used for assaults, while fourth-digit codes can be used to identify the location of the incident. Sexual assaults, neglect and abandonment, and maltreatment have their own separate categories. Maltreatment includes mental cruelty, physical and sexual abuse, and torture, and, unlike most other assaults, the ICD codes do include a series of subcodes to identify the perpetrator, including various types of individuals, such as relatives and government authorities.

Classification by the type of weapon used for a homicide provides important information for development of preventive interventions. The strong association between the availability of firearms and civilian homicides, and of land mines with civilian casualties during and after war operations, are powerful arguments for strict controls or complete bans on such weapons. Unfortunately, in the ICD 10, deaths and injuries from land mines do not have their own category and are lumped together with many other types of explosive weapons of war.

Another important element in homicide and assaults is the identity of assailants and their relationship, if any, to the victim. Thus, other classifications have been proposed that emphasize this variable (Jeanneret and Sand, 1993; Chesnais, 1981, 1985). The identity of the assailant can be a charged political issue, which perhaps accounts for its neglect in most standard classifications of morbidity and mortality. The observation by one physician with extensive experience in war refugee camps that "one person's terrorist is another's freedom fighter" is a concise expression of often dichotomous views of the etiology of violence (Robert Frey, Johns Hopkins School of Public Health, personal communication, 1987).

Thus other possible classifications of violence include the following:

Individual violence:

- Domestic, within the family or household, such as spouse against spouse, parent against child, or child against parent;
- By strangers or acquaintances;

Collective violence:

- Citizens against authorities, such as terrorism, revolutions, or strikes;
- Authorities against citizens, such as state terrorism or police violence.

Violence has been classified under several categories that are oriented more towards identity of the victim or type of assault than the identity of the assailant (Rosenberg and Fenley, 1991). They are as follows:

- General assaults;
- Spouse abuse;
- Child abuse;
- Elder abuse;
- Rape and sexual assault.

In surveys of domestic assaults of spouses and children, careful definition of the nature of injuries and classification of their severity is important in order to provide comparability with other surveys and an objective gradation of different levels of assault. Terms such as beating, battering, pushing, slapping, hitting, and shoving are often used. While such categories may be useful to describe the type of behavior involved in domestic violence, they describe neither the resulting injuries, their severity, nor the underlying determinants.

Violence reporting problems are widespread, particularly for collective violence in which the state is guilty and has the power to suppress or modify reports, or domestic violence in which injuries are misreported as unintentional for a variety of reasons. Underreporting or misreporting probably explain at least some of the remarkable differences in infant homicide rates among countries (Belsey, 1993). In certain developing countries where the number of reported infant homicides is low or zero, there are large numbers of infant deaths from injury of undetermined origin. While the United States has one of the highest reported infant homicide rates in the world, it has a relatively low rate of infant deaths from injury of undetermined origin.

While war casualty figures show that the vast majority of victims are civilians, these figures often include only the victims of war wounds. If deaths from other direct and indirect effects of war, such as famine and disease, are included in the overall death rates from war-related violence, rates can easily double (Kloos, 1993). These deaths, together with war disabilities, should be counted in any comprehensive assessment of the total impact of violence. As military expenditures increase, health budgets often decline precipitously. Therefore, the impact on mortality and morbidity of the resulting loss of already minimal health care and preventive services should also be included.

There may be reasons for particular subgroups in society to exaggerate the numbers and/or the severity of assaults in order to advance a particular agenda. While the categories of a classification system for violent injuries can aid or hinder the development of effective interventions, the impact of underreporting and positive or negative misclassification biases must also be carefully considered.

Examples of Mortality Data for Homicide

Homicide rates in developing countries that have recently reported to the World Health Organization are summarized in Table 13.1. In virtually all countries, males have higher homicide rates than females. These rates have not been adjusted for age differences, since age-adjusted rates were not available for all countries; however, age-adjusted rates based on a world population do not differ substantially from the crude rates for most countries. Unfortunately, very few countries in Africa or Asia report to WHO.

In 17 of 27 countries in the Americas that reported to the World Health Organization during the 1980s, homicide was among the five leading causes of death (PAHO, 1990). In several countries, class warfare and state terrorism are endemic. In the early 1980s, in the three small Central American countries of Guatemala, El Salvador, and Nicaragua, homicide, including war death, was among the top two or three causes of lost years of potential life before age 65 for persons 1–64 years of age, and was often the most common cause of death for young adult males (PAHO, 1986). During 1981 in Guatemala, homicide accounted for 11 percent of all deaths in the country, while in England and Wales homicides made up only 0.03 percent of all deaths (Anywar et al., 1986). In Colombia, homicide, particularly assassination, is reported to have been the leading cause of death among men 15–46 years of age since 1981 (PAHO, 1990; Zwi and Ugalde, 1989).

Homicide rates are also high in rural subsistence villages of some countries, even where state terrorism and murder by armed forces and police have been less prevalent. For example, in a population under continuous epidemiologic surveillance in the isolated Tari valley of the highlands of Papua New Guinea, during 1971–86, the homicide rate among men was 31 per 100,000 population per year. The rate of homicide among females was also very high at 20 per 100,000 (Barss, 1991). When these rates were age-adjusted to the world standard population, they were even higher, 39 and 25 per 100,000, respectively. In subsequent years, homicide rates further increased; during 1987–89, the unadjusted male homicide rate was 76 per 100,000 per year (Barss, 1991). The homicide rate for males in Papua New Guinea was higher than the overall homicide rate of 53 per 100,000 for black males during 1987 in the United States. However, among males 15–44 years of age, homicide rates for United States African Americans were higher than for Papua New Guineans, while among older males, the rates in rural Papua New Guinea exceeded those in the United States.

Not all countries have high rates of homicide. In China in 1987,

Table 13.1. Reported rates for homicide and other assaults in various developing countries, with other countries for comparison

	*Deaths/100,000/year**				
	Homicide		*Other violence*		
	m	*f*	*m*	*f*	*Year*
AFRICA					
Mauritius	2	2	0	0	1994
SOUTHEAST ASIA					
China, rural	3	1	0	0	1994
China, urban	4	1	0	0	1994
Sri Lanka	12	2	6	2	1986
EASTERN MEDITERRANEAN					
Egypt	1	0	24	17	1987
AMERICAS					
Guatemala	5	1	52	7	1984
El Salvador	74	6			1984
Colombia	168	13	4	1	1991
Chile	5	1	51	11	1992
Mexico	32	3	5	1	1993
Guyana	0	0	31	8	1984
Ecuador	18	2	1	0	1988
Paraguay	12	2	5	2	1987
Panama	12	2	10	2	1987
Argentina	7	1	15	4	1991
Costa Rica	7	2	4	1	1991
Uruguay	7	2	0	0	1990
Surinam	8	2	8	2	1985
COMPARISON					
Russian Fed.	53	14	59	14	1994
United States	16	4	2	1	1992
Sweden	2	1	7	3	1993

Sources: World Health Statistics Annual 1986–1995 (WHO, 1986–1996).

*Rates not adjusted for age.

homicide was only the eighth most common cause of death by injury. The urban rate was 2.1 per 100,000 per year for males and 1.0 for females, and the rural rates, 1.8 and 0.6, respectively (WHO, 1990). By 1989, however, the urban rates had increased by almost 50 percent, to 3.1 for males and 1.4 for females (WHO, 1991). Nevertheless, homicide rates in China are far lower than those in most countries in the Americas and comparable to rates in Sweden (Table 13.1).

Homicide rates in urban China in 1986 were only about one-tenth the rates in United States cities (Li and Baker, 1991).

In indigenous populations in some of the developed countries, levels of violence are also high. In Greenland, which has an Inuit population that was colonized by Denmark, the rate of homicide increased from less than 2 per 100,000 per year during 1946–50 to 30 per 100,000 in 1985–90, while the rate in Denmark remained stable at around 1 during the same period (Bjerregaard, 1991).

Among indigenous peoples of Alaska, rates of homicide for males and females in 1950 were reported to be 11 and 6 per 100,000 per year, respectively, while during 1980–89 the rates were 40 and 17 (Middaugh et al., 1991). Homicide rates increased markedly among indigenous peoples during the interval between 1950 and 1980–89, but fell among others. Among Canadian Indians in British Columbia between 1953–78, homicide rates were ten times the rates for non-Indians (Hislop et al., 1987).

In some countries, the level of violence has increased alarmingly. In São Paulo, Brazil, by the early 1980s, murder had become a more important cause of death than traffic injuries. In 1984, 50 percent more residents of São Paulo died from homicide than from traffic injuries (World Bank, 1989). In Rio de Janeiro, the homicide rate is reported to have tripled between 1983 and 1989 and the situation worsened in the early 1990s. There was an unprecedented increase in the male homicide rate in São Paulo state during the 1980s (Fig. 13.1) (Rosenthal, 1990).

Figure 13.1

Trend in unadjusted homicide rates per 100,000 males per year in São Paulo state, Brazil, 1945-90.
Source: Adapted from Rosenthal CB. *A Study of Violent Death in the State of São Paulo, Brazil; Homicide, Suicide, and Motor Vehicle Accident Mortality from 1945 to 1990 (Dissertation). Baltimore MD: John Hopkins School of Hygiene and Public Health, 1995.* Reproduced with permission.

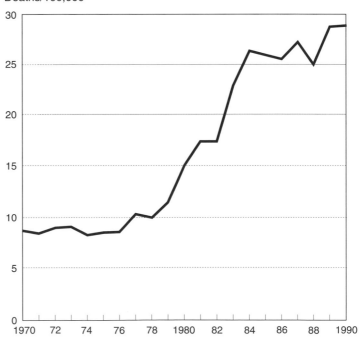

Deaths/100,000

Examples of Morbidity from Domestic Violence

A majority of homicides and general assaults involve males attacking males; however, in the domestic environment, women are the most frequent victims because of the greater strength and dominance of most males.

The incidence of domestic assaults on women varies with the definition and severity of violence. Reports from many developing countries indicate that about one-third to two-thirds of women have been beaten or battered by their partners, and, in some countries, up to 75 percent of women state that they are beaten frequently (Heise, 1993). Developed countries are not immune from such problems. In the United States, wife abuse has been reported as the leading cause of injury among women of reproductive age, and accounts for up to a third of visits to emergency rooms by women. Many abused women are at high risk of various psychiatric problems and suicide attempts.

Data are scarce on the underlying determinants of domestic assaults, since surveys tend to focus mainly on women rather than both partners. The severity and nature of injuries is recorded either in a variety of methods or not at all, making comparisons among prevalences in different surveys difficult. Similarly, in many surveys, the retrospectively reported incidence of assault during widely different periods such as a month, a year, or an entire lifespan is recorded. Lifetime incidence is obviously a function of age, as well as of other determinants. In a survey of marital violence in East New Britain, Papua New Guinea, alcohol consumption by the husband was cited by 71 percent of respondents as the principal marital problem leading to assault of a wife; the next most cited factors were suspicion by the wife about other women, and by the husband about other men (Bradley, 1985).

Although a zero level of violence may be theoretically desirable, norms must be assessed, and more severe degrees of violence identified. With such information, existing norms could be challenged. In some cultures, marital violence is considered "normal" and acceptable by many boys and girls, although most do recognize the importance of alcohol intoxication and other factors in triggering assaults (Bradley, 1985).

In the case of children, physical, emotional, and sexual abuse, as well as neglect, must be considered (Belsey, 1993). Various reporting systems exist for such injuries under child and welfare or law-enforcement agencies. Screening and detection may involve the use of special survey questionnaires, as well as training health professionals to recognize possible abuse of injured children who are brought to health facilities. As for spousal assault, the nature and severity of injuries must be objectively recorded, preferably using standardized questionnaires that have been developed for this purpose. Multiple, severe injuries are not uncommon in such cases.

For abused children, both parental and child characteristics associated with abuse must be discerned to identify high risk children and parents. One method of doing this is to compare parents of abused children and the children themselves with suitable controls. In a study of abused American Indian children, alcohol abuse was found to be a necessary, but not sufficient, condition for child abuse and neglect (DeBruyn et al., 1992). Other parental risk factors were a history of child abuse and domestic violence. Children with single parents were at greater risk of abuse. When personal factors of abused and non-abused children were compared, a significant proportion of abused children were found to be handicapped; however, while certain handicaps may have heightened the risk of abuse, others may have been a result of it.

Political Violence

"Prisoner, tell me who was it that wrought this unbreakable chain?"
"It was I," said the prisoner, "who forged this chain very carefully. I thought my invincible power would hold the world captive leaving me in a freedom undisturbed. Thus, night and day I worked at the chain with huge fires and cruel hard strokes. When at last the work was done and the links were complete and unbreakable, I found that it held me in its grip."
—*Rabindranath Tagore,*
Gitanjali, *1912*

In addition to the problems of homicide at the individual and community level, homicide and other violence from war or oppression at a national or international level are major sources of morbidity and mortality. State terrorism occurs when a government uses its power to terrorize its peoples into submission (J.R. White, 1991). State terrorism has been a major source of violent injuries in many areas of the world, such as the Middle East, Central America, Africa, and Asia (Cock, 1989; Chomsky, 1988, 1991; SKEPHI and ORIGIN, 1990), and is, unfortunately, often funded by strategic aid from developed countries (Lundgren and Lang, 1989; Ugalde and Vega, 1989; Garfield, 1989; Zwi and Ugalde, 1989). Genocide of racial or ethnic minorities is also a serious problem. The number of governments controlled by the military more than doubled, to about 57 percent between 1960–90 (Kloos, 1993; Sivard, 1991).

Serious underreporting of homicides from state terrorism often occurs. In some countries, the military clandestinely dispose of the bodies of victims of state violence by burying them in common graves, by dropping them into the ocean from military planes, or by incinerating them (Ugalde and Vega, 1989). Thus, the status of many disappeared victims is left in limbo, and the quantitative assessment of the impact of such violence on the overall mortality from homicide is inhibited.

Various types of political violence have been described, including structural, repressive, reactive, and combative (Zwi and Ugalde, 1991; Cock, 1989). *Structural violence* is an effect of severe inequities in a society or an attempt to preserve them, and involves various types of discrimination against relatively powerless segments of society.

Repressive violence may be used systematically by governments or other groups to achieve policy objectives, and can involve the use of instruments, such as torture and political death squads.

Reactive violence may include violence against the state in response to repressive violence or may be used by conservative opposition parties as a means of discrediting more progressive ruling authorities. The *intifada* in the occupied territories of Palestine was an example of reactive violence in response to structural and repressive state violence.

Combative violence involves militarization and the use of war within or between nations as a means of bringing about change or preventing it. Unfortunately, the proportion of civilians among war deaths has increased in recent wars, with civilians accounting for 85 percent of war deaths in the 1980s and nearly 90 percent in 1990 (Sivard, 1991; Aboutanos and Baker, 1997). The total number of war deaths in developing countries has also increased markedly during recent decades (Zwi and Ugalde, 1989).

In addition to causing many deaths and acute injuries among civilians and the military, certain types of warfare leave many persons permanently disabled. In Nicaragua, about 1 percent of persons are estimated to suffer from a physical disability, many of which resulted when arms, hands, and legs were blown off in Contra attacks and bombings (Garfield, 1989). The prevalence of disabilities from land mines is stated to be higher than this in countries that are plagued with a legacy of millions of these explosives, including Cambodia, Afghanistan, and Angola (Table 13.2.) (International Committee of the Red Cross, 1993, 1992; Chabasse, 1993). Other regions with large numbers of amputees from land mines include Mozambique, Djibouti, Iraqi Kurdistan, Ethiopia, and Laos. In countries most affected by land mines, the prevalence of amputees is estimated at between 150 and 200 per 100,000 population—that is, as much as 0.2 percent of the population. However, in certain districts, the reported prevalence is much higher, with 3.5 percent of the population mutilated and 2 percent killed by mines in the Spin Boldak district of Kandahar Province in Afghanistan. Land mines lay waste to vast areas of a country's land for generations and continue to maim thousands of civilians long after any conflict has ended (International Committee of the Red Cross, 1992, 1993).

The distribution of land mines by strewing them over wide areas of agricultural land using remote delivery from aircraft or artillery, rather than in mapped minefields on battlefields, is relatively recent (Chabasse, 1993). It began with the United States air drops of "bombies" over Laos and escalated with the Soviet invasion of Afghanistan in the 1980s. Mines were used not only to deny area to enemy troops, but also to control movements of civilian populations in large areas, including entire countries. Mining of agricultural land to deny food to the enemy and to the civilian population has become accepted as a normal strategy (McGrath, 1993a, 1993b; Anderson, 1993). The nature of these weapons has been eloquently summarized as follows (de Preux, 1993):

> Mines may be described as fighters that never miss, strike blindly, do not carry weapons openly, and go on killing long after hostilities are ended. In short, mines are the greatest violators of international humanitarian law, practicing blind terrorism.

It has been stated that the development of weapons such as mines, together with their current inhumane pattern of use, is now

We are mad, not only individually, but nationally. We check manslaughter and isolated murders; but what of war and the much vaunted crime of slaughtering whole peoples?
—*Lucius Annaeus Seneca,* **Epistles,** *95, 30, 4 B.C.E.– 65 C.E.*

Table 13.2. Estimated prevalence per 100,000 population of amputees from anti-personnel mines, by country

Country	Prevalence/100,000
Cambodia	450
Afghanistan	
Country average	170–300
Spin Boldak	3500
Angola	170–230

Source: Chabasse P. In: Symposium on Antipersonnel Mines, International Committee of the Red Cross, Geneva, 1993.

driven more by manufacturers and designers than the military. Metallic detection inserts are installed only as an option and are not used in most mines, making them very dangerous to find and remove after hostilities have ended.

In Afghanistan, the United Nations has begun a mine clearance program, which is a slow and dangerous process. It is estimated that it could take 4,300 years to clear 20 percent of the country's land at a rate of 30 square kilometers per year. There were 16 deaths and 20 injuries among United Nations staff during clearing of the first 68 square kilometers. The cost of removal averages $300–$1,000 per mine (Economist, 1994), and is not included in purchase prices, which are as low as a few dollars per mine.

In areas where people depend upon cattle or oxen, land mines can further destroy the basis for rural agriculture by killing animals that are essential for food or for tilling fields (Kloos, 1993). Many other deliberate strategies of war also lead to widespread famine by disrupting agriculture.

In addition to civilians, many young soldiers are left disabled by war. About one-third of 300,000 Ethiopian prisoners of war returned home injured or disabled (Kloos, 1993).

Determinants of Homicide and Assault

Personal Factors

Some of the most dreadful mischiefs that afflict mankind proceed from wine; it is the cause of disease, quarrels, sedition, idleness, aversion to labor, and every species of domestic disorder.
—*François de Salignac de la Mothe Fénelon,* **Télémaque,** *bk VII, 1699*

Age and sex are important determinants of violence. Homicide is a leading cause of injuries to young adult males in many developing countries. In certain ethnic groups where male dominance is particularly strong, as in the highlands of Papua New Guinea, homicide rates are also high among adult females (Barss, 1991). In rural Bangladesh, homicide accounts for about 2 percent of deaths in women of childbearing age (15–44 years), with a rate of 5 per 100,000 per year (Fauveau and Blanchet, 1989). In this population, high death rates in women from homicide, suicide, and induced abortion are attributed to male dominance and lack of educational and employment opportunities for women.

Infanticide is an important cause of infant mortality in many countries, but may be camouflaged by misclassification and under-reporting. In reports from Ethiopian health facilities, rates of homicide and assault were high among all ages of children. During 1990–91, 17 percent of cases of victims of assault and homicide were children under 15 years of age (Larson and Dessie, 1993).

In some cultures, jaw fractures are frequently associated with interpersonal violence against women. In Greenland, the incidence of jaw fractures is reported to be the highest in the world (Thorn and Hansen, 1984). A similar association between jaw fractures and forearm fractures in women and interpersonal violence has also been observed in the highlands of Papua New Guinea (P. Barss, unpublished data, 1991).

Alcohol and other drugs are often strongly associated with homicide and family violence, although a cause and effect relationship is not always clearly demonstrable (May, 1992; Rosenberg and Fenley, 1991; Breinholdt, 1991; Thorslund, 1990; PAHO, 1990; Secretary of Health and Human Services, 1990; Young, 1988; Bradley, 1985;

Lowenfels and Miller, 1984; Jarvis and Boldt, 1982; Kraus and Buffler, 1979). Alcohol abuse may reflect other underlying problems such as poverty, unemployment, cultural disintegration, and loss of self-esteem. However, the impact on alcohol abuse of the aggressive promotion and marketing of alcoholic beverages should not be underestimated.

It has been estimated that about 80 percent of homicides of indigenous Americans in the United States are alcohol associated (May, 1992). In Ungava, northern Canada, alcohol or other drugs were associated with 68 percent of fights among Inuit victims treated at nursing stations during 1991–93 (Brian Schnarch, Kativik, personal communication, 1994).

There is evidence from so-called "natural experiments" for the importance of alcohol in the etiology of violence. In Greenland in 1982, the incidence of jaw fractures nearly doubled in the nine months following deregulation of alcohol. In Brazil, alcohol was reported to be an important factor in many homicides; a drop in the homicide rate was observed prior to an election, when the sale of alcohol in bars was prohibited (World Bank, 1989).

Equipment Factors

The severity of aggressive violence expressed within families and ethnic groups, or intragroup violence, is supposedly limited by social conventions and norms of behavior (Eibl-Eibesfeldt, 1979). However, the fact that family violence and assaults on women and children is so pervasive indicates that either norms have been lost, or that new norms are needed. The introduction of more lethal weapons into the domestic environment can override the preventive effect of existing norms.

Conflict between groups, or intergroup conflict, is more frequently lethal. Such conflicts cannot all be prevented; however, the lethality of conflicts that do occur escalates markedly with the availability of powerful weapons that allow immediate killing at a distance. Such weapons do not provide any window of time to allow for peaceful withdrawal or negotiation by adversaries.

Thus, in countries such as the United States, where lethal and concealable weapons, such as handguns, are widely available, homicide rates are several times higher than in other industrialized nations (Rosenberg and Fenley, 1991). However, it would be an oversimplification to attribute the extreme rates of homicide in the United States only to the large numbers of handguns and ignore other underlying social and political factors, such as poverty, large disparities in wealth, a heterogeneous ethnic mix, and freely available alcohol and other drugs, with large numbers of addicts. Nevertheless, in a majority of homicides in the United States, the assailant is a family member or acquaintance. The ready access to lethal firearms in the domestic environment undoubtedly contributes to the likelihood of a fatal outcome for many conflicts (Kellermann and Reay, 1986; Sloan et al., 1988).

In tribal fights in the highlands of Papua New Guinea, the number of fatal injuries was low. Conventions were generally observed that prohibited the use of modern, highly lethal weapons such as firearms. Battles using spears and arrows without feathered vanes demand a high degree of skill and allow the release of pent-up hostili-

Though boys throw stones at frogs in sport, the frogs do not die in sport, but in earnest.

—Bion, in Plutarch, **Water and Land Animals,** *325–255 B.C.E.*

> **Violence in television and films is an international problem that is often exported for profit.**

Violence in television and movies can result in increased physical aggressiveness and imitation of violent behavior (Lancet editorial, 1994; Centerwall, 1992; Rosenberg et al., 1992). Countries need to develop effective means of monitoring and controlling violence portrayed in films made locally and in those imported from other countries.

Although production costs for one hour of a violent television program such as Miami Vice can reach $1.5 million, such programs are sold to television networks in developing countries for as little as $500 (Walker, 1990).

In India, many inhabitants of a large apartment building destroyed their own televisions by throwing them out of windows into the street, as a protest against media violence transmitted into their homes. This is a dramatic example of individual community action against media violence when bureaucrats and regulators fail to act.

The most potent weapon in the hands of the oppressor is the mind of the oppressed.
—*Steve Biko, Statement as witness, 1976*

ties and aggression between factions with a minimum loss of life (Dyke and Barss, unpublished data, 1993). A battle often ended if there was a single death. In contrast, in more "developed" countries where commercial marketing of firearms has been highly effective, even minor interpersonal conflicts often have a fatal outcome.

At an international level, militarization and the sale of lethal armaments to developing countries has substantially altered the potential for sustained conflicts and massive loss of life among civilians as well as among the military. As with the export of other dangerous products, such as tobacco and alcohol, the sale of armaments in developing countries allows populations in developed countries to enjoy the profits, while escaping the social and public health costs. The most pernicious of the armaments exported to developing countries are land mines, already discussed above. A number of prestigious universities in some developed countries are heavily subsidized by the defense industry for their activities in the development of complex weapons systems, and thereby silenced as potential critics of the military (Beardsley, 1987).

Environmental Factors

Poverty is an important risk factor for homicide. Homicide rates in Rio de Janeiro and São Paulo, Brazil, are much higher among the poor than among the middle class (World Bank, 1989). In São Paulo, death rates from murder were five times as high among industrial and manual workers as among professionals. A temporary improvement in economic conditions resulting from a development plan was associated with a decrease in the homicide rate of 40 percent.

In Canada, mortality rates from homicides are over five times greater among the lowest income quintile than the highest (Wilkins et al., 1989). Homicide and suicide were the only types of fatal injuries where the differences in mortality rates between the poorest and richest groups actually increased during the period 1971–86.

Cultural acceptance of violence is also believed to be an important factor in the etiology of violence in Brazil. The media have a powerful influence in normalizing violence. "Screen violence" is now an international threat to public health (Centerwall, 1992; Lancet editorial, 1994). Television and film from western countries, particularly the United States, are marketed at far below cost in developing countries, effectively stifling local production (Walker, 1990). This can be done because once the costs of production are recouped in the large United States market, sales at low cost to small countries simply add to corporate profits. Some form of antidumping legislation is needed to prevent marketing of violent media products in small countries at prices that destroy local production of alternative screen programs.

The impact of television violence on harmful aggressive behavior has been documented in 40 years of research and over 3,000 studies. Since adolescents and young adults are the main instigators of violence (Manciaux, 1993), the frequent exposure of children to screen violence is of great concern. During daytime viewing hours on about ten channels accessible to children in Washington, DC, there were a total of about 160–190 violent acts per hour. By the age of 11 years, an average child will have witnessed 8,000 murders and 100,000 other violent acts. It is difficult to imagine that such exposure does not induce new norms of behavior among the young people of a country.

The export of such norms to other countries requires urgent preventive action to avoid a pandemic of violence. Although most developed countries have relatively open, independent ratings systems for visual media, with open membership, this is not the case in the United States. Unfortunately, most developing countries do not have the resources to rate the film products that are marketed to them. Multilateral international action is needed to deal with the issue.

In Colombia, Bogota's two main television stations showed 1,259 violent acts during a single weekend (Vincent, 1993). Children in Colombia were reported to view an average of 27 hours of television per week, with an average of about seven violent acts per hour, as compared to 32 per hour in the United States. A survey of Colombian parents showed that 71 percent said their children imitated violent television characters, and that 77 percent of their children believed that gunshots, punches, and murders were effective means for solving problems. One mother who found that her sons behaved violently after viewing Venezuelan soap operas and United States serials succeeded in obtaining an injunction against several programs when a judge ruled that television violence contributes to real-life violence. Colombian criminals were also interviewed, and 90 percent reported that their ideas for hold-ups and other assaults came from television.

Crowding associated with rapid population growth also appears to aggravate violence (Eibl-Eibesfeldt, 1979). Rapid social change, such as has occurred in many indigenous communities in North America, has also been associated with high levels of homicide and other violence (Young, 1983, 1988; Jarvis and Boldt, 1982; Kraus and Buffler, 1979).

Scarcity of renewable resources, such as water, land, fuel, and forests, has been identified as an etiologic factor in violent conflicts (Homer-Dixon et al., 1993). Rapid population growth and overcrowding, together with maldistribution and export of vital resources are potentially modifiable determinants of scarcity.

Since family homicides are a major cause of mortality in many countries, it is important to consider specific factors associated with such injuries. These include stress resulting from lack of resources to obtain one's goals, social isolation of women or families, lack of protective services for victims of domestic violence, and the cultural belief that it is appropriate to strike women or children to express feelings or to alter behavior (Rosenberg et al., 1987).

Implications for Prevention

Documentation

An important aspect of prevention is the documentation of the existence and magnitude of a health condition, and improvements or deterioration as reflected in the incidence of new events. In addition, to implement primary prevention, it is important to determine the factors that contribute to the problem. Public health professionals can play an important role in these aspects of prevention, since they have generally received special training in methods of measuring the extent of diseases and injuries, as well as in delineating the associated circumstances, including underlying causes and high risk groups, and in evaluating the effectiveness of prevention programs.

The accurate documentation of various types of fatal and nonfatal assaults poses considerable challenges for surveillance and investigation of alleged episodes of violence (Herman and Chomsky, 1988; Armenian, 1989; Barss, 1992). Nevertheless, surveillance and documentation of the incidence, nature, and severity of injuries, together with their determinants, are essential for understanding, preventing, and controlling violence (Foege, 1986). Prospective cohort studies have been suggested for studying violence (Jeanneret and Sand, 1993). In view of the high reported incidence of violence, this may be preferable to retrospective case-control studies. Awareness and categorization of different types of violence, including violence against specific community subgroups, such as women, children, the elderly, the poor, ethnic minorities, and political victims, should help to standardize and facilitate the surveillance of violence. Investigating the underlying political, social, and economic causes of violence can be challenging and dangerous, and many public health workers and injury control professionals hesitate to take this step, or sometimes fail to appreciate its importance.

The correction of important underlying factors for violence, such as poverty and large social and economic differentials within a society, require intervention and sustained commitment at the highest political level. Controlling violence using only repressive means and imprisonment does nothing to correct the underlying causes of violence and is analogous to the former reliance on curative medicine to control immunizable infectious diseases. Accurate documentation of the extent and sources of violence may help to bring about more lasting change by highlighting problems and their sources and by increasing the pressure for change. The process of disseminating such information is obviously not without risk in many societies, as witnessed by numerous recent deaths of journalists in the Americas.

Alcohol

The importance of alcohol must be considered in any preventive intervention for violence aimed at altering personal factors. Alcohol is a substance with strong addictive properties and its use is frequently associated with interpersonal violence, suicide, unintentional injuries, and many medical and social problems (Secretary of Health and Human Services, 1990; WHO, 1985a). In the United States, poor minority groups and their neighborhoods are often the targets for aggressive advertising of alcoholic beverages and cigarettes (Ewert and Alleyne, 1992).

The use of alcohol has been rapidly increasing in some developing countries (WHO, 1985a). For example, during the period between 1960–81, annual per capita consumption of beer increased from 5 liters to 33 in the Cameroon, 4 to 43 in the Congo, and 12 to 135 in the Gabon. While overall levels of consumption still tend to be less than in developed countries, large quantities may be rapidly ingested by young adult males, who are particularly prone to drunkenness, violence and unintentional injuries, as well as marital assaults. Since the demand for beer is highly sensitive (elastic) with respect to price, increases in price by taxation can reduce consumption, especially among high risk groups of young adults. However, in some rural areas, large quantities of beer are home-brewed from crops such as millet.

When substantial increases in alcohol consumption occurred in developed countries, many adverse effects were demonstrated, and it became necessary to develop national policies to balance public health and economic objectives (WHO, 1985b). There are powerful economic incentives for increased sales by companies that wish to increase profits and by governments that have become dependent upon revenues from taxation of alcoholic beverages.

In view of the known adverse effects of alcohol and its potential for causing addiction, it is generally considered unwise to allow the laws of supply and demand to regulate marketing and sales. As in developed countries, national policies to balance public health objectives with the economic interests of producers and governments are needed. Thus, each country requires an appropriate national organization to monitor the adverse effects of alcohol on the population and to recommend appropriate legislation to modify consumption patterns, thereby countering the adverse health and social consequences in its communities.

It has been noted that countries that profit by export of alcoholic beverages to other countries reap the economic benefits of increased sales abroad, while incurring none of the adverse health and social costs of increased domestic sales (WHO, 1985b). Unfortunately, although levels of alcohol consumption in many developing countries have increased dramatically, often through establishment of local subsidiaries of breweries from developed countries, policy measures to deal with the public health effects of alcohol are limited or completely absent in most of these countries (WHO, 1985c). Effective policies are needed to reduce levels of consumption and deter binge drinking and alcohol dependency, as well as to correct the social, cultural, and economic conditions that encourage inappropriate use. Examples of interventions that have been implemented to control consumption include increases in taxation, restrictions on advertising, and restrictions on the times and locations of sales.

Although heavy taxation of alcohol and restriction of advertising may help to reduce consumption, when implementing such remedial measures, it is important not to ignore serious social and economic problems that are underlying long-term factors in the abuse of alcohol and other drugs.

Since young males are often the perpetrators and targets of violence, measures that increase meaningful employment and responsibility among this segment of the population should help to reduce their involvement in violence, including both assault and suicide. In the crowded cities of many developing countries, where ever increasing numbers of bitter and unemployed young people roam the streets (Cohen, 1989), the control of crime may require interventions by multiple sectors.

Psychosocial Environment
In societies where violence against females is a serious problem in rural villages, policies to reduce isolation of women and alter patterns of male dominance, while difficult to implement, may be helpful. Better education and more opportunities for women may also gradually reduce the male dominance that appears to be an important factor in unusually high rates of homicide and suicide among women.

To reduce the risk of child abuse, associated parental problems such as alcohol abuse must be addressed at national, community,

Nonviolence is the answer to the crucial political and moral questions of our time; the need for man to overcome oppression and violence without resorting to oppression and violence ... Man must evolve for all human conflict a method which rejects revenge, aggression and retaliation. The foundation of such a method is love.

—Martin Luther King Jr, Speech accepting the Nobel Peace Prize, 1964

and individual levels. Parents who have been abused or exposed to domestic violence appear to be at high risk of injuring their spouses and children, and may need special attention to break intergenerational cycles of domestic violence. Similarly, one-parent households may require special attention.

Complex psychosocial environmental factors underlie much violence. Since rapid increases in crowding appear to increase the risk of conflict and violence, effective means of stabilizing the population of communities and promoting only sustainable development should reduce the potential for violence and conflicts over renewable resources (Homer-Dixon et al., 1993; Last, 1993). Given the importance of endemic class warfare and structural violence in many developing countries, measures are needed to improve social equity by decreasing extreme disparities in wealth, education, and employment. A more equitable distribution of resources is urgently needed. Improved living conditions in rural areas might slow uncontrolled migration to cities. Education of women and family planning may help to reduce family sizes and provide better educational and employment opportunities for young people in both rural and urban areas.

Equipment

Equipment factors are an important determinant of violence. Access to highly lethal weapons, such as firearms, escalates the severity of violence and can initiate an ongoing cycle of retribution for previous fatalities. Thus, measures to decrease access to lethal means of resolving conflict are needed at international/national, community, and household levels. The sale of concealable weapons such as handguns and land mines is particularly reprehensible.

Efforts to restrict the sale and possession of weapons will be vigorously opposed by the arms industry. Nevertheless, in many industrialized nations, citizens and politicians have managed to place strict legal controls on the availability and access to lethal weapons.

This is, unfortunately, not the case in many developing countries. For example, in many African countries, there have been massive increases in military spending, compared to expenditures on social services such as health care (Ityavyar and Ogba, 1989). As much as 20 to 40 percent of central government expenditure goes to the military. Collective international action is necessary to redirect state funding and foreign aid towards more beneficial sectors of local economies (Overseas Development Council, 1988).

International sanctions and class action legal suits are needed against companies in developed countries that market weapons that kill many civilians. In Italy, for example, three companies that produce land mines for export have been responsible for maiming dozens of civilians each day in developing countries (McGrath, 1993a). Other major exporters of land mines have included China, Brazil, and the former Soviet republics. While such weapons are often marketed for a few dollars each, if the manufacturers were made legally responsible for the lifetime costs of all civilian victims and for removal of mines once hostilities had ended, they would soon be too expensive to buy (Ashtakala and Barss, 1996). The United States commendably introduced a moratorium on the export of these weapons (Anderson, 1993; Economist, 1994); this must be made permanent and extended world-wide.

Weapons, however beautiful, are instruments of ill omen, to all creatures. Therefore he who has Tao will have nothing to do with them.
—*Lao Tzu*, **Tao Tê Ching**, *604–531 B.C.E.*

Our weapons are space age, but our diplomacy is stone age.
—*Haroutune Armenian*, **Comment at meeting at the Johns Hopkins School of Public Health on public health impact of Gulf War**, *1994.*

Education

Although the impact on injuries of educational approaches has been difficult to verify, education may be useful in conjunction with other types of intervention. Techniques of non-violent conflict resolution involve the use of learned techniques of negotiation with an appreciation for the interests of all parties. The principles of conflict resolution are well documented in a number of publications and are taught in formal courses (Fisher, 1981; Fisher and Brown, 1988; Fisher and Ury, 1991; Laue, 1988; Moore, 1986; Susskind and Cruikshank, 1987).

Although the long-term effectiveness of training in conflict resolution remains to be demonstrated, the method has been applied to conflicts between family members, businesses, nations and other groups, both intragroup and intergroup conflicts. In Greenland, teaching non-violent conflict resolution in schools has been suggested as one means of reducing high levels of violence in the indigenous population (Breinholdt, 1991).

Unfortunately, the recent tendency to rely mainly upon military force for the resolution of international conflicts suggests that the leaders of some developed countries are unaware of the elementary principles of non-violent conflict resolution, or alternatively, that violence is their preferred method for settling differences of opinion.

Some of the measures recommended by a panel of United States psychologists to control screen violence include the portrayal in programs of non-violent methods of resolving conflicts, programs that educate children to prevent violence, restriction of dramatized violence to times when children are unlikely to be viewing, and rating programs by the level of violence portrayed (Reuters, 1993). Colombia passed legislation that bans the depiction of graphic murders, armed assaults, and car crashes from television before 10 P.M. (Vincent, 1993). A group of 22 censors screens shows for violent material and has canceled some Latin American soap operas and censored violent scenes from United States programs.

Education and improved personal contacts between members of different cultural groups as a result of improved communications and transport systems may help to reduce the ethnocentricity that is often a source of violence both locally and between nations. This should contribute to more effective negotiations between different nationalities and ethnic groups.

Measures such as multilateral international investigations and economic sanctions and boycotts may help to control state terrorism and genocide that affect internal minorities, such as the Kurds and Palestinians, and entire nations, such as the Cambodians and Timorese. Such interventions could also help to limit the damage from combative wars between nations.

The 1948 Genocide Convention was adopted by The United Nations General Assembly for the prevention and punishment of the crime of genocide (Geissler, 1986). More effective means of reporting and verifying violations and of punishing offenders are needed to ensure that the convention can fulfil its objectives. Fisher (1981) has discussed methods of modifying undesirable behaviors of governments. For effective control of state terrorism, the ultimate causes of such violence must be explored. In many countries in Latin America and other developing regions, the military has been identi-

> **Prevention of homicide and suicide includes social measures and restricted access to lethal agents and alcohol.**

Since homicide and suicide are often associated with poverty, class disparities, and alienation from society, primary prevention in the broadest sense often requires fundamental political and social change.

The environment can be also be modified by appropriate policies to provide some protection against suicide and homicide. These policies include limiting access to agents such as lethal pesticides, potentially lethal medications, and handguns. Since media portrayals of violence have been linked with both aggression and suicide, better methods of control are also required.

The depressive and disinhibiting effects of alcohol and other addictive drugs are also important in the etiology of violence, including suicide (Hayward et al., 1992), and controls on the marketing, sale, and use of such drugs are needed.

fied as the "immediate" cause of state violence and the ensuing physical injuries and mental illness of the victims of state terrorism. However, the underlying or "ultimate" cause of state violence has often been external support of the local military by foreign policy makers of western nations (Ugalde and Vega, 1989; Zwi and Ugalde, 1989).

The destruction of ethnic or racial minorities, such as indigenous inhabitants of tropical rain forests, may occur not only by direct assault, but also by indirect violence, as when the cultural and environmental conditions necessary for the physical and spiritual survival of these communities are damaged by powerful majorities. A better understanding of the destructive effects of ethnocentrism may help to protect such vulnerable minorities.

SUICIDE

My life, my real life, was in danger, and not from anything other people might do, but from the hatred I carried in my own heart.
—*James Baldwin*, Notes of a Native Son, *1955*

Suicide is a major cause of loss of potential life in industrialized countries and many developing countries, and has often increased as other causes of injury death have begun to be controlled. Suicides, both completed and attempted, are acts of violence against the self. However, the underlying determinants and motivations of this act vary from a true wish to end life to a desire to communicate anger or hopelessness (Diekstra and Gulbinat, 1993). Thus, while suicide may be used as a convenient diagnostic category, this should not obscure the search for underlying individual or community diagnoses, the proximal determinants. Similarly, although in some countries depression often includes several diagnostic categories strongly associated with suicide, depression itself is often a symptom of an underlying individual, family, or community disturbance.

Suicide is frequently an individual response to intolerable conditions; however, the conditions that precipitate persons to take their own lives are often specific to their family and/or local culture. Thus, where there are marked differences in culture and the environment, it may be misleading to generalize from data on suicides from one country to another, or even from one region or community to a neighboring area. In some cultures, preventing suicide may involve developing new societal norms for dealing with interpersonal crises and shame and for addressing certain underlying determinants if change is feasible.

While suicide is sometimes endemic within specific age and sex subgroups of a population, epidemics of suicide also occur in certain demographic subgroups. Such epidemics may be evinced by a sustained increase in incidence over several years (Rubinstein, 1983), or they may manifest as clusters of suicides in a community (O'Carroll et al., 1988; Young, 1988). In some cultures, both features may be present, as noted in Micronesia, where a sustained rise in incidence and clusters of suicides occurred among young males (Rubinstein, 1983). Clusters appear to be a feature of many suicides in North American indigenous communities (May, 1991).

Classification and Reporting of Suicides

The ICD classification system for suicide is based upon a detailed grouping by the method of suicide (WHO, 1992). These data are useful, since restriction of access to highly lethal methods appears to be one approach that is successful in preventing suicide (Marzuk et al., 1992). Of particular relevance to many developing countries is the number of suicides that result from highly toxic pesticides, and the high risk groups by age, sex, occupation, and rural/urban residence.

However, a classification of suicide based only upon the method of self-destruction is limited. Classification and study of suicide should not be restricted to deaths (Diekstra and Gulbinat, 1993). A somewhat broader focus includes consideration of mortality and morbidity, and may include suicide, parasuicide, and suicidal ideation.

Suicide involves a fatal outcome that may result from positive or negative acts, or from deliberate risk-taking behavior. Parasuicide includes attempts to cause self-harm by various methods that include physical force and ingestions. Habitual ingestion of excessive and potentially lethal quantities of alcohol and other drugs or habitual self-mutilation are not classified as parasuicides. Suicidal ideation includes thoughts that range in severity from intermittent feelings that life is not worth living to organized plans for suicide.

It has long been recognized that there are difficulties in obtaining valid mortality rates for suicide (Sainsbury, 1983). At least some of the differences among countries in reported rates may be because of variability in the completeness and accuracy of reporting. In ten mainland countries in the Americas for which data were available, reported age-adjusted suicide rates ranged between 0.5 (Guatemala) and 19 (Suriname) per 100,000 population per year, with a median rate of 5 (PAHO, 1986).

In some countries, most suicides are reported in the category of undetermined intent, or as unintentional or "accidental" injury deaths (Diekstra and Gulbinat, 1993). There are often substantial pressures on coroners and lay juries at coroners' inquests to report a suicide as an unintentional death (Jacobson et al., 1976). Such pressures can result from religious and social considerations, as well as from the financial impact of a verdict of suicide on life insurance payments.

In Greenland during 1977–86, it was found that suicides among the Inuit and other residents were accurately classified as such. Death certification was based upon joint examination of each case by the police and the district medical officer (Thorslund and Misfeldt, 1989). This joint assessment is required by law. However, in Alaska during 1979–84, suicides among indigenous Americans were frequently found to be misclassified, with only 5 out of 38 suicides classified as such in both coroners' files and in records of vital statistics (Marshall and Soule, 1988). In both Greenland and Alaska, police reports were found to contain the essential elements of a "psychological autopsy"; however, there appeared to be greater communication problems between departments in Alaska than in Greenland.

Despite reporting problems, national mortality data have in general been found to be valuable for epidemiological purposes (Diekstra and Gulbinat, 1993). Hospital admissions can be studied to document parasuicides, but underreporting may be severe. Other sources of data include records of various types of practitioners and confidential population surveys. The latter show much higher suicidal ideation and parasuicide than would be expected from hospital data. In such surveys, the incidence of suicidal ideation may be studied for a defined retrospective period or as a lifetime incidence.

In surveys of suicide, parasuicide, and suicidal ideation, it is pertinent to study not only the personal characteristics of affected individuals, but also those of other significant members of their family or community. These characteristics should be compared with those of unaffected controls. If a particular sex and/or age group is already known to be at high risk, then controls might be matched on age and sex. Mortality and/or morbidity interview questionnaires can be developed that include not only general determinants of suicide, but also factors specific to the local culture. For example, by comparison with controls, suicidal ideation among Zuni Indian adolescents was found to be associated not only with individual drug use, lack of communication skills, and other factors, but also with drug use by their parents (Howard-Pitney et al., 1992). The choice of interviewers is critical for such a sensitive topic.

Examples of Mortality from Suicide

Suicide rates from developing countries that report to the World Health Organization are included in Table 13.3, with a few industrialized countries as comparisons. The rates included in the table are probably underestimates because of the reporting problems discussed above. Most of the least developed countries were not able to provide any data at all. Cuba is not included in the table, but in 1988 the overall suicide rate for both sexes combined was high, 23 per 100,000 (PAHO, 1990). Low rates cannot be assumed simply because there are no officially reported data or public outcry; extremely high rates of suicide were found in special surveys from an undeveloped rural area of Papua New Guinea, as discussed below under personal factors (Barss, 1991; D. Smith, 1981). The fact that such findings were not an aberration has been confirmed by recent data from a much larger population in rural China, also discussed below (WHO, 1991).

Suicide can account for a large proportion of all deaths, and is sometimes the leading cause of death among young adults. Sri Lanka is an example of a developing country with a high suicide rate, mainly from ingestion of pesticides; in 1981, suicide accounted for 5 percent of all deaths (Anywar et al., 1986). As a comparison, in England and Wales, suicide accounted for 1 percent of deaths.

In women of childbearing age (15–44 years) in rural Bangladesh during 1976–86, the suicide rate was moderately high, 13 per 100,000 per year, and accounted for 5 percent of all deaths in this age group. Two-thirds of suicides resulted from the use of a herbicide or other poison and one-third from hanging (Fauveau and Blanchet, 1989). In this population, the highest suicide rate was noted among the youngest women, with a rate of 23 per 100,000 per year for 15–24-year-olds; the rates for 25–34-year-olds and 35–44-year-olds were 6 and 2 respectively. In teenagers 15–19 years of age, suicide and complications of induced abortion accounted for 94 percent of all deaths during pregnancy.

In the Americas, the highest suicide rates are found in the oldest age groups. However, recent trends have shown substantial increases in suicide among adolescents and young adults, and, in developing

Table 13.3. Reported suicide rates in various developing countries, with other countries for comparison

	Deaths/100,000/year*		
	males	*females*	*Year*
AFRICA			
Mauritius	20	4	1994
SOUTHEAST ASIA			
China, rural	24	31	1994
China, urban	7	7	1994
Sri Lanka	47	19	1986
EASTERN MEDITERRANEAN			
Egypt	0	0	1987
AMERICAS			
El Salvador	17	7	1984
Uruguay	17	4	1990
Argentina	9	3	1991
Chile	8	1	1992
Costa Rica	7	1	1991
Ecuador	6	3	1988
Colombia	5	1	1991
Panama	6	2	1987
Mexico	5	1	1993
Paraguay	3	2	1987
Guyana	2	1	1984
Guatemala	1	0	1984
Surinam	32	12	1985
COMPARISON			
Russian Federation	74	13	1994
Sweden	22	10	1993
United States	20	5	1992
Great Britain	12	3	1994
Kuwait	1	1	1987

Sources: World Health Statistics Annual 1986–1995 (WHO 1986–1996).

*Rates not adjusted for age.

countries in the Americas, suicide has become a severe problem for 15–24-year-olds (PAHO, 1986, 1990). In Ethiopia, 38 percent of suicides reported by government health facilities involved children below the age of 15 years, and may be related to pesticide ingestion (Larson and Dessie, 1993).

Suicide rates are extremely high in many indigenous communities in the Americas and Greenland. In Greenland during 1985–90, the rate of suicide was 138 per 100,000 per year, while in Denmark in 1989 the rate was 26 (Breinholdt, 1991). Similarly, in Canada, suicide rates are high among young aboriginals (Young, 1983, 1992; Muir, 1991; Trovato, 1988; Hislop et al., 1987; Mao et al., 1986; Boldt, 1985), as they are in the United States (Baker et al., 1992; Middaugh, 1992; Middaugh et al., 1991; Marshall and Soule, 1988; Kraus and Buffler, 1979). However, there are significant differences in suicide rates between indigenous populations. For example, rates among the Cree of eastern James Bay, Canada, are similar to those in the general population, while among the nearby Inuit, rates are much higher (Damestoy, 1994; Barss, 1998a; Boyer et al., 1994a, 1994b; Petawabano et al., 1994).

Suicide rates among indigenous Greenlanders have increased markedly from 3–4 per 100,000 per year during the first half of this century to 93 for males and 78 for females during 1968–85 (Bjerregaard, 1991). During substantial portions of the latter period, suicide was the most frequent single cause of death among males, followed by drownings. Young males aged 15–24 were at especially high risk. Thus, suicide among young people accounted for about 10 percent of all deaths in Greenland (Misfeldt and Senderovitz, 1989). Among indigenous Alaskans, suicide rates increased from 28 per 100,000 per year for males and 12 for females in 1950 to 84 and 14, respectively, during 1980–89 (Middaugh et al., 1991).

Very few countries have reported decreases in suicide rates; however, there were actual declines in suicide rates in Japan for all ages and in Great Britain among the elderly (Diekstra and Gulbinat, 1993). When known, the reasons for these changes and for differences between the rates for various indigenous populations could be useful to other countries.

Examples of Morbidity from Suicide

Data are scarce on morbidity from suicide attempts in developing countries. As a possible indication of the relative frequency of suicide attempts and completed suicides, it is illustrative to consider data from a few developed countries and from one of their indigenous populations.

In developed countries, parasuicides or suicide attempts are reported to be from 10 to 50 times more common than completed suicides and are generally more frequent among young females (Diekstra and Gulbinat, 1993; O'Carroll, 1992; Boldt, 1987). Although the seriousness of such attempts varies markedly, their frequency indicates the general severity of the problem in the population.

In a large multisite survey in the United States, it was found that three out of every 1,000 adults had attempted suicide in the previous year (Moscicki et al., 1989). A survey in Calgary, Canada, revealed that 13 percent of adults had made plans for suicide in their lifetime, 6 percent had deliberately harmed themselves, and 4 percent had attempted suicide. In the year preceding the survey, 4 percent had made plans for suicide and 2 percent had deliberately harmed themselves or had attempted suicide (Ramsay and Bagley, 1985). In a population-based survey of several Cree indigenous nations of northern Canada, it was found that 4 percent of the population aged 15 and over had attempted to commit suicide at some point in their lives

(Boyer et al., 1994b). This prevalence figure was similar to that for the general population of the same province. About 3 percent of Crees aged 15–44 years had a history of a parasuicide in the preceding 12 months, while in the age group of 45 and older there had been no parasuicides. Among Navajo indigenous Americans in the United States, nearly 15 percent of 7,524 students in grades 6 through 12 who were surveyed in 1988 reported a previous suicide attempt (Grossman et al., 1991).

Determinants of Suicide

While there are many factors associated with suicide discussed below, there are a few that have been cited as being particularly amenable to public health intervention (Diekstra and Gulbinat, 1993), including the following:

- Psychological risk factors, including mental and physical illness, alcoholism, financial problems, and interpersonal disputes;
- Easy access to a lethal agent;
- Publicity about suicidal acts.

Personal Factors

Personal factors such as age, sex, mental and physical illness, and alcoholism are important considerations in deaths from suicide. While alcoholism and binge drinking are frequently associated with suicide, they may not always be the underlying cause (May, 1991, 1992; Grossman et al., 1991; Breinholdt, 1991; Thorslund, 1990; Marshall and Soule, 1988; Lowentels and Miller, 1984; Hudgens, 1983; Jarvis and Boldt, 1982; Kraus and Buffler, 1979). Alcohol abuse may be a result of other underlying community, family, or personal disturbances. Nevertheless, inappropriate use of alcohol can be a major contributor to suicides. Although after initial ingestion of alcohol, brain serotonin levels rise and the individual may experience a sense of well-being; this is followed by a drop in serotonin, which has been associated with suicide and aggressive violence among a substantial proportion of populations (Wright, 1995; Kotulak, 1993). Among indigenous Americans in the United States, it was estimated that alcohol was involved in 75 percent of suicides (May, 1992).

High rates of suicide among males or females at different phases of the life cycle appear to reflect stresses specific to the local culture rather than an intrinsic effect of gender. Thus, age and sex-specific rates of suicide, parasuicide, and suicidal ideation can provide important clues concerning potential environmental stressors that should be investigated more intensively by special surveys, as well as case-control and/or cohort studies.

In developed countries, completed suicide tends to be more common among males, and attempted suicide among females. This is not always the case in developing countries, where suicide rates are sometimes very high among rural females. Examples are found among subsistence cultivators in the highlands of Papua New Guinea (D. Smith, 1981), in villages in China (WHO, 1991), in Delhi, India (Singh et al., 1971), and among Indians living in Fiji (Price and Karim, 1975).

The suicide rate in rural China among women aged 15–24 was

Alcohol is a factor in many suicides in indigenous communities in developed countries.

In developed countries, the depressant and disinhibiting effects of alcohol on persons who are already depressed from a personal loss or other crisis are known to be particularly serious. The importance of alcohol in suicides in developing countries must be clarified, especially for adult males. The adverse effects of alcohol may have a much greater negative impact in communities that have been destabilized by loss of traditional social structures and support, as observed in many indigenous communities in developed countries and in poor populations in inner city slums of the United States.

Even in communities with high overall suicide rates, the most severe impact of alcohol may be concentrated among a minority of families that are at unusual risk because within the households there exist severe social problems exacerbated by alcohol (May, 1987).

Community interventions to limit the use of alcohol during temporary depression resulting from interpersonal crises could help to prevent many suicides in indigenous communities in developed countries.

48 per 100,000 during 1989 (WHO, 1991) and among 20–24 year olds in 1986 was 78 per 100,000 (Li and Baker, 1991).

Suicide is especially common among elderly males in developed countries. The potential importance of suicide as a cause of death among the elderly in developing countries appears to have been underestimated, possibly because of the smaller populations at risk, a lack of data or, in some countries, the greater respect shown the elderly, placing them at lower risk. However, even if in certain countries the elderly may formerly have been accorded respect and special treatment, demographic and social change have important effects on the numbers and status of the elderly. As more data become available, suicide among the elderly may be found to be a serious problem in many of the developing countries.

In China in 1989, suicide rates were higher among the elderly than for any other age group. In rural areas, suicide rates for the age group of 75 years and older were 141 per 100,000 for males and 98 for females, compared to overall suicide rates for all ages of 23 for males and 32 for females. In urban areas, suicide rates for the elderly were 60 for males and 47 for females, while the rates for all ages were 8 for males and 10 for females (WHO, 1991). As an external comparison, the suicide rates for the 75 and older age group in the United States in 1988 were 58 for males and 6 for females (WHO, 1991).

Extreme rates of suicide among specific subgroups of a population by age or sex are often the result of adverse psychosocial and environmental conditions in a culture rather than a specific propensity for persons of a particular age or sex to take their own lives, as discussed below. Nevertheless, certain subgroups of a population may be at particular risk because of personal factors. For example, in Brighton, England, it was found that there appeared to be at least three distinct types of victims of suicide (Bagley et al., 1976). The first included elderly persons of the middle class who were living alone and depressed; many had lost a spouse. They tended to kill themselves by an overdose of drugs. The second group included persons from a deprived background with early disruption of family life, difficulties with employment, social isolation, and sociopathic personality. A third group included persons suffering from chronic depression, often with a history of psychiatric treatment and previous suicide attempts.

Further study is needed in developing countries to better define the reasons for suicide and its meaning for different age and sex groups in specific cultures and communities. While in some cultures various types of untreated mental illness are probably important determinants in a substantial proportion of suicides, in others, social and environmental factors such as isolation, shame, poverty, family stress, and alcoholism may be more common as underlying causes for high rates of suicide.

Thus, where clusters of suicides or endemic high rates of suicide occur among certain demographic subgroups of the population, suicides are often more clearly linked with characteristics of the local society than with specific mental illnesses of individuals. For example, for all suicides in Greenland between 1977–86, the investigating police were able to find problems that might have triggered the suicide in 90 percent of cases, but in only about 30 percent of cases was there psychological background information to explain the suicide (Thorslund and Misfeldt, 1989).

In the highlands of Papua New Guinea, where the incidence of suicides of young women is among the highest in the world, psychological autopsies rarely found psychological risk factors or mental illness as a determinant of suicide. Marital conflicts were often precipitating factors for female suicides (Dyke and Barss, unpublished data, 1993).

Equipment Factors

Poisoning is the most common method of suicide in many countries. In some of the least developed areas, hanging is the most common method, while in certain parts of India, burning and drowning are more frequently used. In developing countries, commonly used poisons include the herbicide paraquat, organophosphate insecticides, and certain medications (see the section on poisonings in chapter 10). Natural plant poisons such as rotenones (derris root) are also sometimes used. Paraquat is extremely toxic and is a major agent in both suicide and unintentional poisoning; in many countries, it continues to be sold at small shops to illiterate individuals in unmarked containers, such as soda bottles. Inexpensive and highly lethal tablets of an insecticide, aluminum phosphide, are often used for suicide by members of poor farm families in India, especially women (Joshi, 1991). In a village survey, pesticides were the only method used in all recent suicides (Mohan, 1993).

The ready availability in rural households of extremely toxic pesticides, including insecticides, has made it easy for young people who are suffering temporary stress to obtain these chemicals for suicide attempts. Such cases are frequently fatal, whereas they would less often have ended in death if extremely toxic chemicals had been unavailable.

Many therapeutic or prophylactic medications are widely available in developing countries without a prescription. Some, such as the antimalarial chloroquine, are lethal in quantities only slightly greater than a therapeutic dose. In Papua New Guinea, chloroquine tablets are increasingly used for suicide in place of other methods such as hanging (Sengupta et al., 1986).

In communities where firearms are widespread, access to such weapons in a household can increase the risk of suicide (O'Carroll et al., 1991) by as much as tenfold in the 15–24 year age group (Kellermann and Reay, 1986). In the United States, firearms, particularly handguns, are the most commonly used agent for suicide (O'Carroll et al., 1991; Baker et al., 1992). The presence of a gun in the home has been found to be associated with a significant increase in risk of suicide. Firearms are often used for suicides in aboriginal communities in developed countries. In countries where firearms are less available, other agents are favored. Nevertheless, the increasing militarization and sales of firearms in many developing countries may lead to increases in suicide by firearms in the future, as weapons and ammunition are stored in households and as familiarity with the method grows.

Environmental Factors

Suicide has been conceptualized as an individual response to intolerable life conditions (Boldt, 1988). These conditions most often arise during certain critical periods of the life cycle, during late adolescence or early adult life, and middle or old age (Sorensen, 1991).

Poverty is one factor associated with the risk of death from suicide. In both the United States and Canada, the risk of suicide is twice as high among the lowest quintile of income as among the highest (Baker et al., 1992; Wilkins et al., 1989). Since the data were not adjusted for other confounding factors, it is possible that other factors associated with poverty are more significant than poverty itself as a risk factor for suicide. Poverty among retirees has also been reported as a factor in suicides in Argentina (Nash, 1992).

As discussed above, on first impression many suicides appear to be a result of personal risk factors such as a vulnerable age or sex or particular individual circumstances. Further study, however, may show that a majority of these deaths were associated with a more generalized adverse psychosocial environment in the community or in the family. Nevertheless, the deleterious effects of an unhealthy psychosocial environment may exert their greatest impact on the most vulnerable individuals in the community. Thus, suicides in known high-risk age and sex groups should be considered as potential sentinel or warning events indicative of social pathology in the family, community, or nation.

Marked differences in the environment from one culture to another are often evidenced by widely disparate high risk groups for suicide by age and sex. For example, in remote subsistence communities with a patrilineal kinship system in the highlands of Papua New Guinea, the suicide rate was very high among young females during the early years of marriage, as discussed above (Barss, 1991). High rates of female suicide occurred in a cultural milieu of extreme male dominance and violence, on a geographical background of remoteness and isolation in small hamlets.

In contrast, in matrilineal communities in Micronesia, very high rates of suicide have been observed among adolescent males, with low rates among females (Rubinstein, 1983). In Sri Lanka, suicide rates are high among both men and women.

Suicide rates among young males in Micronesia were highest in periurban villages and lower in remote communities. Among young women in Papua New Guinea, on the other hand, suicide rates were significantly lower in periurban villages than in remote subsistence villages (Barss, 1991). In China, suicide rates were high among young women living in rural villages and much lower among urban women (WHO, 1991; Li and Baker, 1991).

Such large differences in suicide rates among cultures can be confusing to a policymaker searching for universal causes amenable to standard programmatic interventions. However, local answers may come from a better understanding of culture-specific meanings of suicide and of the conditions that render life intolerable for certain high risk groups in the local culture(s) (Boldt, 1988).

For example, high rates of suicide among young females in isolated villages in rural patrilineal societies appear to reflect the impossibility of escape from the overwhelming stresses of marriage for females in such communities. On the other hand, high recent rates of suicide among young males in Micronesian communities are reported to be a result of the uncertain status of adolescent males in a matrilineal society where rapid change has resulted in exacerbations of intergenerational conflicts and loss of the traditionally meaningful activities and socialization for adolescent males. On this environmental background, imitative cluster suicides among young males have been a recurring problem.

Stresses related to the difficulties of coping with rapid social and environmental changes and the ethnocentrism of dominant white majorities appear to account, at least in part, for high suicide rates observed in indigenous communities in North America and Greenland (Thorslund, 1990; Young, 1988; Jarvis and Boldt, 1982; Kraus and Buffler, 1979). Parental lack of self-esteem and other problems, such as alcohol abuse, may account for adolescent suicides, and any study of adolescent suicide must focus on the family unit, as well as the community. Cultural and community problems can have a severe impact on parents that may be expressed indirectly via their children. An adverse atmosphere in the parental home appeared to contribute to the risk of suicide among indigenous Greenlanders; this included disharmony, quarrels, and alcohol abuse (Thorslund, 1990). Suicide was generally associated with poverty. In towns, the suicide risk was highest among hunters, fishers, the unemployed, and persons with unstable occupations.

In the rural Bangladeshi population discussed earlier, the high suicide rate among young unmarried women and high mortality rate from induced abortion were believed to be a consequence of strict control by males over the sexual life of females and reproduction. Also as a result of male dominance, few women in the society were able to attain secondary education, to work, or to move about outside their households. The authors suggested that the provision of safe abortion services at an early stage of pregnancy (menstrual regulation) for unmarried women might help to reduce the high death rate from traditional abortions and suicide (Fauveau and Blanchet, 1989).

The media can contribute to an increase in suicide. Some studies have found an increase in the incidence of suicide related to television stories and movies about suicide (O'Carroll et al., 1991). Exposure to portrayals of suicide as an exciting or glamorous response to personal romantic problems or intergenerational family conflicts would be expected to exert a disproportionately powerful impact on susceptible populations with relatively limited exposure to screen media.

High rates of suicide have been observed among prisoners, especially indigenous males, after incarceration. It has been recommended that prisoners should be interviewed by a psychologist on arrival to determine whether they are at potential risk of suicide.

Implications for Prevention

The prevention of suicide can be undertaken at various levels, including community, regional, or national (Berger and Tobeluk, 1991; Claymore, 1988). Surveillance of risk groups for suicide by age and sex and a more detailed assessment of the circumstances of suicide can be helpful in assessing local determinants and in planning appropriate interventions. Suicide may sometimes have to be considered as a public health emergency when contagious spread to other persons is probable. Thus, surveillance for clusters of suicides may be justifiable, especially for certain high-risk populations, such as many North American aboriginal communities (MMWR, 1990).

At a national level, legislation to limit domestic access to highly lethal agents of suicide has been helpful. Policies to modify marketing,

Sometimes people kill themselves because they have found no one to help them. They have lost hope in mankind. They have found no compassion. When we are truly filled with the idea of reverence for life, all our attitudes, action, thinking change. We must go deep into ourselves to find inspiration. Slogans, publicity, and means of communication don't help us to find this philosophy. Nor is there one formula for everyone. . . .
—Albert Schweitzer, Answer to a journalist's question about suicide, 1959

> **Multisectoral collaboration can prevent or control suicide clusters in young people.**

Some communities have found it useful to prepare a plan in advance. Then, when someone harms or tries to harm himself or herself, the people already know what to do. This plan includes collaboration of the schools, media, health workers, police, counselors, and others. It involves helping the affected person, their family, friends, and the community before the harmful behavior spreads to others. People have found it helpful to share the responsibility of coping with and preventing these tragic events. Public health agencies may be able to play a coordinating role (Centers for Disease Control, 1988).

sales, and consumption patterns of alcohol should be considered. The impact of media portrayals of suicide may need to be monitored.

At national, regional, and community levels, social policies to reduce severe stress on certain highly vulnerable subgroups of the society may be helpful. Examples of such vulnerable subgroups include young adult females in rural China and Papua New Guinea, adolescent males in Micronesia, and young adults in indigenous communities in Canada, the United States, and Greenland.

Culture-specific interventions and programs for vulnerable minorities may need to be developed in close cooperation with the local community, as has been suggested for indigenous communities in Canada (Boldt, 1985). Where specific mental illnesses are shown to account for a major proportion of suicides, better recognition of the signs and symptoms of mental illness, especially depression, and improved access to treatment of underlying causes of depression may help to reduce suicide rates among affected individuals.

A reduction in the availability of a locally favored method or agent of suicide can reduce the incidence of suicide. While it might be expected that persons intending to commit suicide would simply switch to another method, generally this does not appear to be the case, since the majority of persons who kill themselves do so during a severe, but temporary, crisis and may not switch to a different method if the favored agent is unavailable (Seiden, 1977).

Barbiturates used to be the leading means of suicide by drugs in many countries; however, as safer alternatives were developed, physicians changed their prescribing patterns to less toxic medications with the result that fewer drug ingestions eventuated in completed suicides. Strict controls on the dispensing of especially toxic drugs, such as the antimalarial chloroquine, could be useful in developing countries, but may be difficult to implement where such products are widely used by households for personal and family prophylaxis and treatment.

The adverse effects of alcohol and the need for national policies to control quantities and patterns of consumption of this addictive and toxic substance have already been discussed above under prevention of homicide and other violence. Similar considerations apply to the prevention of alcohol-associated suicides, since both chronic alcoholism and acute binge drinking are frequently associated with suicide. The importance of avoiding the use of alcohol during depression and personal crises must be emphasized to physicians, as well as to families.

Reductions in suicide and unintentional deaths have sometimes occurred when changes in the availability of lethal agents occurred for reasons unrelated to public health objectives. An example is the change in the composition of household cooking gas mentioned above. Natural gas contains no carbon monoxide, while coal gas contains about 20 percent (Lester and Abe, 1992; WHO, 1982). A business decision to convert from coal gas to natural gas for domestic use in the United States in the 1950s and in Japan in the 1970s had a marked impact on deaths from suicide and unintentional poisonings. In Great Britain, suicide rates fell by about one-third after this change and there did not appear to have been a switch to other methods.

Similarly, the introduction of emission controls and the use of catalytic converters on automobiles in the United States was associated with a decline in car exhaust suicides, while in Great Britain, where emission controls were not introduced, suicides by this method increased (Clark and Lester, 1987). Thus, control measures on sales and packaging implemented to prevent unintentional poisonings from lethal agricultural chemicals should also help to prevent suicides from these agents. A special training program for vendors of pesticides and farmers has been developed in Sri Lanka (Cormier, 1993). Pesticides must be stored in appropriate containers and locked away from teenagers and other vulnerable individuals. However, new societal norms may need to be established in communities where suicide is an acceptable response to interpersonal crises.

In industrialized countries, it has been reported that the early diagnosis and effective treatment of various types of mental illness, such as depression, can prevent many suicides (WHO, 1982). Suicide prevention programs in developed countries sometimes promote a medical model of prevention with the emphasis on early detection and treatment of depression and other mental illness by health professionals, such as psychiatrists. However, it has been suggested that this "mental illness conception of suicide" may inhibit prevention by defining suicidal behavior as a problem for mental health professionals (Boldt, 1987).

Mental health personnel are in very short supply in developing countries, and their training is generally focused on dealing with individual clinical problems rather than with the development and implementation of public health approaches of primary prevention directed towards modifying the psychosocial environment in the community. The recognition and treatment of specific mental illnesses in developing countries may be less important overall for the prevention of suicides than in developed countries. In any case, a clinical approach based on individual treatment is generally less feasible than a public health approach because of limited resources and scarcity of mental health professionals.

If depression is found to be an important factor in suicides in a region, it could be useful to develop programs to improve the early recognition and management of severe depression and its underlying determinants by families and health professionals and to promote increased public awareness of the preventability of suicide and recognition of its early warning signs and symptoms, particularly among the most vulnerable subgroups of the population.

When suicide is defined as a community problem, shame and stigma for individuals may be reduced, and the efforts of the community can be focused on understanding and correcting the problems and stressors that engender suicidal behavior among certain high-risk groups, such as adolescent males, young married females, or elderly widowed males. A "life-enhancement" conception has been recommended with a shift in the moral onus for prevention of suicide from the individual to society (Boldt, 1987).

Where the underlying determinant for adolescent suicide lies with the parents and/or the community, parental and community distress must be addressed. In some aboriginal communities, children who were sent away by the government to residential schools at an early age have had little experience of normal parent-child interactions. Many find it difficult to communicate with and discipline their own children.

> **Innovative population and community approaches are needed to control suicide.**

A policy emphasis on altering adverse social influences at a community or population level rather than an individual clinical approach based upon classical psychiatric medical models may be most appropriate for resolving the suicide problem in many developing countries and indigenous communities. Interventions that address only an effect of a disturbed community, such as suicide, rather than the underlying causes in the community may not provide long-term improvements (Rodgers, 1991).

In any case, the number of mental health professionals is extremely limited in most developing countries and indigenous communities and a public health approach is essential.

Rural societies in developing countries where young adult females are at high risk of suicide provide an example of the importance of community factors in raising the risk of suicide among subgroups of the population.

Special resources may be needed to help remote communities gain local control of their suicide problem.

In the United States, the Indian Health Service organized a Special Initiatives Team to act as a resource group to disrupted communities suffering from suicide and other violence (De-Bruyn et al., 1988). They provided consultations to communities upon request and helped them to identify problems and possible solutions, while leaving the decisions and interventions up to the community itself.

In an extensive bibliography of suicide among American aboriginals, the following four general approaches to suicide prevention were suggested for these populations (May, 1991):

- Socioeconomic improvement;
- Enhancement of self-esteem;
- Specific intervention protocols for communities with crises of multiple suicides;
- Monitoring and evaluation of various suicide prevention programs.

Other promising approaches include correcting determinants, such as alcohol and drug abuse and poor interpersonal communication skills (May, 1986).

Better education and employment opportunities for women could help to reduce suicide among young females in rural communities where male dominance persists. Communities that are affected by high female suicide rates may need help in organizing themselves to understand and deal with the attitudes and domestic factors that make the lives of so many women intolerable. Reducing the isolation of women in remote villages could have a useful effect in reducing the stresses and domestic tensions that lead to suicide (Barss, 1991). Family planning may also have a role as suggested in the study from Bangladesh described above (Fauveau and Blanchet, 1989).

chapter 14

Choice and Development of Injury Prevention Programs

Injury control becomes a possibility when at least one person recognizes that injuries are an important problem in the community. However, recognition alone is not enough.

An essential insight is an awareness that the probability of specific types of injuries is significantly increased by certain exposures and combinations of risk factors. Such insights often occur first among health providers who take a few moments to inquire about the external causes for the injuries sustained by their patients, or by coroners who make similar inquiries during investigations of fatal injuries. However, this process of professional awakening generally requires that an individual health provider see many cases of specific injuries and maintain systematic records. In some countries or regions, a substantial proportion of injury victims are never seen by a health provider.

A more systematic approach to the epidemiologic surveillance of rates and circumstances of specific injuries has gradually developed in recent years. Compilation and analysis of the details of large numbers of injury events rapidly dispels the notion that injuries are purely random events. High risk groups, hazardous equipment and environmental factors, and dangerous activities can be identified. The results of injury surveillance should provide important insights for policy makers who have already realized that injuries are an important problem in their community, but who may not have recognized that something can be done to prevent them.

Policymakers must be convinced that most injuries are predictable and preventable before they can shed traditional fatalistic attitudes that injuries are a result of bad luck, acts of God, or sorcery. A similar process of awakening had to occur before policy makers could begin to prevent the extensive damage to health that results from cigarette smoking. Although not every cigarette smoker develops lung cancer, and the exact moment when a cancer develops is not predictable, it is now clear that the risk of cancer and many other diseases is greatly increased by inhalation exposure to tobacco smoke.

Similarly, not every drunken driver is involved in a crash on any

It is more important and more sensible to materialize our minds than to try to spiritualize matter. If mind cannot find expression in material form, or in some action or achievement in life, it remains a mere thought or a vague emotion that remains within our heads or hearts and never finds any expression in words, deeds, or works of art.
—*Lama Anagarika Govinda,* **Buddhist Reflections,** *1991*

specific day, but the probability of a crash is greatly increased in the presence of the central nervous system impairment that results from alcohol. Nor does every member of a family that uses open flames in the home for cooking, heating, or lighting die or be maimed by burns or smoke inhalation; nevertheless, the probability or risk of these injuries is substantially greater in the presence of daily household exposures to open flames.

A final step in the development of individual and community awareness that injuries can be controlled is knowing some of the successful interventions that have been developed in other communities, regions, or countries. Sharing experiences at meetings and dissemination of information about successful interventions can be instrumental in generating enthusiasm to initiate change.

DEVELOPING AN INJURY CONTROL PROGRAM

The first steps in developing a public health program include the identification of specific health problems in a population and the setting of priorities by ranking these problems in order of importance (Pineault and Daveluy, 1986). Programs or countermeasures then must be developed and implemented to deal with the selected priority problems. Finally, the impact of the program(s) on the health problem should be measured.

Ideally, one would like to measure health positively instead of studying only negative adverse outcomes. Nevertheless, in the case of injuries, positive changes in the harmful impact of injuries, as reflected in improvements in various indicators of mortality and morbidity, do provide tangible measures of improvement.

High-Risk Group and Population Approaches to Prevention

The principle of management by exception suggests that regions, communities, or population subgroups with unusually high injury rates should be identified so that they can be targeted for special interventions. The circumstances of the most common injuries among high-risk individuals or groups must be determined, since they may differ from the general population. For example, young children in villages with unenclosed wells must be protected against falling in, even though the problem is specific to one age group and to villages with open wells.

On the other hand, most of the population attributable risk, or the greatest proportion of the total burden of all injuries, may come from the larger low-risk portion of the population. Thus, other interventions should be considered for the general population. Measures may be needed to protect all persons at risk and not only those individuals at highest risk (Rose, 1992). Often, however, interventions that are introduced to protect high-risk individuals also provide the most effective protection for the general population. In illustration, signs and road markings that are designed to be obvious to elderly drivers with reduced night vision are seen more easily by all drivers.

Multisectoral Nature of Injury Control

Injury prevention programs often require the cooperation of various government departments and private organizations. The planning and implementation of injury control programs may demand greater coordination and communication than a typical vertical health program, such as an immunization campaign. Departments of public health and health ministries should be considered potential coordinators for a multisectoral program to deal with injuries (Gosselin et al., 1991). Public health staff are usually highly motivated and well situated to carry out comprehensive ongoing surveillance of injuries and their causes and circumstances, and to provide a balanced portrait of the effect of different types of injuries on a population.

Many effective interventions for the control of injuries, be they directed towards modification of environmental, equipment, or personal factors, ultimately derive from legislation and regulation. Sectors other than health often have greater authority to develop the legislation and regulations needed to prevent injuries. The expertise of professionals from multiple disciplines must be integrated to develop the most effective and efficient solutions for specific injury problems. For certain types of injuries, such as traffic injuries, drownings, or sports injuries, departments or organizations other than those involved with public health may be more efficient in coordinating prevention activities by multiple organizations. Public health epidemiologists can provide technical assistance to such groups in the development of surveillance and research.

Politicians often have the ultimate say in whether funds are allocated to study and prevent injuries, and they develop and approve legislation. Politicians tend to be driven more by economic pressures than by those issues of human health and suffering that motivate health professionals.

Thus, health and other sectors should collaborate with economists to clearly and forcefully document the short and long-term economic impact of injuries. This involves analysis of the direct and indirect costs of premature mortality and morbidity, including temporary and permanent disability.

Steps to Develop an Injury Control Program

The main steps in developing a program to control injuries are outlined in Table 14.1. These include prioritizing injuries and populations or regions, investigating and identifying local determinants of specific injuries, applying criteria of efficacy, efficiency, and feasibility of potential interventions to select determinants to be targeted for modification, developing programs and interventions, and evaluating the interventions.

Identify and Prioritize Injury Problems

To identify which types of injuries should be prioritized for prevention, it is necessary to determine the health indicators to be used in setting priorities. Measures of mortality, of morbidity, and of the economic impact of injuries were discussed in Chapters 1–5.

The health sector, with its epidemiological focus and experi-

No great thing is created suddenly, any more than a bunch of grapes or a fig. If you tell me that you desire a fig, I answer you that there must be time. Let it first blossom, then bear fruit, then ripen.

—Epictetus, **Discourses,** *bk 1, ch 15, 55–135 C.E.*

Table 14.1. Steps to develop an injury control program

1. **Identify injury problems**
   - Assess size of the problem for different specific injuries in mortality, morbidity, and cost.
   - Define high-risk subgroups of the population.

2. **Determine specific circumstances of injury**
   - Ascertain where, when, and how incidents occur.
   - Compile data on associated activities, as well as personal, product or equipment, and environmental factors.

3. **For each injury problem**
   - Identify all possible preventive measures.
   - Consider modifiable personal, equipment, and environmental factors for preevent, event, and postevent phases.
   - Determine feasibility, acceptability, and cost of all measures likely to be effective.

4. **Prioritize interventions based upon**
   - Size of the problem.
   - Likelihood of success in reducing it.
   - Constraints—political, economic, other.
   - Possibility of additional beneficial effects.

5. **Implement interventions**
   - Design both the program and its evaluation.
   - Involve relevant sectors, such as health, transport, police, labor, finance, and education.
   - Secure backing of influential groups.
   - Identify individuals to play key leadership roles.
   - Obtain commitments of funding, manpower, and other resources.
   - Educate media, legislators, other decision-makers, and the community.

6. **Evaluate effect of intervention(s):**
   - Measure changes in health outcomes.
   - Measure changes in process objectives such as knowledge, attitudes, and practices.

ence in processing health data, can play an important role by providing objective information needed to guide policymakers in various sectors. Police and coroners' departments may also maintain records that can be valuable sources of information about intentional and unintentional injuries. Priorities should be based not only on the relative size of various injury problems, but also on the degree to which the particular injuries can effectively be prevented or reduced.

A focused program that can successfully prevent childhood burns from open fires or oil lamps by providing enclosed stoves, more stable lamps, or other safe heating or lighting may deserve priority over a larger, more widespread injury problem with no promising solution.

Identify Determinants of Injuries

After deciding which injuries to target for prevention, the major determinants of these injuries must be ascertained. Certain determinants, such as alcohol or poverty, may have an important impact on several types of injuries, as well as on many other health conditions; such determinants could be given a higher priority for intervention, if there are promising preventive strategies.

Special local, regional, or national surveys may be needed to identify the major risk factors, exposures, and geographic distributions of targeted injuries.

Develop Programs

To assess the choices of possible countermeasures directed towards modifying determinants of a specific type of injury, it is important to consider the feasibility, acceptability, effectiveness, and cost of any interventions proposed to modify risk factors, activities, and exposures. Different interventions should be considered to modify personal, equipment, and environmental factors in each of the pre-event, event, and post-event phases, as discussed in Chapter 2. By considering a variety of approaches in a systematic manner, one may avoid becoming locked into a single approach that is the most obvious, but not most effective, intervention.

Interventions for specific injuries may be highly focused. For example, traffic injuries can be prevented by introducing enclosed buses for public transport to replace open-backed vehicles. On the other hand, more general programs, such as "Safe Communities," may include multiple interventions designed to prevent various types of injuries throughout the community (WHO Collaborating Centre, 1992). Activities of intermediate specificity could include special programs to establish a water-safe or road-safe community.

Where a single determinant, such as alcohol, is associated with many different types of injuries, a highly specific intervention targeting that factor may have a broad general impact.

Implement Programs and Specific Interventions

Programs may be undertaken at various levels, including international, national, regional, or local. Interventions may involve single sectors such as health, transport, police, labor, or finance, or they may include multiple sectors working cooperatively towards shared objectives.

Appropriate means of intervention must be selected and the necessary resources obtained; some examples are discussed below under Social and Political Considerations. Once the countermeasures have been selected and funding sources identified, much more remains to be done. For example, the technical and financial feasibility and acceptability of the program and the most appropriate strategy for implementing it must be determined. Many of the most effective interventions are backed by legislation and regulation.

Evaluate the Effect of Interventions

Management by objectives is a basic principle of health management. In order to facilitate evaluating a program or intervention, objectives should be specified at the time the program is being developed. These objectives are generally intermediate steps to achieving broader goals. Objectives ideally should be measurable changes in health outcomes of morbidity and/or mortality, as discussed in Chapters 3 and 4. Other outcomes, such as changes in knowledge, attitudes, or practices, are sometimes used in evaluations, and are discussed below.

INTEGRATING RESEARCH INTO INJURY CONTROL PROGRAMS

Surveillance Versus Research

Once data collection on injuries becomes a relatively routine recurring procedure, monitoring these data for important trends or changes represents a form of surveillance activity. Injury surveillance is the ongoing collection and monitoring of data on mortality and morbidity from injuries. Such data, if available, can be helpful in identifying injury problems, following trends, and evaluating outcomes of interventions. Surveillance data can be used to prioritize specific injuries for further intensive research and the collection of new primary data. Surveillance data acquired from secondary data sources seldom provide detailed information on the circumstances of injuries, and even the external cause of injury may be missing. However, research can be used to improve the validity and utility of routine data sources for injury surveillance.

Research to Identify Injury Problems

The first step in developing a public health program includes the search for and discovery of significant public health problems (Dab and Abenhaim, 1984). Until recently, injuries were underrecognized as an important problem, and funding for research in injury control was very limited compared to other health conditions. In some countries, research to document the health and economic burden of injuries on society has helped to bring about a rethinking of public health priorities and financing.

The share of health resources allocated for injury control is, in most cases, still far less than the proportion of morbidity, premature mortality, and direct and indirect economic costs attributable to injuries; however, a gradual reorientation of priorities is occurring among political leaders and public health professionals as they begin to comprehend the magnitude of the health and economic impacts of injuries.

Once injuries in general, or a specific injury, have been identified as a public health problem, it is useful to determine their relative importance with respect to other health conditions or other specific injuries. This is the second point at which research may be needed; the analyses should include both health and economic indicators.

Research to Elucidate the Health Problem

This includes identification of important determinants of injuries, such as the following:

- Personal addictions and substance abuse, including alcohol and smoking;

There are very few human beings who receive the truth, complete and staggering, by instant illumination. Most of them acquire it fragment by fragment, on a small scale, by successive developments, cellularly, like a laborious mosaic.
—*Anaïs Nin,* **Diary,** *vol III, Fall, 1943*

The whole of science is nothing more than a refinement of everyday thinking.
—*Albert Einstein,* **Physics and Reality,** *1936*

- Personal medical problems, such as epilepsy, dementia, and mental retardation;
- Psychosocial and physical environmental factors;
- Hazardous equipment and activities.

Comparing rates of different injuries among communities or regions can be helpful in setting local priorities. Knowledge of the specific circumstances of injuries is invaluable. Examples are the findings that grass skirts, open fires, or kerosene stoves were important risk factors for burns in certain communities.

The most suitable interventions for a specific injury may be unclear. An integrated systematic evaluation of alternatives by a multidisciplinary team of professionals with public consultations may help to identify the most promising approach (Gielen, 1992).

Research to Establish Specific Objectives and Evaluate Programs

It is important to establish specific objectives for an intervention in the planning stages, as discussed above. Researchers should be able to assist in this process of establishing objectives. The objectives may be based upon the measures used to establish the importance of the specific injury problem and upon its major determinants. The objectives provide staff with a tangible goal to work towards in their daily activities, as well as a means of evaluation.

Finally, the intervention or program must be evaluated to determine whether it has had a beneficial impact in reducing the numbers or severity of injuries. The indicators to be used for evaluation should be established at the time of program planning in conjunction with program planners, and should be closely linked with program objectives. The costs of intervention may be weighed against the direct and indirect costs of deaths, hospitalizations, and disabilities that were prevented.

Changes in the prevalence of risk-taking behavior or the use of safety devices, such as helmets or safety belts, are a measure of possible modification in the level of individual risk for certain specific injuries, but may not always be reliable as proxy outcome measures. An example is the proportion of individuals in a population or community who are observed to use automobile safety belts or motorcycle helmets (Sugarman et al., 1992).

In general, observation of actual practices provides a better reflection of reality than questionnaire surveys of self-reported behavior (Robertson, 1992). For example, the proportion of motor vehicle occupants who are observed to use automobile safety belts is usually substantially less than the proportion who say that they do so.

Surveys of observed behavior can often be completed more rapidly and less intrusively than interview surveys. On the other hand, a potential advantage of interview surveys is that the results of self-reports of behavior can be linked with other personal characteristics of the respondents, such as age, sex, occupation and consumption of alcohol.

In some cases, while the general population at minimal risk adopts a safety measure, individuals at greatest risk of injury, such as alcoholics or young males, may fail to change their behavior. Thus, the observed effect on health outcomes is less than what might be expected if the safety measure had been adopted by the same propor-

It is sometimes possible to combine interviews and observations.

Canadian recreational boaters were interviewed on the water to find out why they wore or did not wear a flotation device. Their actual wearing practice at the time of interview was also recorded (Masson and Barss, 1996).

tion of persons in all risk groups. For this reason, the ultimate test of efficacy for an injury control intervention remains a measurable improvement in health outcomes.

For relatively small populations, the use of changes in mortality as an objective may be impractical. Fatal injuries are often rare events, and an excessively long observation period could be necessary to demonstrate a statistically significant change in injury death rates. Significant changes in morbidity rates, as reflected in hospitalizations for specific injuries, may be measurable over shorter time periods, provided hospitalization patterns did not change. If there have been substantial demographic changes during a study period, age-adjustment of injury rates may be necessary when comparing rates during different years.

The use of suitable control or comparison groups should be carefully considered in any study. Comparisons may be made of individuals, as in case-control and cohort studies, or of populations, as in ecologic studies. The choice of appropriate control or reference groups demands good judgement and a careful consideration of the characteristics of the study population and possible control populations.

Many of the issues involved in choosing controls or referents have been worked out in greatest detail for case-control studies (Wacholder et al., 1992a, 1992b, 1992c), but similar considerations often apply to prospective studies (Rothman, 1986). An example of using an ecologic study to evaluate an injury control intervention is the study by Robertson and Zador (1978) to evaluate the effect of school driver education programs on death rates among teenage drivers, as discussed by Kelsey et al. (1986).

For injury control in developing countries, it appears that the greatest research need at the present time is for relatively, simple, basic, descriptive, and etiologic epidemiologic data to show the extent of morbidity and mortality from specific injuries, and to identify the causes, specific circumstances, and high risk groups for specific injuries. It is first necessary to determine which injuries are the greatest sources of mortality and morbidity. The next step is to define the most important causes of these injuries and the age, sex, and occupational groups at highest risk of injury. More complex and expensive controlled studies are unnecessary for most planning and prevention purposes. However, the use of controls may be indicated for investigating the importance of personal factors, such as alcohol consumption, in the etiology of specific injuries, such as pedestrian injuries, drownings, or suicides (Haddon et al., 1961; Honkanen et al., 1983). Controlled studies have also been used to investigate equipment and environmental factors.

Data Needs

Necessary epidemiologic data must be obtained by each country, region, and community to meet its specific local needs. Appropriate staff must be trained to collect the data and carry out the relatively simple analyses that are needed. Some of the steps in obtaining and using such information are outlined in Chapters 2–4. A few practical examples of how injury data were collected and analyzed at a provincial hospital and health centers in a rural province in a developing country are described at the end of Chapter 4.

Not all research requires collecting new or primary data. In locations where there are adequate routine service data on deaths, hospitalizations, or visits to health providers, it may be possible to use such existing sources of secondary data to establish priorities.

Whenever data from health facilities are used for epidemiological research, it is important to consider whether the facilities are readily accessible to and trusted by the study population. One also needs to know whether similar proportions of patients with different types of injuries and illnesses use the health facility for treatment. There can be severe underreporting, miscoding, and other biases in data from routine death registers. Problems with routine data sources are discussed in more detail in Chapters 3 and 4.

Unfortunately, routine collection of data is often so deficient that special surveys are needed to establish the relative importance and specific circumstances of different types of injuries, especially for fatalities such as drowning and suicide. It is helpful that in surveys information can often be collected from proxy respondents (Halabi et al., 1992; Gray, 1989; Gray et al., 1990) and that verbal autopsies are particularly sensitive and specific for deaths from unintentional injuries (Snow et al., 1992).

In some cases, the process of data recording may need minor improvements to make the records useful for injury research. For example, if health providers have not consistently recorded the external causes of injury for their patients, it should be possible to modify clinical history forms and summary sheets so that the essential information is more likely to be included as routine. Information on acute alcohol intoxication and smoking as contributing factors to another diagnosis should also be recorded as a routine in health records and death reports. Medical records clerks or coders can be directed to refuse to accept a clinical record for filing if the essential details have not been provided, or they may contact the health provider concerned to obtain the missing item(s) of information.

In some cases, simple questionnaires or group surveys using key informants from each location of interest may provide valuable details about the most important injuries and the main preventable factors for each type of injury. The generation of data from key community informants during such a group session can also help to convince the participants that the local problems are really their own and not simply something abstract described by an outside researcher or health provider. Such recall techniques would be most helpful in small communities, where significant local injury events tend to be well-known to most inhabitants.

Research on Cost

To assist governments in their decision making about whether to fund and implement specific measures for injury control, there is a need to demonstrate the efficacy and cost-effectiveness of proposed interventions. Information about costs is often unavailable, even in industrialized countries; however, as a result of a detailed report to the United States Congress on the cost of injuries, some cost-effectiveness and cost-savings information are available for a limited number of prevention strategies that have proven to be effective in the United States (Rice, MacKenzie, et al., 1989).

Example of using key community informants to obtain data on circumstances of fatal injuries in indigenous communities.

At a meeting of local community health and safety officers from a group of remote First Nations communities in northern Québec, Canada, it was possible, in a period of 30 minutes, to identify most of the major causes, risk groups, and preventable factors for fatal injuries that had occurred in their communities during the previous decade.

This was accomplished by drawing systematically upon the collective memories of the representatives from each community. Each person listed the key details for his or her community, including the age and sex of the victim, year of death, external cause of death, and preventable factors.

The results were then combined to provide a regional profile of the types of injuries, together with the high-risk groups and modifiable risk factors for each injury. The retrospective information obtained in a single meeting equalled, and in some ways surpassed, service data collected on an ongoing basis at considerable expense during the previous ten years.

It would be useful if the costs of locally appropriate injury control programs and interventions could be evaluated in representative developing countries. One such analytical framework was proposed in a paper presented at a World Bank symposium on road safety (Hills and Jones-Lee, 1983). Methods for costing road injuries for developing countries are described in a manual from the Overseas Unit of the British Transport and Road Research Laboratory, discussed under Traffic Injuries.

Anderson (1991) has provided a cost-benefit analysis of different approaches to dealing with disasters in developing countries, including a comparison of prevention and recovery. Her economic analysis suggested that prevention is as economically justifiable in developing countries as it is in developed countries.

Other Research Needs

In addition to the need for the data discussed above, there are research needs specific to the prevention of particular types of injuries. Some suggestions are outlined in Chapters 7–13.

Many research projects could help define optimal treatment and rehabilitation systems of tertiary prevention to reduce adult morbidity, mortality, and disability from injuries; some examples are outlined in Chapter 15. Special economic initiatives for financing primary and secondary prevention and treatment systems also requires research and evaluation.

Another important area of needed research is documentation on the importance of good living conditions for good health (Health Situation and Trend Assessment Program, PAHO, 1991). Problems such as violence and drug addiction often appear linked to a deterioration in living conditions, poverty, alienation and hopelessness. A number of studies in developed countries have found an association between adverse environmental factors in socioeconomically deprived neighborhoods and an elevated risk of unintentional and intentional injuries (Wilkins et al., 1989).

The World Health Organization's Ottawa Charter for Health Promotion cited the close correlation between health and living conditions for various population groups (Canadian Public Health Association, 1986). Fundamental resources for health were stated to be peace, shelter, education, food, income, a stable ecosystem, sustainable resources, social justice, and equity. Studies are needed in various developing countries to determine the relative importance of such factors in the prevention of intentional and unintentional injuries.

Research programs and prevention policies should be linked to ensure that research is carried out in the best interests of the people. For this reason, policy and research issues for specific injuries should be considered together in subsequent chapters.

Examples of some of the issues involved in assessing a research program for unintentional injury and in providing appropriate recommendations at a national level in a developed country can be found in *A Review of Research on Unintentional Injury: A Report to the Medical Research Council of New Zealand* (Langley and McLoughlin, 1987) and in the United States National Academy of Sciences Report, *Injury in America: A Continuing Public Health Problem*

(Committee on Trauma Research, 1985). Several European countries have a long history of injury research dating back to as early as 1930, and their initiatives may provide useful examples (Linwood, 1988).

Participatory Action Research (PAR)

Since prevention of many injuries involves citizens and professionals from sectors other than health and research institutions, participatory action research is a vital approach to injury surveillance and research. This is especially so at the community level, but PAR can also function at regional and national levels.

Participatory action research has been defined as "an approach to research that brings together investigation, education, and action at the community level to allow people to look at health concerns in their lives and their communities" (Wotton et al., 1997). While still unknown to many traditional researchers in industrialized countries, and only recently studied for health promotion, it has a longer history in many developing areas (Organisation for Economic Co-operation and Development, 1995). Because most researchers have little or no power to actually initiate prevention programs other than by providing information, the involvement of non-researchers can provide enormous leverage in prevention programs (Boyce et al., 1997).

SOCIAL AND POLITICAL CONSIDERATIONS

Many unintentional and violent injuries result primarily from environments of poverty and hazardous personal lifestyles. Positive or negative changes in equity and poverty within a society could have a major impact on the risk of injuries for deprived groups in the population. Discussion of the importance of these sociopolitical factors and a consideration of possible interventions have been scarce in literature on injury control from the United States. This is understandable, since the fundamental changes implicit in such interventions would be politically unacceptable and even unthinkable to many national policy and decision makers.

All animals are equal, but some animals are more equal than others.
—*George Orwell*, **Animal Farm**, *ch 10, 1945*

Technical innovations and changing individual behavior provide relatively "safe" topics for research and intervention and are unlikely to seriously threaten or alarm the political establishment and status quo. Nevertheless, many technical innovations were initially resisted by powerful economic interests, such as the automobile industry, because of the potential negative implications for corporate profits (Nader, 1991).

The planning and implementation of fundamental changes in society are beyond the scope or capacity of the duties of professionals in most sectors. Nevertheless, the underlying importance of socioeconomic factors and the psychosocial environment should never be forgotten in discussing the overall injury problem with key decision makers who have the power to implement basic political and economic changes.

Many professionals are key providers of information and developers of research methodology. A research priority is to develop im-

Programs of micro-credit, which have stimulated self-sufficiency among economically disadvantaged people, could help to reduce injury risks.

"With access to credit, we can invest in small livestock instead of brewing beer (bili-bili) which is no good for our husbands!" Village woman in Chad (Bedard, 1997).

proved methods to assess the importance of factors, such as social justice, equity, and education, in the control of adverse health conditions, such as addiction, violence, and various diseases (Health Situation and Trend Assessment Program, PAHO, 1991).

Well-researched information in the form of public health data on morbidity and mortality in different subgroups of society, such as socioeconomic differences in injury mortality and morbidity among deprived minorities, can ultimately have a powerful effect in bringing about societal changes that might otherwise not occur. An example of potentially useful data can be found in a study from Great Britain (Walsh and Jarvis, 1992). The relative risk of death from unintentional injury was 7.5 times as great (95 percent confidence limits, 1.8 and 32.6) for children from the most socioeconomically deprived neighborhoods of Newcastle-upon-Tyne as it was for children in the most affluent neighborhoods. The risk of severe nonfatal injuries was 3.6 times as great (95 percent confidence limits, 1.3 and 9.5) for children in the poorer neighborhoods.

Useful concepts for a more general social and community approach to the prevention of injuries appear to be evolving in some of the Scandinavian countries (Svanström et al., 1991; Svanström, 1991; Bjärås, 1991; Schelp, 1987). The approach to injury control known as "Safe Communities" was developed in Sweden.

Safe Communities programs appear to be particularly feasible in the socio-political situation in the Scandinavian countries, where populations are relatively homogeneous and class disparities have been modulated by egalitarian tax and economic policies. These programs are also being used in some deprived urban neighborhoods in Glasgow, Scotland (Morrison et al., 1992; Graham, 1992).

The World Health Organization has begun to promote the concept of safe communities, with an emphasis on equity and community involvement (Romer, 1991; WHO Collaborating Centre, 1992; WHO Collaborating Centre, nd.a, nd.b; Klang et al., 1992). Up-to-date information on developments in Safe Community programs is available from the World Health Collaborating Centre on Community Safety Promotion, Department of Social Medicine, Karolinska Institute, S-172 83 Sundbyberg, Sweden. Several criteria must be met by the community in order for a city, town, or neighborhood to be declared a "Safe Community" (Table 14.2).

Indicators for monitoring the progress of Safe Community programs have been developed and research projects undertaken in Sweden (WHO Collaborating Centre, 1992). The community approach has also been used in Thailand (Svanström and Svanström, 1989) and adapted for other developing countries (Havanonda et al., 1989, 1991; Tucker, 1991).

It may be possible to integrate or coordinate the Safe Community approach with more general programs for "Healthy Cities" or "Villes et villages en santé" (Duhl, 1986; Healthy Cities Symposium, 1990). Evaluation of the effectiveness of such broad multisectoral health promotion projects poses significant challenges for research (Milio, 1990; Hayes and Willms, 1990). The community approach to prevention may be particularly important for the primary prevention of intentional injuries, including suicide, homicide, and domestic violence (Rodgers, 1991).

While the development of local community programs for safe

Table 14.2. Qualification as a safe community

Criteria for admission

- A cross-sectoral group responsible for injury prevention must exist.
- The local community network must be involved.
- A program must cover all ages, environments, and situations.
- The program must show concern for high risk groups and high-risk environments and aim particularly at ensuring justice for vulnerable groups.
- Those responsible must be able to document the frequency and causes of injuries.
- The program must be a long-term program rather than a short-term project.

The community must agree to undertake certain other measures

- Utilize appropriate indicators to evaluate processes and the effects of change.
- Analyze the community's organizations and their possibility of participation in the program.
- Involve the health care organization in both registration of injuries and the prevention program.
- Be prepared to involve all levels of the community in solving the injury problem.
- Disseminate experiences both nationally and internationally.
- Be prepared to contribute to a network of safe communities.

Source: WHO Collaborating Centre, 1992.

communities is desirable, it should not be used as a politically palatable excuse to avoid implementing, or to downscale, regional, national, and international programs for development and regulation of safer products and environments. Although social and economic changes or various types of community programs may be necessary for the control of certain types of injuries, technical and equipment changes that are implemented at a national or international level have been proven to be highly successful in preventing many injuries. Environmental changes that provide "passive" automatic protection and do not require repetitive vigilance or "active" protection by the individual have the best record of proven efficacy and are favored by many injury researchers.

Automatic protection, such as a household fuse or a safety guard on the moving parts of a machine, can prevent injuries or reduce their severity, even among persons who lose control of a vehicle or machine because of intoxication or fatigue. Thus, the passive protection provided by the permanent modification of an equipment factor can sometimes overcome the harmful effects of an adverse personal factor. Since it is impossible to control and regulate human behavior 100 percent of the time, it is important to provide "user-friendly" environments to protect people during moments of vulnerability.

Development and application of safer products and environments often require political decisions, ranging from the allocation of financial resources to competing demands regarding the location of a new highway. It is often difficult, moreover, to convince legislators and other decision makers that, where possible, it is preferable to provide automatic protection for the community rather than attempting to persuade all individuals to alter their behaviors.

INTERVENTION STRATEGIES FOR INJURY CONTROL

The implementation of the many intervention strategies discussed in Chapter 2 can be organized into five broad areas: education and individual behavior change, taxation and other economic incentives, legislation, product design, and environmental modification (Rice et al., 1989). There is some overlap, since changes in product design, behavior, and the environment often result from legislative initiatives. Economic incentives may also stimulate product design changes.

Political, economic, and social changes are more fundamental and could be most effective in the long run for the prevention of many injuries, especially intentional injuries. The details and mechanisms for implementing such structural changes are, however, beyond the scope of this publication.

The most effective interventions to prevent injury are not always directed towards the most obvious risk factor. To illustrate, excessive speed might appear to be the most important causal factor in motorcyclist injuries in rural areas, yet the most effective preventive measure could be a motorcycle helmet law. This does not imply that enforcement of speed limits is unimportant, but rather that the same benefit may not be achieved, especially in rural areas where speed enforcement is prohibitively costly. To determine which combination of countermeasures is most useful in preventing a particular injury, a systematic assessment process has been suggested. The assessment process may involve the contributions of a multidisciplinary team to consider epidemiologic, legal, engineering, and economic aspects of proposed solutions. Surveys of the public may help to establish how well they understand the problems and what preferences they have for various countermeasures. Information from various sources must be integrated by a policy-making body in order to formulate guidelines for decision makers. The technical and economic feasibility of the proposed countermeasures, together with their political and public acceptability, should be considered when promoting different interventions. Published studies of the efficacy of specific interventions are relatively uncommon, but can be very helpful when available.

Education for Individual Behavior Change

This strategy relies on education to encourage people to change their unsafe behaviors. Evaluation of educational programs has shown that our ability to induce significant behavior change is often limited. An example is a special educational program to encourage seat belt use in a United States community. Robertson et al (1974) showed that the extensive television advertising used in the program had no effect on local rates of seat belt use. Prior to the enactment and enforcement of legislation that mandated the use of seat belts in the United States, rates of use had remained at about 12–14 percent for years, despite extensive promotional campaigns.

Although it can be difficult to change behavior through educational efforts alone, an important function of educational efforts is to inform the public and modify their knowledge and attitudes about injuries. Appropriate educational campaigns may create the public support that is needed for adoption of other more effective interventions.

Education may be particularly helpful prior to the introduction of interventions that involve regulation of personal behavior, since otherwise some individuals consider enforcement of the regulations to be an infringement upon their personal liberties. On the other hand, legislation and enforcement can help to reinforce and sustain any short-term behavior changes that may result from educational campaigns (Gielen, 1992).

One of the most important functions of education is modifying the attitudes of key decision makers and professionals who design and modify products, equipment, and the environment. Managers, engineers, and architects who are familiar with the principles of injury control have tremendous power and potential to ensure that safety is an essential component of basic product design and the environment.

Many hazards can be predicted and addressed with design or engineering solutions. Policy makers and politicians can contribute to this process by developing appropriate legislation to modify products, the environment, or behavior. Such interventions would help to provide permanent automatic protection for the public.

Taxation and Other Economic Incentives

Taxing hazardous products has been suggested as an important means of controlling injuries. Price increases of harmful products frequently associated with injuries can decrease their use. Examples include, alcoholic beverages, tobacco, and hazardous equipment.

The effects of price increases on sales and consumption of harmful products is affected by the price elasticity of demand. Price elasticity is a function of various factors, including the inflation rate, and may be confounded by changes in income and the effects of income elasticity (Maynard, 1986).

Certain vulnerable groups, such as teenagers and young adults, may be more susceptible to the effects of price elasticity. However, the elasticity of demand for highly addictive products, such as cigarettes, may be somewhat less than for other products. Heavy taxation of addictive but legal drugs, such as tobacco and alcohol, may encourage illegal black markets or cross-border shopping, if tax policies in neighboring jurisdictions are not jointly coordinated.

It has been suggested that a 35 percent tax on the retail price of alcoholic beverages could reduce alcohol-related fatalities by 50 percent, and that a 50 percent tax could reduce fatalities by 75 percent (Phelps, 1988). Such large effects might occur if price increases of alcohol had the greatest impact on reducing consumption among young persons who are at greatest risk of crashes. Alcohol and tobacco advertising often target young people who are not only vulnerable to the effects of such propaganda, but also at high risk of injuries. Transportation taxes on hazardous modes of transport can also shift users to safer products, as discussed in Chapters 7 and 8.

Insurance discounts for cars and homes with automatic safety features are another type of economic intervention that can motivate consumers to purchase safer products. In the United States, insurance fees for personal injury protection have been discounted up to 60 percent for cars equipped with full front airbags and up to 30 percent for automatic seat belts (Insurance Institute, 1990a). Similarly, insurance rates may be lowered for homes with safety features such as automatic sprinkler systems for prevention of housefires.

Legislation and Regulation

Many effective interventions have included the enactment of laws that encouraged or coerced safer behavior, together with adequate enforcement to ensure compliance. Education helps to improve compliance with new regulations.

The passage of automobile seat belt or motorcycle helmet-use laws has significantly increased usage rates in countries where the laws are enforced (National Committee for Injury Prevention and Control, 1989). Lower speed limits on highways have saved many lives in the United States and could also be effective in developing countries, at least in areas where implementation and enforcement are feasible.

Regulations to prohibit the sale, or even possession, of alcohol have been introduced in India (Bang and Bang, 1992) and in many indigenous communities in North America (May, 1992). The effects of prohibition have not always been as predicted, however, and such programs must be carefully monitored and studied to be sure that they do not have an adverse impact on the incidence of injuries. This is particularly likely to occur if alcohol is available in nearby jurisdictions. Persons from "dry" areas may travel to "wet" areas and rapidly consume large quantities of alcohol, leading to brawls or road injuries (Gallaher et al., 1992; Lujan, 1992a, 1992b). Prohibitions on alcohol sometimes appear to be associated with the substitution of other dangerous practices, including sniffing of neurotoxic solvents such as gasoline.

Product Design

Many governments have recognized the importance of injuries caused by poorly designed and unsafe consumer products. Some countries have established special organizations to set standards, monitor the safety of consumer products, and advise the government about products that should be modified or withdrawn from the market to protect the public. The need for costly development of safety standards, whether for cars, farm machinery, pesticides, or other potentially hazardous products, can be eliminated if a developing country adopts and/or adapts standards developed by other countries. The example of the European Union is instructive. In drafting common safety standards, member countries with high standards have generally refused to compromise on safety, and the effect has been to raise the standards in countries with lower standards.

It is often easier and more effective to change the design of a product to make it safer than it is to teach everyone to be careful whenever they use it. An example is the development of enclosed cooking stoves in Nepal to reduce the risk of burns from open fires. Such an intervention can protect a number of different high risk groups, including children, women, and people with epilepsy, and may also provide other health and social benefits, such as control of smoke-related lung diseases. Other simple products to prevent injuries include the long-handled devices used in some countries to

Law is order, and good law is good order.
—*Aristotle*, **Politics**, *bk VII, ch 4, 384–322* B.C.E.

Even when laws have been written down, they ought not always to remain unaltered.
—*Aristotle*, **Politics**, *bk II, ch 8*

The more laws and order are made prominent, the more thieves and robbers there will be.
—*Lao Tzu*, **The Way of Lao Tzu**, *604–531* B.C.E.

Laws are like cobwebs, which may catch small flies, but let wasps and hornets break through.
—*Jonathan Swift*, **A Critical Essay upon the Faculties of the Mind**, *1707*

prune mango trees and harvest the fruit, thereby eliminating the risks associated with climbing.

Possible undesirable effects of an intervention must be anticipated and addressed to ensure acceptance. Otherwise, a promising intervention may be rapidly discredited and rejected by the community. In illustration, while enclosed stoves can prevent many severe injuries and diseases, the elimination of smoke may result in increased numbers of flies, bedbugs, and other insects in unscreened village huts. This is not only an annoying nuisance, but also can increase the risk of certain diseases, such as trachoma (Sahlu and Larson, 1992). Thus, a comprehensive ecologic approach to intervention may be necessary in some cases.

In certain countries, legislation and regulations or litigation against the manufacturers of unsafe products have been the driving forces behind product safety changes. Demand and purchasing preference for safer products by informed consumers has been an increasingly important factor in developed countries.

Environmental Modification

Many highway design interventions rely on the modification or removal of hazardous environmental features, such as rigid roadside structures. Road networks can be modified to divert high speed traffic away from areas with large numbers of unprotected people, such as pedestrians and cyclists.

Other examples include preventing drowning by constructing barriers around bodies of water to prevent small children from falling in or by providing footbridges over hazardous river crossings. Fatal head injuries from falling coconuts can be avoided by planting coconut palms in areas away from homes and busy village trails (Barss, 1984a). In some developed countries, legislation and the fear of litigation are important incentives for many environmental changes, as they have been for product safety.

CASE STUDY: COST EFFECTIVENESS AND COST SAVINGS FROM PREVENTION OF TRAFFIC INJURIES IN THE UNITED STATES

Few data are available on the cost-effectiveness of injury prevention or control measures in developing countries. Examples of estimated cost savings from injury control measures in the United States are presented here as examples of the types of economic analyses that can be helpful to policy makers when they are asked to allocate funds for injury prevention programs; naturally, the expected cost savings and the availability of the necessary data would differ substantially in developing countries.

This case study is based upon an extensive study (Rice, MacKenzie, et al., 1989) which demonstrated that substantial cost savings can be achieved from a number of injury prevention strategies. The researchers estimated potential reductions in both fatal and nonfatal injuries and calculated cost savings using 1985 United States estimates. Readers are referred to their document for further details.

While many injury prevention measures have proven to be effective, complete information to determine the net cost savings to society was often not available, even in the United States. For the calculation of cost savings, information is needed about the effectiveness of the intervention, including the degree of reduced injury severity to be expected, the estimated coverage by the intervention, and the estimated cost of implementing the intervention or providing increased coverage.

Rice, MacKenzie, and colleagues calculated the potential cost savings for a limited number of interventions for which good data were available, using both the human capital and the willingness-to-pay methods. The human capital approach to calculating costs of an acute injury considers both the direct treatment costs, including rehabilitation, and the indirect costs, including lost earnings. The costs of subsequent disability and premature death are added to the estimate. The human capital method does not include several other important costs such as pain and suffering, reduced productivity of family and other helpers, voluntary services, property damage, and legal costs. The willingness-to-pay method provides an estimate that is based on the amount that individuals say they would be willing to pay for a change to reduce the probability of an injury, illness, or death; this method does include a value for estimated pain and suffering.

Examples of cost savings from injury prevention strategies are considered for each of four areas: individual behavior, legislation, product design, and environmental modification. Examples for three of the areas are shown in Table 14.3. (It should be noted that the beneficial effect of eliminating driver education programs and raising the minimum age of drivers to 17 years was due to reducing the number of vulnerable teenage drivers on United States roads.)

Table 14.3. Estimated annual cost savings from selected injury prevention strategies using 1985 United States data

Intervention	Savings (millions of US $)	
	Human capital	Willingness to-pay
Individual behavior change		
Child pedestrian injury campaign	58	180
Bicycle helmet promotion	183	284
Elimination of high school driver education programs for teenagers	863	2,230
Legislation		
Minimum age of licensure 17 years	1,446	4,267
Motorcycle helmet use laws	97	1,200
Product design changes		
Reduced ignition potential of cigarette paper	187	1,100
Air bags on all new cars for the year	4,650	19,491
Side-crash protection	0	1,529
Automatic vehicle running lights	0	534

Adapted from Rice et al., Cost of Injury in the United States: A Report to Congress, 1989.

Where possible, the applicability of these findings to developing countries is briefly discussed. Many of the findings are more pertinent to vehicle occupants than to vulnerable road users, and researchers in developing countries should be encouraged and funded to investigate the cost-effectiveness of interventions for pedestrians, bicyclists, motorcyclists, and open-backed vehicles.

Individual Behavior Change

Child Pedestrian Injuries

Children and the elderly are at particularly high risk of pedestrian injury in the United States (Baker et al., 1992). The cost savings in excess of program costs for nationwide implementation of a successful local program to prevent children from darting out between cars were estimated to be $58 million, using the human capital method (Rice et al., 1989). The situation differs somewhat in developing countries where all ages are at high risk of pedestrian injury; however, it may be possible to develop locally appropriate strategies.

Bicycle Helmet Promotion

Head injuries from bicycle crashes are increasingly recognized to be an important preventable cause of death and long-term disability. On the basis of effective bicycle helmet promotions in Australia, it is estimated that the implementation of a similar program in the United States could save about $183 million per year. While few data are available from developing countries, the development of low-cost and effective bicycle helmets, together with their effective promotion, is likely to result in considerable cost savings in countries with high rates of bicycle use.

Driver Education

Not all educational efforts are effective, and occasionally interventions that are proposed to reduce certain injuries may have the reverse effect and increase injury rates. The importance of careful evaluation of the effectiveness of any new intervention was emphasized by a study of the effects of a program of high school driver education in the United States. Driver training was adopted in many schools prior to an objective evaluation. The program had been established under the untested assumption that it would help to reduce the high rates of motor vehicle injuries and deaths among United States teenagers. When evaluation was eventually carried out, however, it was found that there was no significant reduction in crash rates for teenage drivers in areas with driver education, compared to control areas (Robertson and Zador, 1978). Driver education did, however, enable more students to obtain their driver's license and to drive at an earlier average age, when there is a much higher risk of crashing per mile traveled. Sixteen-year old drivers have a fatal crash rate per mile driven that is over 11 times greater than that of 35–39 year olds (Robertson, 1983). It was estimated that 666 motor vehicle injury deaths per year (1982–1983) could have been prevented in the United States if those children encouraged by driver education programs to obtain their license before age 18 had instead been driven over the same distances by their parents (Rice, MacKenzie, et al., 1989). This research showed, therefore, that both students' lives and public funds could be saved by reducing the funding for high school driver education, with an estimated cost savings in 1985 of $863 million. Elimination of school-based programs shifted the decision of when a teenager should commence driving from the school back to the parents. An economic aspect that perhaps should have been considered is the value that parents place on the time that they use transporting teenagers who might otherwise have been able to transport themselves.

The relevance of this research is difficult to determine for developing countries where few teenagers have access to automobiles. There may be a greater need for publicly funded driver education in developing countries, and the age of licensure may be less affected by high school driver education. Nevertheless, Robertson's research illustrates the need for careful evaluation of the efficacy of potential interventions that may be theoretically appealing, but have unexpected effects.

Legislation

Raising Licensing Age for Drivers

In the United States in 1985, 2,014 deaths occurred in crashes where a driver was a 16-year-old. An increase in the legal driving age from 16 to 17 years has been estimated to reduce motor vehicle fatalities involving 16-year-olds by 75 percent (Williams, et al., 1983). It is assumed that young drivers may have similarly high risks of fatal crash involvement in developing countries; some countries minimally regulate driving age. A high rate of young drivers involved in crashes has been noted in a number of countries, even those with little alcohol use, such as Qatar in the Arabian Gulf (Eid, 1980). The effectiveness of restricting driving age depends on whether strict licensing requirements can be established and enforced, since this may be more difficult in developing countries. In Saudi Arabia, 45 percent of drivers involved in crashes were found to have no license (Hamour, 1982); however, it would be useful to know the percentage of all drivers who were unlicensed.

Motorcycle Helmet Laws

Several United States studies have estimated that laws requiring the use of helmets can reduce deaths of motorcyclists by 30 percent (Watson et al., 1980). The calculations were based on an assumption of pre-law helmet use of about 50 percent; in many developing countries helmet use is well below this figure. The mortality rate in crashes of motorcyclists who do not wear a helmet is almost double that of those who do use one (Watson, et al., 1980). The cost savings of mandatory helmet use were estimated to be $97 million using the human-capital approach and $1,200 million by the willingness-to-pay method.

In spite of high death rates among motorcyclists and the large reductions in mortality and cost savings known to result from helmet laws, motorcyclists in the United States have often lobbied successfully to block implementation of such laws, and even to repeal successful legislation, on the basis that such laws limited their personal freedom. A disproportionate share of treatment and rehabilitation costs for injured motorcyclists is paid for by taxpayers, since many injured riders do not have adequate medical insurance to cover the great expense of treating their injuries (Rivara et al, 1988).

Lack of compliance could be a problem when such laws are enacted in developing countries; sometimes riders use a helmet, but their passengers do not. Improper use of helmets without chin straps was reported to have nullified the effect of a helmet law in one state in Nigeria (Asogwa, 1980a). The expected benefits of helmet laws in developing countries could be substantial, however, since motorcycles are used by so many people.

Product Design Changes

Simple design changes can dramatically reduce the risk of injuries from using a product. Some of the most effective and efficient injury prevention strategies are changes in products that make them safer to use. For example, a simple change in the porosity of cigarette paper could reduce the number of housefires caused by smokers and result in considerable savings (Table 14.3)

Unsafe at Any Speed. The Designed-In Dangers of the American Automobile.
—Ralph Nader, 1965, 1991

Airbags

Airbags are an effective way to reduce automobile-related injuries. They are devices that automatically inflate and provide an air cushion to protect occupants in crashes. Lap-shoulder belts can reduce automobile fatalities by up to 50 percent when used by everyone in a vehicle (NHTSA, 1984). However, there is considerable resistance to using them in many countries, and even in U.S. states with laws requiring the use of safety belts, usage rates were often less than 40 percent. High-risk drivers, such as alcoholics, tend to use safety belts at even lower rates. Safety belt usage rates in many non-industrialized countries are low; for example, in Saudi Arabia, use was reported to be only 7 percent, while in Sweden it was over 80 percent (Mufti, 1986) and in Canada is now over 90 percent. The low rate of use was attributed to the lack of legislation to enforce the use of belts; informational campaigns appeared to have little effect on rates of use.

Airbags provide a partial technical answer to the low rates of seat belt use and may protect even occupants who do not wear belts. They also provide additional protection, especially to the face and head, even for belted drivers. Estimates of the efficacy of airbags alone for the reduction of automobile fatalities, assuming no belt use, are 32 percent for drivers (Ferguson, 1996) and 23 percent for right front passengers (Braver et al., 1997) (their efficacy is less than belts because they are only effective in frontal or front angle crashes, and they do not prevent ejections). All new cars sold in the United States must provide automatic protection. Some use automatic belts, but most use airbags, which have proven to be cheaper and more effective.

Hundreds of children are killed every year in the United States because they are unrestrained or not restrained correctly; a very small number of these deaths have involved airbags. Despite the thousand of lives saved by airbags, recognition of their potential hazard to incorrectly restrained infants and young children has raised questions about the safest way to transport youngsters. The basic fact to remember is that children should always be correctly restrained so they cannot be close to an airbag when it deploys. Rear-facing infant seats on the front seat place a baby's head too close to an airbag, and young children who lean forward may also be at risk of head injury.

Therefore, children should be restrained in the back seat. An infant seat or child seat should be secured to the vehicle by an adult seat belt, with the child buckled into the seat For similar reasons, adult passengers should sit as far away from airbags as possible. Deactivation or on/off switches are rarely advisable (Insurance Institute for Highway Safety, 1997).

Rice, MacKenzie, et al. (1989) estimated the cost of airbags to be $365 per car for full-front airbags, which includes the life-time energy costs of the added weight of the vehicle. Since about 10 percent of the U.S. fleet is replaced annually, the effects are incremental. Airbags were the most cost-effective injury intervention studied, and should provide estimated savings of $4,650 million by the human capital approach and $19,691 million by the willingness-to-pay method.

Given the large cost savings of this single intervention in the United States, it is likely that a requirement for airbags on all new cars imported into developing countries would also be cost-effective, although it will take much longer to replace all of the older cars. Nevertheless, in countries such as India where only about 5 percent of traffic victims are occupants of cars, interventions directed towards other road user types may be of higher priority.

Once all new cars are available with airbags, individual governments will be faced with a decision as to whether all imported cars should be required to meet the same standards as in the United States. It is likely that the cost savings of purchasing a vehicle without airbags will be minimal, if most cars are already being manufactured with airbags for the large U.S. market. Given the high costs of new cars, the reduction in vehicle price from not including airbags would be only a small part of the total cost of the vehicle. Thus, it is recommended that all new cars imported to developing countries should be made to the same safety standards as in the United States and include airbags. Retrofitting of airbags is technically difficult and not economically viable.

Side Crash Protection

Side impacts were responsible for 32 percent of car occupant fatalities in the United States in 1985 (NHTSA, 1988). A proposal to increase protection from side collisions to occupants by reinforcing vehicle doors and frames would reduce passenger car occupant fatalities in side crashes by about 16 percent at a maximum cost of about $185 per car. There were no net cost savings using estimates prepared by the human capital approach, but with the willingness-to-pay method the estimated savings were $1,529 million in 1985 dollars. This modification to car design would affect all models sold in the United States and thus should also provide protection for new cars in developing countries. However, some models not sold in the United States may not offer the same protection. Where possible, all cars imported to developing countries should be built to resist side impacts.

High Seat Backs

A U.S. Federal standard requires head restraints to protect against neck injuries in rear-end crashes. However, adjustable head restraints, which are often left in the lowest position, only reduce injuries in rear-end collisions by 10 percent, compared to a 17 percent reduction in injuries observed with immovable high seat backs (Kahane, 1982). Despite the fact that using immovable high seat backs could result in a price reduction of $28 per car, manufacturers were slow to adopt the more effective design. The presence of high seat backs in 100 percent of U.S. cars was estimated to save about $14 million in injury costs, excluding the costs of pain and suffering. As with the case of side-impact protection, this intervention is beyond the control of most developing countries, but should be considered when drafting safety regulations for imported or locally-assembled cars.

Automatic Vehicle Lights

The risk of collisions with other vehicles can be reduced by increasing the visibility of vehicles. A controlled experiment found a 22 percent reduction (compared with unaltered control vehicles) in daytime multiple-vehicle collisions in the cars of a corporate fleet equipped with relay switches that automatically turned on the front parking and rear tail lights with the engine ignition (Stein, 1985). Studies in other countries have shown similar results, and it is estimated that on average a reduction of about 20 percent in injuries could be expected from this intervention. The costs of modifying vehicles at the time of manufacture would be less than the $7.50 per car that the changes cost in the experimental vehicles. More dramatic reductions (up to 50 percent) in daytime crash involvement have resulted from laws that require motorcyclists to drive with their headlights on (Muller, 1982; Zador, 1983).

In developing countries with high pedestrian injury rates, an increase in the visibility of vehicles may also help to reduce pedestrian deaths. Automatic daytime vehicle lighting would also help to prevent crashes by motorists who forget to switch on their lights at dusk, are unaware that they should do so, or who deliberately leave their lights off. In some countries, such as Ethiopia, many drivers are reluctant to turn on their lights until total darkness forces them to do so (J. Pickering, McGill Ethiopia Program, personal observation, 1994).

Other changes in vehicle visibility have also been shown effective in reducing crashes. An important example is the addition of a high center-mounted brake light at eye level, which has been shown to reduce rear-end collisions by more than 50 percent (Rausch et al., 1982). This simple innovation, which costs only a few dollars per car, is now standard on new vehicles.

Environmental Modifications

Minimum Road Width

A number of modifications to highways can reduce the risk of crashes, and decrease the severity of a crash should it occur. Mortality rates per mile traveled on U.S. interstate highways are one-third of those on other roads, despite the higher speeds on the interstates. The principle reasons for this are improved road design, such as elimination of intersections, reducing access, and separating lines of oncoming traffic. Unfortunately, such major highway changes may not be possible in the immediate future in developing countries, where most major roads are two-lane undivided highways; however, other modifications to such roads may reduce the crash rate on them. For example, an important environmental intervention that could be useful in developing countries is the separation of high speed motorized vehicles from the large numbers of slow moving and vulnerable pedestrians and bicyclists.

A recent committee of the Transportation Research Board (1987) estimated that a 40 percent crash reduction on federally funded two-lane rural roads could be achieved by increasing the minimum lane and shoulder widths. The estimated average cost per crash prevented was $32,000. There were net cost savings, however, only when the willingness-to-pay method was used in calculating the potential savings. Targeting changes to roads with higher traffic volumes and particularly to curved sections would increase the cost savings per mile of road modified (Bissell et al., 1982). Further targeting by redesigning a relatively small number of easily identifiable locations, such as particularly hazardous corners, downgrades, bridge abutments, and utility poles could considerably improve the return on any safety investment (Robertson, 1983; Wright and Robertson, 1976; Wright and Zador, 1981).

In many developing countries, improvements in roads have led to much higher travel speeds with concomitant increases in fatalities. Therefore, when roads are widened or improved in other ways, it is essential that appropriate preventive measures be undertaken. Some examples include the enforcement of reasonable speed limits and use of safety belts, the construction of shoulders at the edges of roads to accommodate pedestrians, disabled cars, etc., and the use of engineering safeguards, such as guardrails next to steep drop-offs and other hazards.

A major limitation of these U.S. cost studies is that property damage costs were not considered, only human damage costs. The inclusion of all costs in such estimates would considerably improve the cost-effectiveness of many injury interventions, particularly estimates of potential cost savings from primary or pre-crash prevention.

There is a need for more detailed studies in developing countries to determine injury costs. Cost studies could provide a strong economic incentive for prevention, as discussed in earlier chapters. A publication of the Transport and Road Research Laboratory (1994), *Costing Road Accidents in Developing Countries*, should help to meet the specific requirements of developing countries for cost studies. Their situation differs from that in industrialized countries, with many more vulnerable road users and fewer vehicle occupants at risk.

INJURY PREVENTION AT THE INTERNATIONAL, NATIONAL, REGIONAL, AND LOCAL LEVEL

With regard to excellence, it is not enough to know, but we must try to have and use it.
—*Aristotle*, Nicomachean Ethics, *bk 10, ch9, 384–322 B.C.E.*

Policy development, research, and implementation of injury control programs can be undertaken at international, national, regional/provincial, and community/local levels. Maximum effectiveness requires communication and cooperation among staff working at these different levels, as well as with other sectors relevant to injury control.

Because of their importance in the etiology of many types of injuries, alcoholic beverages receive extensive discussion. This has been limited mainly to national policy and research considerations, but interventions to control the adverse impact of alcohol on injuries are possible at all levels.

Similarly, the adverse impact of socioeconomic disparities may need to be addressed at all levels. This controversial topic is considered only briefly here, since it is discussed in earlier chapters.

International Level Initiatives

International policy and research initiatives often concern issues such as implementation and standardization of national surveillance of injuries, coding, and reporting. Injury coding classifications must be prepared with special consideration for the needs of developing countries.

We have learned that we cannot live alone at peace; that our own well-being is dependent on the well-being of other nations, far away.
—Franklin Delano Roosevelt, Fourth Inaugural Address

For countries with limited resources and national institutions, international assistance could help in the development of national and local programs and in appropriate training of staff in injury surveillance, coding, and research methodology. Systems must be established for reporting and collecting data from representative rural and urban populations and for analyzing and publishing data using standardized codes to facilitate international comparisons.

Injury surveillance may have to be developed in collaboration with surveillance of other health conditions. However, special attention must be given to essential requirements of injury surveillance, including accurate records of the external cause and circumstances of all injuries that result in a hospitalization or death.

Appropriate working groups and staff are needed to monitor the impact of various specific injuries on mortality and morbidity. An ideal team would include personnel such as an epidemiologist and a demographer, as well as at least one person with a clinical background. All should have received at least some specialized training in the principles of injury epidemiology and control.

It is also necessary to regularly reassess the overall importance of injuries with respect to other health conditions, and to follow trends in rates of specific injuries. In addition, changes in the major determinants of injuries must be monitored.

Creative national or local initiatives in injury prevention can be encouraged, evaluated, and communicated to other countries. International meetings with multisectoral participation can be helpful in exchanging ideas about the success of local initiatives. Since many developing countries cannot afford extensive holdings of professional journals and books, research findings must be disseminated to appropriate agencies and staff at low cost.

A mechanism must be developed to regularly inform developing countries about unsafe products that are marketed internationally, and assist them in developing consumer protection bureaus to monitor the safety of products used and sold within the country. Examples from developed countries include the Consumer Safety Institute in the Netherlands and the Consumer Product Safety Commission in the United States. This area will probably develop rapidly within the European Union with the additional resources that are available from the collaboration of so many countries.

Product safety standards are important for consumer protection (Van Weperen, 1993). Groups of countries may wish to collaborate to draft product safety legislation and to organize regional institutes to develop essential safety standards for products and materials that are marketed in the region. European examples of standardization institutes include CEN (Comité Européen de Normalisation) and CENELEC (Comité Européen de Normalisation Electrotechnique).

International organizations can assist with the development of research initiatives to document the effect of large socioeconomic disparities, lack of equal opportunities for education, and deprived neighborhoods on rates of intentional and unintentional injury. Since research of this nature could be politically unpopular and even dangerous, special international support may be necessary to assist such research in many countries.

National Level Initiatives

God—I don't know why— wanted me to be a Czech. It was not my choice. But I accept it and I try to do something for my country because I live here.
—Václav Havel, Interview, 1988

While the prevention of many injuries often involves injury-specific interventions, there are also broad general initiatives that could potentially prevent many types of injuries. For example, alcohol consumption and poverty are risk factors for many types of injuries and diseases. National policies to address alcohol abuse, the extent or the effects of poverty, lack of education, and substandard general living conditions, such as housing and neighborhoods, could help to prevent a variety of injuries and diseases.

National initiatives are also needed for the following:

• To establish injury surveillance;
• To train personnel for research and intervention;
• To develop consumer product protection;
• To provide needed regulation and legislation.

Alcohol and Injuries

Thanks be to God, since my leaving drinking of wine, I do find myself much better, and do mind my business better, and do spend less money, and less time lost in idle company.
—Samuel Pepys, Diary, January 26, 1662

Alcohol ingestion is associated with many types of unintentional and intentional injuries (MMWR, 1992; Jones et al., 1992; Secretary of Health and Human Services, 1990; also see Chapter 6). Alcohol acts as a depressant on the brain, slows reaction times, and can inhibit the perception of risks. Thus traffic injuries, drowning, falls, and burns are often associated with the ingestion of alcohol, either by the victim or by another individual responsible for the incident.

The depressant and toxic effects of alcohol on brain function may increase the perceived importance of relatively minor interpersonal problems. Such effects, together with the suppression or loss of normal inhibitory controls on violent behavior, may result in assaults on others or in suicide (Hayward et al., 1992).

Alcohol Policy

Controlling the sale, advertising, and use of alcohol within a country should be a high priority in any injury control program. Other reasons for national and local alcohol control programs include the harmful effects of alcohol on other health conditions and social problems, together with its property of inducing addiction or dependency.

Cheap alcohols, including methanol, are sold in some developing countries and are responsible for many poisonings, some of which cause death or blindness (see Chapter 10). While consumption of alcohol is associated with many types of injuries, the combined use of alcohol and tobacco has a more specific synergistic impact on burns and smoke inhalation by greatly increasing the risk of fatal house fires (Runyan et al., 1992).

Aggressive advertising of alcohol and tobacco products is often

directed towards the poor and illiterate, who may be completely unaware of their addictive properties, toxic effects, risk of injuries, and
medical and social complications. Tobacco advertising is also targeted to young people, since the tobacco industry needs to maintain a steady supply of new addicts (Maynard, 1986). Since the markets for alcohol and tobacco are decreasing in many developed
countries as educated and aging populations become more health
conscious, manufacturers of these profitable products view developing countries as important markets with substantial potential for expansion in sales.

The effects of controlling aggressive marketing of alcohol by advertising bans may need to be evaluated in developing countries
where alcohol has an important negative impact on health and society. Total bans on advertising of tobacco appear to have been effective in reducing consumption in a number of industrialized countries (Townsend, 1992).

Alcohol use has rapidly increased in some developing countries
(WHO, 1985a; Ritson, 1985). The adverse effects of these increases
may be even greater than expected from the quantities sold, since
there is a tendency for the consumption of alcohol to be heavily concentrated among young adult males. Young men may be more prone
to binge drinking than other community members. Rapid consumption of alcohol often leads to drunkenness and violence, as well as to
various unintentional injuries.

Because of the strong addictive properties of alcohol and its association with many injuries and other problems, it is unwise to allow the marketing and sale of alcohol to be regulated only by the
laws of supply and demand. National policies and organizations are
needed to monitor the adverse effects of alcohol and to balance
public health and economic objectives. Otherwise, powerful incentives for corporate profit and government tax revenues will tend to
work against the general interests of society. Since addiction to tobacco is often associated with abuse of alcohol, there should be coordinated policies and interventions for control of alcohol and tobacco products.

May (1992) has provided an extensive review of policy options to
contain the damage caused by alcohol to indigenous communities in
North America. He cautions against the adoption of simplistic solutions or the expectation of immediate results, and suggests that a combination of interventions may be most effective.

Some communities in developing countries have chosen to completely ban the sale of alcohol (Bang and Bang, 1992). For example,
Gadchiroli is an undeveloped district in India with 650,000 inhabitants, about one-half of whom are aborigines. A quick survey revealed that this population included about 20,000 alcoholics, of
whom 1,000 died annually. The total annual costs associated with alcohol were found to exceed the entire development and welfare budgets for the district.

A community ban on alcohol was initially applied in 200 villages
in Gadchiroli. The effect spread and eventually the state government
agreed to stop the sale of all alcoholic beverages in the district. Public campaigns in several other provinces, states, and cities of India
have also led to restrictions on the sale of alcohol and the closure of
many liquor shops.

Impact of alcohol exports on developing countries and successful control measures.

The export of alcoholic beverages to developing countries, or
their production in local subsidiaries, can be highly profitable for companies in developed countries. By exporting
the product together with its
harmful side effects, foreign exchange and profits are maxi-
mized in the exporting country,
while avoiding all of the social
and health costs of increased
domestic sales (WHO, 1985b).
Similar considerations also apply to unsafe devices such as
motorcycles. Unfortunately, national or local policy measures
to deal with the public health
effects of alcohol are poorly developed or completely absent in
many developing countries
(WHO, 1985c).

Policies to contain the damage
caused by alcohol include heavy
taxation, control of location
and time of sales, and restriction of advertising. For motor
vehicle injuries, suicide, homicide, and other injuries, legislation to raise the legal age for
drinking and to mandate severe
penalties for driving under the
influence of alcohol can be useful (Jones et al., 1992) and has
been used in various countries
(Ross, 1984).

The long-term effect of this intervention on morbidity and mortality must be monitored and reported, since the results could be useful for other jurisdictions. Similar measures of alcohol prohibition have been enforced in many indigenous communities in Canada (May, 1992) and in some provinces in Papua New Guinea.

Prohibition in indigenous communities in Canada and the United States is generally confined to a reserve or to single villages, rather than to large districts, as in some areas of India. Vehicles have to be searched for alcohol when they enter or return to the dry community. However, drinkers often travel to outside towns and rapidly consume large quantities of alcohol, leading to many fights and to road injuries on the return trip (Gallaher et al., 1992).

For many communities, careful monitoring of the adverse effects of alcohol coordinated with strict control of conditions for its sale and use may be more feasible and acceptable than total prohibition. Controlled local sales of alcohol may also help to reduce the harmful effects of travel by road immediately following rapid consumption. Taxation of local sales can provide a source of local financing for community prevention and education programs, rather than allowing profits to be siphoned off into neighboring areas. An effective means of recovering the full economic costs of alcohol abuse to society at the point of distribution or sale must be established.

It is also important to consider means of altering the adverse social and economic conditions, including lack of education, that may contribute to binge drinking, alcoholism, and other addictions such as cigarette smoking (Crum et al., 1992). Attention to issues of soul, spirituality, communication skills, and the harmony of individuals and families within their communities has helped many people to eliminate their dependency on mind-altering substances, including alcohol.

Alcohol Research

Alcohol control efforts could be spurred if total national costs attributable to alcohol were determined for damage from each specific type of intentional and unintentional injury. This would require estimates of the proportion of mortality and temporary and permanent disability from each type of injury. Estimates should include not only direct costs of treatment and rehabilitation, but also the indirect economic and social costs of death and time lost from work. Costs of the police and courts must be considered. Such comprehensive data on the negative economic impact of alcohol on society are rarely available (Maynard, 1986).

An appropriate level of taxation simply to recover the costs of the damage from alcohol-related injuries could then be established. Corresponding proportions of the costs recovered should be directly allocated to the primary, secondary, and tertiary prevention of injuries associated with alcohol. Such cost recovery would provide self-financing to prevent or repair damage from alcohol, with immediate funding from profits as alcohol was sold.

Pricing policies for alcoholic beverages and tobacco should not only ensure full cost recovery of all damage to society, but attempt to reduce consumption among vulnerable high-risk groups and avoid the creation of new addicts among young people. Thus, studies of the price and income elasticities of different types of alcoholic beverages among young males could be useful.

Research can define the extent to which advertising of alcohol is used to portray false and misleading images of the effects of alcohol consumption to vulnerable subgroups in the population. The types of neighborhoods and individuals targeted by different types of advertising could be studied to determine whether national, regional, and/or local controls on advertising are needed.

Other National Injury Control Initiatives

Surveillance, training, consumer product standards and monitoring, and special initiatives, such as the safe communities program, represent examples of other general injury prevention activities that may be suitable for sponsorship or organization at a national level. Appropriate laws and regulations usually must be drafted at a national level, although for certain types of injuries, municipalities or states are a more suitable locus of legislative initiatives.

A system for the general epidemiologic surveillance of all injuries is needed to establish the relative importance of different causes of injuries and to identify regions with unacceptably high injury rates. Such expertise may be established in injury programs within national and regional or provincial departments of public health.

It may also be desirable to encourage the development of more specialized monitoring within other departments or sectors. For example, departments of transport and/or police may compile and analyze data on traffic injuries and factors important to their prevention. The departments of justice and/or police may be involved in compiling detailed data on homicides, assaults, and suicides. Private organizations, such as the Red Cross, could compile data on water-related fatalities or on morbidity and mortality preventable by basic first-aid.

Regional or Provincial Level

Regional or provincial staff may provide direction and funding for local initiatives in injury surveillance and prevention. Public health departments need to take the lead in providing good injury data to guide other sectors, and should consider developing the capacity to serve as a coordinating center for injury control. The coroner's department may provide a useful link between some of the other departments and public health, particularly where coroners are medical staff with a link to district health services (Thorslund and Misfeldt, 1989).

Many coroners have had no training in public health or epidemiology, yet their records are a potentially valuable source of information for injury prevention. Often their focus is only on legal aspects of their work, including determining the intent of injuries. To stimulate awareness of the public health potential of their investigations and to maximize their contributions to injury control, coroners should receive brief courses to familiarize them with the basic principles of injury coding and control. This training should include a review of Haddon's injury matrix, together with a structured approach to recording the details of circumstances surrounding different types of injuries.

Coroners have powerful tools for initiating change through their annual reports, special directives, and appropriate media coverage. They may require epidemiological assistance to develop appropriate check lists to investigate different types of injuries and highlight important risk factors and activities with periodic analyses. When coroners are made aware of the importance of carefully documenting details of environmental, equipment, and personal risk factors and hazardous activities, their reports are a valuable source of data for the prevention of fatal injuries. Well-publicized reports by coroners on specific injury topics can be a stimulus to change, affecting the purchase of safer motor vehicles and equipment and the elimination of specific environmental hazards.

Meetings of local safety officers and public health officers can be effective in initiating discussion of the injury problem, in comparing their local injury situation with other areas or national averages, and in initiating community-based research and programs. Data on high rates of severe and fatal injury in low income neighborhoods may help to identify other hazards in these high-risk neighborhoods and target them for intervention.

Local Level

A community is like a ship; everyone ought to be prepared to take the helm.
—*Henrik Ibsen,* **An Enemy of the People,** *act I, 1882*

Multisectoral safe community initiatives can be based upon local data collection and analysis (Bjärås, 1993). Public health units, police, schools, industry, and private organizations such as the Red Cross/Red Crescent may cooperate to identify and deal with specific local hazards, alcohol, or social problems. Local data on morbidity and mortality from specific injuries can help to facilitate public acceptance of enforced legislation and municipal regulations.

Documentation of high injury rates among certain minority groups or poor neighborhoods may stimulate appropriate countermeasures. Examples of local programs could include identifying environmental hazards at specific locations. This might be followed by interventions, such as redesign of traffic flow to protect children and the elderly in poor crowded areas, or fencing of ponds and ditches in residential areas to prevent drowning of toddlers.

Large family size and reliance on older children for child care appear to be associated with increased rates of hospitalization of children for several types of injuries (Bijur et al., 1988) and with drownings (Nixon et al., 1979; Pearn et al., 1979a, 1979b). Special interventions, such as child care, family planning, or environmental changes may be needed to help large families reduce their risk of serious injury. The local importance of these factors could be investigated.

Local educational programs can target problems of concern, such as prevention and treatment of childhood burns, and control of epilepsy and its associated injury hazards. Trained village safety officers are employed in indigenous communities in northern Québec, Canada, and work in conjunction with the local fire department and public health officer.

Aggressive and misleading advertising of alcoholic beverages and tobacco products in poor communities and neighborhoods should probably be banned. If not, local community groups may be able to eliminate unwanted billboards by radical protests, as has been achieved by minorities in some inner city communities in the United States.

chapter 15

Injury Treatment and Rehabilitation: The Role of Health Services and Other Sectors

Preventing injury-causing events or their adverse effects on the human body is clearly preferable to attempting to repair the ensuing damage. Moreover, deaths from certain types of injuries often occur before there is any opportunity for medical intervention. Examples include many drownings, suicides, severe traffic injuries, and smoke intoxication from carbon monoxide poisoning in housefires.

Nevertheless, for many types of injuries, treatment and rehabilitation, or tertiary prevention, is an important part of injury control. Timely, appropriate treatment of injuries prevents many deaths and permanent disabilities and minimizes pain, suffering, and economic losses from inability to work. Tertiary prevention works not only by repairing damage and restoring function, but also by preventing an escalation in the extent and severity of the initial injury. Immediate control of hemorrhage from a penetrating wound prevents the rapid progression of a localized injury to systemic shock and death. Adequate early cleaning and covering of open wounds avoids entry of destructive bacteria into the adjacent structures and bloodstream during the hours and days after the initial injury. Infected wounds can escalate to systemic septicemia and death, or smoulder on to permanent disability by destruction, atrophy, and scarring.

It is essential that community members and primary health care workers be appropriately trained in the initial treatment of injuries to avoid progressive damage. The adequacy of local networks of communications and transport is a key determinant to the outcome of severe injuries. Also critical are subsequent medical and surgical treatments requiring special skills and training in trauma management. Rehabilitation of the injured is also important to avoid progressive damage. For example, therapy for a damaged limb avoids muscle atrophy that can leave an injury victim with a permanent physical malfunction.

This chapter focuses on various sectors that support an integrated system of health care for injuries, together with the levels of the health system as they relate to acute treatment and rehabilitation of the injured.

There is no medicine to be found for a life which has fled.
—Ibycus, Fragment 23, 580 B.C.E.

TREATMENT SYSTEMS FOR INJURY

Efficient management of injuries requires a comprehensive national program and treatment system to minimize the public health impact of injuries on a population. Ideally, injured persons should have access to an adequate hierarchical system of care that can minimize morbidity, mortality, and permanent disability (West et al., 1988; Sklar, 1988; Barss and Blackford, 1983).

The level at which treatment is provided in a hierarchy of services depends upon the severity and complexity of the injury(s), and upon whether trained personnel, communications, and transport systems exist to provide appropriate treatment and, when necessary, referral. Unnecessary referrals to higher levels of the health system substantially increase the direct costs of treatment and may overload secondary and tertiary health facilities to the extent that the overall quality of care suffers. On the other hand, failure to refer serious injuries can be fatal or lead to permanent disability, and represents an inefficient underutilization of higher level facilities (Bhatnagar and Smith, 1989). Delayed or inadequate treatment may also greatly increase the total direct costs of care, if prolonged hospitalization is required to treat complications, such as severe wound infections or osteomyelitis. In Ghana, it was found that long delays in treatment of limb injuries were a significant predictor of disability (Mock et al., 1993).

Serious problems often ensue from incompetent early management of minor injuries. It was reported from the Bhopal Hospital in India that many initially minor injuries became complicated by infection, both because of delays in obtaining treatment and because of inadequate basic treatment of wounds by primary health care workers, and physicians (Sharma and Kumar, 1974).

Natarajan (1978) estimated that 30 percent of trauma deaths in the Tamil Nadu State were potentially preventable by more rapid transport to hospital. Better ambulance services were recommended along with extensive upgrades of hospital facilities.

An issue rarely discussed is the need for better training and equipment for primary health facilities, so that patients could be resuscitated locally prior to transfer, instead of depending on immediate service by ambulance. Mohan (1984) has noted that sophisticated ambulance and helicopter services will not be available to most people in India in the foreseeable future. Simple emergency care measures, such as basic wound cleaning and dressing, pressure to stop bleeding, and cool water application for small burns, must be widely taught. A study of morbidity and mortality among trauma patients at a hospital in rural Ghana found that many complications occurred because of a lack of basic prehospital care and long delays, of 24 hours or more, before treatment was obtained (Mock et al., 1993). It was suggested that better care at a local level and/or more rapid transportation to hospital represented more essential needs than sophisticated hospital facilities and equipment.

The fact that many large hospitals in developing countries are overcrowded, understaffed, and reservoirs of exotic and lethal antibiotic-resistant bacteria underscores the fact that the simpler injuries should be managed away from such facilities. Skills at the community and primary health care levels must be upgraded to increase self-reliance and reduce dependency on large hospitals, except for the most severe cases.

HIERARCHICAL LEVELS OF INJURY CARE

The levels of injury management within an organized hierarchy of care are described below, including basic logistical requirements at each level and the essential linkages between levels. A well-organized hierarchy of care is useful not only to control injuries, but also to prevent maternal mortality and morbidity from complications of childbirth.

Individual and Household Level

Self-reliance in basic injury treatment is an important competency for individuals and families, especially in remote subsistence communities. There has been inadequate publicity about how to give immediate treatment to injuries in the home or village that do not require expensive medicines and the expertise of health professionals.

Often family members, neighbors, or co-workers are responsible for important early decisions about management and referral. Simple first-aid, such as direct pressure to a wound or elevation of an injured limb to control hemorrhage, can be effective and life-saving. Relatives may make the decision to not seek hospital care for a seriously injured patient because of local beliefs that injuries are caused by sorcery or because of previous dissatisfaction with local health facilities. The need to improve household care is evident because there are still many deaths caused by hemorrhage or infection from relatively minor wounds.

Another important principle of first-aid is to clean and cover wounds that otherwise can become infected and contaminated by flies. Such infections can end in death from septicemia or may cause disability from scarring of vital structures, such as tendons in the hands, or from chronic tropical leg ulcers (Manson-Bahr and Bell, 1987). When neglected for many years, tropical ulcers often progress to malignant carcinomas requiring amputation (Foster and Webb, 1988). A permanently disabled adult is the end-product of many of these processes, often after a relatively minor initial injury.

In other cases, lack of basic communications or transport, or lack of funding for the emergency use of such systems, prevents transfer to a primary health care facility or hospital. The spatial distribution of health facilities is frequently inequitable and inefficient. The construction of a health facility in a particular location implies a long-term commitment of resources to that area, but denies services to other sites. The choice of location should meet both local and integrated regional criteria. If local politicians or competing religious groups are allowed to unduly influence decisions about the most appropriate site, serious long-term damage to a treatment system often results. The result is that rapid access to care remains an impossibility for many villagers (Akhtar and Izhar, 1986).

Drafting an agreement of rational criteria for regional site selection for health facilities before conflicts arise can help to minimize waste and maximize efficiency. Nevertheless, if a community's previ-

During a village health patrol, one of the authors was asked to attend to an adult male subsistence cultivator who was in shock as a result of uncontrolled hemorrhage from a small axe wound on a leg. A tourniquet of vines applied above the wound had caused constriction of the veins and severe hemorrhage from the wound. Bleeding stopped immediately once the tourniquet was removed, a small pressure dressing applied, and the leg elevated. The patient required intravenous fluids to control shock from the blood loss (P. Barss, unpublished observation).

A letter from a nurse-tutor working at a rural health center contained the following observation: "I must tell you about a recent tragedy within walking distance of the health center— a boy of ten or so who received a cut on his ankle from an axe hemorrhaged to death slowly. This happened in broad daylight, and why did no one carry him to be sutured? . . . because a witch had cut him, so it would not have been right to interfere . . . " (M. Sedgewick, personal communication, 1989). This death resulted from a combination of two factors, namely, failure to apply immediate simple first-aid, and the decision not to refer the patient for primary health care.

A young man who was fishing from an open canoe was speared in the lower chest by a needlefish. The small penetrating wound was sutured by an aidpost orderly. Unfortunately, the possibility of internal injury was not entertained until hours later, by which time the patient's general condition had deteriorated. He was taken to a nearby health center. His blood pressure was not measured and no radio contact was made with the hospital. After several more hours, the patient reached hospital by village boat, but he had died just before arrival. Postmortem showed that the beak of the fish had penetrated the man's stomach, which was full of blood.

This patient could have been saved by a relatively simple operation at the hospital, but only if primary health staff had monitored the vital signs, recognized shock, contacted the hospital, and perhaps given enough intravenous fluids to avoid fatal collapse of his blood volume during transfer.

A girl suffered extensive burns from a clothing fire that had occurred on a remote island. She was taken to the nearest aidpost. The staff radioed the nurse at the nearest health center, which was several hours away by water. The nurse traveled by outboard dinghy to the aidpost. On arrival, he measured the blood pressure and found that the patient was already in shock from fluid loss

ous experience with the treatment provided at a nearby health facility has been poor, or when cultural beliefs lead to fatalistic apathy, the necessary initial contact with primary care providers may never be made, despite proximity to a facility.

It should by now be obvious that appropriate management of first-aid and referral at the individual or household level is essential for good injury care, and deserves more attention from health providers and bureaucracies. Intersectoral planners should make improvements in care at this level one of their priorities, if they are seriously interested in minimizing the negative impact of injuries on the entire population. In many developed countries, non-governmental organizations such as the Red Cross/Red Crescent provide standardized training and certification in first-aid and safety for school children and adults. However, such groups sometimes neglect to include in their teachings the use of simple and effective local remedies and first-aid. Much more must be done to develop and distribute literature and audiovisual materials containing this information, such as the books *Where There Is No Doctor* (Werner, 1977) or *Disabled Village Children* (Werner, 1987). When national curricula and materials are being developed, nature of injury data from representative rural health clinics and district hospitals should be used as a guide to the type and frequency of various injuries to be expected and emphasized in training programs.

Primary Health Care Level

This first level of contact with the established health system generally includes facilities such as aid posts and health centers that provide care for populations ranging from several hundred persons to 10,000 or more. In urban areas of some developing countries, the offices of private health providers or hospital emergency rooms may be the site of primary health care for injuries, while in industrial or plantation settings, there may be a company health clinic.

If the family, neighbors, or co-workers of an injured patient are successful in overcoming all of the potential barriers to referral discussed above, the patient may eventually reach a primary health facility. Primary health care workers who staff such facilities should be well-versed in the same principles of basic first-aid for control of hemorrhage and prevention of infection that are so useful at a household level.

Depending upon the range of training available for health workers, primary care staff may include aid post orderlies, nurse aides, nurses, health extension officers, and physicians. In addition to providing more advanced first-aid, staff at this level should be capable of measuring vital signs to detect early shock or respiratory complications. They should know how to make a general assessment of the patient, including the detection of less obvious internal injuries.

Primary health care workers should also be capable of recognizing cases in which the patient will benefit from rapid referral to secondary facilities. They must be able to clear and monitor the airway and resuscitate patients in shock with intravenous fluids when indicated. They also must be capable of providing definitive treatment for many of the more common injuries, including lacerations, penetrating wounds, burns, and fractures.

Basic supplies such as intravenous fluids, antibiotics, dressings, and materials for splinting fractures must be available at this level. In addition, communications systems, such as two-way radios or telephones, should be available so that staff can obtain rapid advice on assessing and managing the more difficult cases and arranging emergency transfer to hospital when it is necessary. Ideally, primary health facilities of moderate size, such as health centers, should be located near a road, airstrip, or harbor to facilitate evacuation.

Secondary Health Care Level

Secondary care for injuries is generally provided at a district or provincial hospital, typically serving a population of 100,000 or more. The same basic skills and supplies necessary at the primary level are important at the secondary level, together with the additional capacity for complete early assessment and management of more severe injuries, including moderately complex closed fractures and all open fractures, abdominal, thoracic, and head injuries, and large burns. In addition, safe screening and cross-matching of blood must be available at all times, which implies a well-staffed laboratory; physicians must be trained in the safe and responsible use of transfusions.

Physicians at the secondary level should be actively involved in training and updating primary level providers, including initial patient assessment, basic resuscitation, and wound care. They must be available at the hospital end of the primary-secondary communications link to provide suggestions concerning assessment and resuscitation and to help arrange emergency transfers. The importance of adequate communications and transport linkages and cooperation between primary and secondary levels cannot be overemphasized.

Under some circumstances, facilities for air transport are a valuable component of the health care system. A two-year study of all emergency medical air evacuations was made in a widely dispersed population of 130,000 in a province of Papua New Guinea (Barss and Blackford, 1983). Of the 92 patients evacuated, it was estimated that, without emergency air transfer, 63 might have died and another 9 might have been left with a serious disability. Obstetric emergencies accounted for one-half, and surgical emergencies for one-third. Of the 19 surgical evacuations for injuries, only one person died, and it was estimated that of the 18 who recovered, 10 (56 percent) might have died and 5 (28 percent) been left with permanent or prolonged disability in the absence of prompt air evacuation. In descending order of frequency, cases included open fractures, head injury, severe wounds, ruptured spleen, large burns, fractured spine, and infected wound.

The average cost per capita of providing emergency evacuations by charter of light aircraft was US $0.12 per year, and the cost per life saved was US $520. Of all flights, 93 percent were used to transport patients from primary to secondary level within the province, and 7 percent were for transport of patients out of the province from secondary to tertiary level when a doctor with adequate surgical experience was unavailable at the provincial hospital. During the same period, many other emergencies were transferred on regular scheduled flights or by boat at substantially lower costs; charter

into the burns. He was able to start an intravenous drip and stabilize the patient's condition. The following day, it was possible to contact the district hospital by radio to arrange emergency evacuation by light aircraft. The patient eventually made a full recovery, after further resuscitation in hospital and many wound dressings and skin grafts. Without the necessary infrastructure, including transport, communications, and primary health care, this little girl would have died within hours of the burn.

Injury care at the secondary level.

A boy on a remote island fell from a breadfruit tree and struck his head. He awoke for a brief period and then lapsed back into coma. He was carried by his family for a few hours to the nearest health center, where he was found to be in a deep coma with a dilated pupil in one eye. The district hospital was contacted by radio. A physician recognized the typical signs of an expanding intracranial clot and arranged for an air charter to the island. It was too late to return the same day, so appropriate surgical instruments were taken along by the physician to the health center. A simple craniotomy was carried out shortly after arrival, which released a large epidural hematoma that was exerting severe pressure on the brain. The following day the patient was taken back to the hospital, where he received the basic nursing care necessary for an unconscious patient. He regained consciousness after one week, and several weeks later had made a full recovery.

flights were used only when evacuation by a scheduled flight or diversion was not possible within a reasonable period of time, depending upon the urgency of the case.

The results of this study would be most applicable to mountainous or island areas of developing countries with minimal road transport, but with adequate resources to support such transfers. For areas with well-developed road systems, road transport would be substantially less expensive and often much safer.

Injury care at the tertiary level.

A young village man injured by a crocodile while fishing in a mangrove swamp sustained a severe injury of one leg. He was resuscitated at a primary facility and then transported to a secondary facility, where treatment for shock and septicemia and a below-knee amputation were needed. He was subsequently transferred to a tertiary facility for fitting with a below-knee prosthesis. This device was simple and functional, and enabled him to function nearly normally in his community, rather than remain crippled.

Another case involved a young man admitted unconscious to a secondary facility as a result of ingestion of methyl alcohol at a drinking party. The hospital had never managed such a case. The recent installation of a telephone system with microwave towers had linked the national capital with provincial capitals. This made it possible to obtain immediate specialist advice from the national teaching hospital concerning the management of the metabolic acidosis that occurs in such poisonings. The patient eventually made a full recovery.

A third case involved a young plantation worker who had been transferred by air to a secondary facility from a copra and rubber plantation after being bitten by an extremely venomous snake; he was on the verge of respiratory paralysis on arrival. The initial air transfer had been possible because of a good radio link between the

Tertiary Health Care Level

Within an organized system of injury care, the most important role of the university teaching hospital, which is generally a tertiary facility, is probably to train appropriate staff for secondary facilities, to develop sustainable standard treatment protocols and pharmaceutical lists for all levels of the health system, and to provide specialized rehabilitation services, such as construction and fitting of lower limb prostheses.

Skills, protocols, and drugs and supplies must be tailored to the level of development, resources, and the extent of remoteness within any specific country. Since many urban areas lack a well organized hierarchy of health facilities, many "tertiary" hospitals are, unfortunately, so heavily burdened with primary and secondary level functions that they are unable to fulfill their potential as tertiary centers.

In some countries, the development of an organized trauma unit may be economically justifiable if it provides concentrated and efficient periods of staff training, as well as more standardized and efficient treatment for the steady flow of severe injuries seen in many densely populated areas. In any case, simple and sustainable routines and equipment should be standardized and regularly updated. Techniques and equipment should be as simple as possible, so that experience acquired by staff at the larger facility can be transferred to secondary facilities.

Low priority should be given to complex, costly, and intimidating capital equipment. Such items often benefit a relatively small number of patients, are generally unavailable at secondary levels, are usually costly and difficult to maintain, and may even be harmful when inappropriately used. Nevertheless, pressure exerted by sales representatives and various special interest groups within hospitals for purchase of such expensive "prestige" items is often overwhelming.

Other important functions of tertiary level facilities include training nurses and physicians in simple routines for management of various injuries. Some examples include, basic treatment of wounds, including wound irrigation for penetrating wounds and delayed closure for late and infected wounds; simple closed management of common fractures and appropriate routines for handling open fractures to minimize the risk of infection; detection and management of tendon injuries; detection and care of internal injuries of the chest and abdomen; assessment, monitoring, and management of patients with head injury by nursing care, burr holes, and other relatively simple measures; burn care, including resuscitation; wound care to control infection, skin grafting, physiotherapy, and simple procedures for releasing scars to reduce disability. Tertiary staff need to share their technical expertise with staff at isolated facilities and to develop local competency, rather than jealously guarding skills and insisting on referrals.

Two-day practical courses in Advanced Trauma Life Support have been prepared by the American College of Surgeons, and are now widely used in the United States to provide a rapid review of the major principles and procedures for early diagnosis and resuscitation of trauma victims; such courses are offered for all physicians and nurses who deal with severely injured patients and require recertification every four years (American College of Surgeons, 1989; Ali and Naraynsingh, 1987). Similar courses would be useful for health workers in developing countries, although more emphasis and information on definitive care are needed.

Another important role of many tertiary centers lies in providing the specialized skills and facilities needed for the fabrication and fitting of artificial limbs. Simple and robust prostheses must be developed to meet the needs and finances of people who live in remote locations. Wealthier countries may be able to afford special units for the rehabilitation of spinal cord injuries, but the resources of many countries are too limited to sustain effective units. Even if the patient is saved in the hospital, survival after discharge is not certain.

It is obvious that some of the same basic skills are necessary at all levels of the health system, from households to major regional centers. Each step up in the level of an organized system implies the superimposition of several more advanced skills and supplies.

Staff who work in remote areas and in primary and secondary facilities require a broad range of knowledge and skills, while staff who work in tertiary hospitals require more narrow, specialized, and in-depth knowledge and skills. For example, persons who fit and construct artificial limbs have highly specialized skills.

Many minor injuries should be successfully managed at the household level. If tertiary centers have adequately fulfilled their role of training and standardizing care, the vast majority of more seriously injured patients should be managed successfully at secondary or primary levels. This avoids overcrowding and hospital-acquired infections with antibiotic-resistant bacteria that are widespread in tertiary facilities.

Regionalization of services can be beneficial in some countries, particularly where populations are not widely dispersed and where transport and communications services are highly developed. On the other hand, the results of a study in England and Wales suggest that a consequence of highly centralized trauma and emergency service may be relatively high death rates in areas that are far away from such facilities. A concentration of high-technology, expensive facilities in a few areas may lead to inaccessibility in more remote areas, if primary or secondary facilities are downgraded, closed, or never opened (Bentham, 1986).

There is urgent need for research on cost effective trauma care centers suitable for capital-starved hospitals. The only models available at present are from the lavish trauma centers in the metropolises of developed countries.

plantation and the district hospital. Because of the installation of the national microwave telephone links discussed above, it was later possible for a hospital physician to obtain telephone advice from a medical consultant at a tertiary facility regarding the method of ventilating such a patient manually using simple equipment. When respiratory arrest occurred, it was managed successfully at the secondary facility. The patient was intubated and a nurse aide engaged to carry out manual ventilation overnight using a simple resuscitation bag. By morning, the patient was breathing on his own and went on to a full recovery.

A failure may also be illustrative. A young person with a complex open fracture of the elbow was transferred from a secondary to a tertiary facility for orthopedic management, since at that time no one was available with basic orthopedic skills at the district hospital. However, a few weeks later when the patient returned to the secondary facility, it was noted that the fracture was poorly reduced and infected. It turned out that the patient had never been seen by the specialist to whom he had been referred and had received unskilled treatment, which left him with a permanent disability. This problem resulted from the fact that the tertiary facility was so overcrowded with routine cases from the periurban area, that many patients referred with more complex problems were never seen by the specialists to whom they had been referred.

THE ROLE OF HEALTH AND OTHER SECTORS: POLICY AND RESEARCH

Large capital and recurrent expenditures for costly health facilities and staff will be wasted or inefficiently used unless essential communications and transport links are available to facilitate the flow of patients and information between levels of the health system. The link between primary and secondary facilities is essential, and while technical factors are obviously relevant, the importance of personal contact and trust between professionals at different levels of the system is also vital. Professional participation and leadership are needed at local, national, and international levels to develop and sustain effective systems.

At the community and household level, it is necessary to study the local situation and ensure that the solutions developed are feasible and the most suitable for local conditions. Interested health workers and/or groups such as the Red Cross/Red Crescent should be encouraged to provide advice and assist in demonstrations. For example, in some schools in developed countries students are able to obtain basic Red Cross certification in first-aid. The presentation of rarely used and less essential information, often more appropriate for advanced first-aiders and emergency staff, should probably be avoided, except for interested persons at more advanced levels of training.

At a national and/or regional level, decisions about regionalization and financing of treatment and support systems and the development of locally appropriate guidelines for training, equipment, and procedures are needed. Often there is an unmet need for coordination of the communications, transport, education, health, agricultural, industrial, and private voluntary sectors to develop systems for the care of injuries in both rural and urban areas.

In the absence of well-developed national leadership in intersectoral coordination, the World Bank and United Nations organizations, such as the World Health Organization, could provide direction and facilitate the necessary interactions and processes. Economists may be able to suggest options for financing injury treatment systems, such as user taxes on motor vehicles, fuel, and alcohol, that could be adjusted to cover the costs of adequate care for all injuries from motor vehicle crashes. International bodies can also develop general guidelines for training, equipment, procedures, financing, and the types of research needed to guide policy.

Possibilities for action-oriented policy measures are described below under sector headings, together with suggestions for research to guide programmatic activities. These should be considered as mere starting points for initiating discussion and developing locally appropriate programs and research.

Health Sector

Policy

The health sector should take the lead in developing a system that provides adequate treatment and rehabilitation of the injured (Table 15.1).

At a few large urban teaching hospitals, low-technology trauma units could be considered. Such units could be useful to develop and evaluate standard national routines for the initial assessment and management of trauma, and also to provide a rapid training program in such routines and in the care of multiple injuries for physicians who staff district hospitals. If such units are developed, routines, supplies, and equipment should be standardized to a simple and economically sustainable level, so that they are readily transferable nationwide.

Table 15.1 Examples of health sector activities for development of a national system of treatment and rehabilitation of victims of trauma

---

Development of infrastructure and information systems

• Collaborate with other sectors to develop reliable communication and transport links between all levels of the health system.

• Establish information systems that identify the nature, causes and severity of injuries treated at all levels of care from primary to rehabilitation; data from the information system should be used immediately in developing and updating teaching materials and training programs.

Ensure professional and community competence

• Develop standard injury assessment and treatment routines at teaching hospitals appropriate to the country's level of economic development and simple enough to be used at district hospitals.

• Provide short intensive courses at tertiary hospitals for nurses and physicians from secondary facilities, including emergency resuscitation, stabilization, recognition of cases requiring specialized management, and treatment; consider adaptations of programs such as the Advanced Trauma Life Support Course.

• Provide basic training at secondary level district hospitals for primary health workers, including first-aid, assessment, management, and appropriate referral of injuries.

• Incorporate teaching of first-aid into routine job descriptions of appropriate health staff

• Ensure that essential and simple measures of first-aid are taught at the community level, in collaboration with schools and appropriate non-governmental organizations.

Organize and maintain sustainable supply systems

• Develop (and periodically update) supply lists for each level of the health system by central pharmaceutical services and trauma staff from all levels of the system, covering inexpensive basic supplies such as bandages, bandaids, sutures, materials for immobilizing fractures, intravenous fluids, chest drains, surgical instruments, antibiotics, etc.

• Establish distribution systems that equitably supply all levels of the health system (not only hospitals).

• Develop simple, durable limb replacements for amputees that are appropriate to the country's level of economic development; establish a center(s) for making, fitting, and maintaining such prostheses and for on-the-job training.

The tendency to overcentralize care and divert funds from secondary and primary facilities should be particularly resisted, since this may lead to deterioration in the competence of staff and equipment at important district facilities, and contribute to a corresponding deterioration at primary levels. Overcentralization and concentration of resources and staff may reduce accessibility to basic emergency care in most areas, except those near centralized units.

Communications

Policy

Internationally, guidelines to the most appropriate communications technologies for different climates and environments must be made available. National governments should encourage development of networks of appropriate radio or telephone systems, particularly in rural and remote areas where communications are unreliable. At a regional level, communications links should be created between primary and secondary health facilities.

Reliable radio or telephone communications between the primary and secondary levels are essential to improve the initial assessment and management of injuries by primary health workers, and to facilitate transfer to district hospital when necessary. The maintenance and support of such equipment is often considerably more efficient when it is integrated into provincial or regional networks for multisectoral use, rather than performing as stand-alone systems operated exclusively for health purposes. Communications between secondary and tertiary levels tend to be less in need of development, since such facilities are usually in towns or cities and often have telephone links.

The use of communications networks for regular training and updating of health personnel in the management of common injuries should be encouraged. The use of media such as radio for educating families and individuals in the assessment and management of injuries should be developed.

Research

The proportion of health centers, subcenters, and other primary health facilities that have adequate communications links to secondary facilities should be determined and estimates made of the costs of extending such links to all primary health centers within provinces and countries. Patterns of use and utility of communications links for management of trauma should be verified. The availability and use of local media, such as radio, for educating the public in injury prevention and first-aid should be studied. This could include assessment of the effect on knowledge, attitudes, and practices of the public with respect to their assessment and management of common injuries, including the importance and means of controlling hemorrhage and preventing infection in wounds.

In rural areas, where telephones and ambulances are rare, the government may wish to explore the feasibility of training truck drivers in the basic steps to be taken at the scene of a crash or other emergency. Truck drivers in remote areas must be resourceful and are likely to have opportunities to apply such training. Providing trained drivers with transmitting and receiving radios would serve as an incentive to join the program and enable them to transmit information to the hospital and receive instructions.

Transport

Policy

Time is that wherein there is opportunity, and opportunity is that wherein there is no great time.
—*Hippocrates,* **Precepts,** *ch 1, 460–377* B.C.E.

Governments should facilitate the development of efficient low-cost transport systems that would be available on demand for emergency transport. Rapid and relatively inexpensive transfer from primary to secondary level is important; prolonged delays in treatment are highly detrimental for certain injuries, and may adversely affect the morale and status of the primary health workers who make the referrals. As in communications, transport is generally most efficient if integrated into provincial or regional systems. Stand-alone units, such as "flying-doctor" units, provide charisma and often attract external support and staff, but are costly when compared to efficient use of local private and government carriers, since normally only intermittent use is required (Barss and Blackford, 1983).

In countries with difficult geography and limited road systems, small airlines can be encouraged to operate in marginal rural areas; governments should provide adequate funds for diversions and charters, or provide military aircraft for serious emergency cases. Such transfers should be affordable, or could be made affordable, for some developing countries, as discussed earlier; the ongoing expense and risk of aircraft crashes must be balanced against the substantial boost to the confidence and security of both health providers and the population that results when emergency transfers are available for those few life-threatening or disability-threatening emergencies that cannot be adequately treated at a primary health facility or transferred by more economical means.

Unless judiciously managed and sparingly applied, however, air evacuation programs are subject to waste and misuse, as well as high crash rates. Since travel by light aircraft can be hazardous, emergency flights should not be made under adverse flying conditions, regardless of the perceived urgency of the case. Even in areas with established road networks, taxi or truck drivers may demand as payment for transport of patients amounts that are equivalent to several months of subsistence income.

Governments should ensure adequate budgetary support for basic transportation and communications. The construction of costly, "high-tech" health facilities is inefficient for the population if equitable access to primary and secondary care for basic treatment of injuries is unavailable because of poorly developed communication or transportation systems. While direct subsidy of private transport systems might be unwise, allocations of funds for the regular use of such systems for patient and staff transport provides an indirect subsidy in remote areas with low or irregular traffic. Careful monitoring of such travel is necessary to avoid waste and abuse.

Research

At international and national levels, the efficacy, costs, and feasibility of various types of air and land transport for the injured should be compared. The costs, benefits, and unmet needs for routine and emergency transport of injured persons, from primary to secondary facilities within provinces and countries, should be determined. Particularly in rural areas, where the demand for urgent transport is sporadic, the feasibility of using and adapting existing systems of transport for transfer of the injured should be evaluated (Barss and Blackford, 1983).

Education

Policy

At an international level, general guidelines for first-aid curricula should be developed, including criteria for the use of local research data to develop specific locally appropriate materials. This could be carried out by bodies such as the World Health Organization and/or by private organizations such as the Red Cross/Red Crescent.

At national, regional, and local levels, health curriculum staff in departments of education should be encouraged to work closely with groups such as the Red Cross/Red Crescent and with suitable health workers to develop appropriate first-aid training for schools. Special attention should be given to the needs of rural and remote areas, where distances from health facilities and delays in obtaining definitive treatment are greater. As a guide to the emphasis that should be given to different types of injuries, during curriculum development injury epidemiologists or other health professionals should be encouraged to provide data on the numbers of different types of injuries, using nature of injury data from clinics and hospitals.

School systems could incorporate basic first-aid training into their curriculum, with an emphasis on development of simple practical skills for control of hemorrhage and prevention of infection. Students should be encouraged to discuss these topics with their parents. Adult education efforts could include instruction for parents in the evenings or on weekends.

Simple local surveys of the types of injuries that present to various types of health facilities and the most common complications of inappropriate home treatment would provide a basis for the development and updating of curricula. Health curriculum writers should be expected to regularly verify that the instruction provided is simple and up-to-date, and that information and demonstrations are repeated in successive years to ensure learning retention.

All teachers should be encouraged or required to maintain basic certification in first-aid, and certification should be provided for all students who successfully complete a basic first-aid course. Regular recertification should also be required. Schools should be helped to conduct first-aid courses for adults, particularly in rural areas where they may be unavailable otherwise.

In areas at high risk for natural or technological disasters, communities and individuals should be trained to prepare and respond, since action at the local level is generally the most appropriate and feasible in the early stages of a disaster.

Short spots on television were shown to be effective in promoting simple first-aid measures for burns in India (Mohan and Varghese, 1990). Such items should be repeated periodically as part of regular programming on national networks.

Research

Studies should determine rates of morbidity and chronic disability from complication of wounds and fractures that result from inadequate first-aid and primary care of wounds and injuries. These data should be used in developing locally appropriate first-aid curriculum materials.

The current status and unmet needs for first-aid training should be determined, particularly in schools and in remote communities. The costs of expanding such activities to all unserved areas within provinces and countries should be estimated.

In areas at high risk of disaster, awareness of the appropriate responses to common scenarios could be assessed for individuals and key decision makers. Appropriate training or education could be developed to remedy problems identified by the research.

Agriculture and Industry

Policy

Agriculture and industry often involve exposure to special hazards, including heavy machinery and toxic chemicals. First-aid programs for workers and health staff may, therefore, need to be more complex than for general households. These sectors should be encouraged to ensure the provision of adequate first-aid and primary health care for their workers in an integrated program for both prevention and management of injuries. Some companies may be able to provide various types of logistical support to communities and the health system, but cannot be regularly depended upon to do so, since this would generally be done on a voluntary basis to generate public good will and support. Treatment of injured workers should not be emphasized at the expense of primary prevention, since some industrial injuries are so severe that prevention is the only real answer to the problem of life-long disabilities from injury.

Special attention must be given to the injury problems of subsistence cultivators who work on their own or on small farms, often in remote locations. Such workers are ignored by most existing occupational injury prevention and safety programs.

Research

The extent of unmet needs for first-aid and basic management of injuries at companies and agricultural plantations should be surveyed within provinces and countries, and cost estimates prepared for the expansion of such activities.

The knowledge, attitudes, and practices of subsistence cultivators and farmers, with respect to management of injuries, together with the types of injuries and complications they are most subject to, need careful study. This should facilitate development of appropriate public educational programs to meet their needs.

Finance

Policy

The finance sector must ensure that the costs of providing treatment and rehabilitation of specific product-related injuries are recovered in the costs of the products. For example, alcoholic beverages are implicated in the etiology of many types of unintentional and intentional injuries. Products such as automobiles and motorcycles also cause many deaths and injuries. Treatment costs could be recovered in a variety of ways, including taxation on the initial sale of the product, mandatory no-fault insurance to cover treatment costs, and fuel taxes. Taxation and insurance should contain specific components designated to cover the estimated average costs of treatment per product item during the lifetime of the product. Similar taxes on cigarettes are already used by some countries to finance the treatment costs of illnesses and injuries resulting from nicotine addiction. Lawsuits are also being undertaken by some governments to recover costs of treating victims at public health facilities from the manufacturers of hazardous products such as cigarettes. This could be a useful approach to discourage the sale of other dangerous products.

Research

At a national level, the direct and indirect costs of all injuries resulting from motor vehicles, including motorcycles, should be estimated. The feasibility of compensatory user taxes on vehicles and fuel as a potential source of financing for the treatment of traffic injuries should be evaluated. This would necessitate preliminary investigations to estimate the numbers of patients treated for injuries from such crashes and related cost estimates. Such estimates should reflect the total costs of treatment and rehabilitation for the country, and not just the costs to the individual patient, which in nationalized health systems may be minimal.

A related study could investigate the costs of motor vehicle injuries resulting from alcohol. Since up to 50 percent of such injuries may result from alcohol, treatment costs can be financed by a user's tax on alcoholic beverages, applied at the point of manufacture or importation. If possible, the cost burden of other injuries related to alcohol should also be determined and covered by taxation.

Other hazardous products, such as the herbicide paraquat, could be considered for similar taxation, if health data suggest that the treatment costs are high enough to justify the administrative costs of a new tax.

Nongovernment Organizations

Policy

At an international level, non-governmental organizations should consider the widespread need for better education in the basic principles of assessment and management of acute injuries among households and individuals in remote villages. Governments should ensure that organizations such as the International Red Cross/Red Crescent and other groups are provided with political and, where needed, financial support.

Such organizations should be encouraged to expand their first-aid activities in developing countries, particularly into remote and underserved areas. They could work with national education curriculum units and health systems to ensure that all school children, teachers, and health providers are certified and regularly recertified in basic first-aid. They could also train suitable instructors to work with rural communities to develop adult programs in first-aid and, where appropriate, disaster response.

Remote communities should receive priority for first-aid and training at the household level, since it is in such places that the needs and potential benefits would be greatest. Special attention should be given to the high incidence of untreated or poorly managed injuries in rural subsistence agriculture.

Research

Non-governmental agencies, including missions and other service organizations, often have an important role in providing both education and treatment services in areas underserved by the government. The most effective ways to make use of their services must be determined. The utility and appropriateness of the services provided also need careful assessment based upon surveys of local health conditions and the most common and/or serious complications (Table 15.2).

Table 15.2 Examples of research to be undertaken by the health sector

HOUSEHOLD, PRIMARY AND SECONDARY LEVELS

Research for improving treatment practices for injuries

- Assess the knowledge and practices of first aid for common injuries by individuals and households in typical rural and urban locations; reassess these attributes after programs of public education by the health sector or non-government organizations.

- Use health facility data to identify the most common injuries treated at different levels of the health system, including severity and cost as assessed by the mean, median, and mode for duration of hospital stay.

- Assess the proportion of health facilities at primary and secondary levels that have adequate numbers of staff with appropriate training and skills to provide competent injury care at their level.

- Assess whether primary care staff are able to recognize and treat hemorrhagic shock and provide basic care of wounds, including control of hemorrhage and prevention of infection.

- Assess the proportion of secondary facilities having at least one physician with a year or more of postgraduate training in essential surgical and orthopedic skills.

- Measure the prevalence of depression and suicide in the community and the extent to which health workers and families are trained to recognize and manage risk factors for suicide.

Research for improving basic supplies for health facilities

- Assess the availability of standard up-to-date pharmaceutical supply lists and purchasing systems for basic equipment and supplies for management of injuries at primary, secondary, and tertiary level facilities.

Research for improving management decisions for allocation of resources for injury care and prevention

- Assess the proportion of hospital discharges with the External Cause of injury recorded in their record by a health provider and determine whether this is properly recorded in the discharge summary so that External Cause codes can be assigned; if unavailable, develop methods of improving data.

- Assess appropriateness of location of primary and secondary facilities in providing equitable and timely access to basic injury care.

- Assess the proportion of total hospital admissions and bed days that result from all injuries combined and from the most important specific injuries.

- Collaborate with health economists to estimate the direct and indirect costs of treating both common and severe injuries at different levels of the health system.

- Measure the prevalence of disability from injury in various subgroups of the adult population and estimate the proportion that might have been avoided by better prevention, treatment, or rehabilitation.

TERTIARY LEVEL

Research for improving treatment practices for injuries

- Assess ability and willingness of specialist units within tertiary facilities to train staff for secondary level facilities.

- Assess knowledge among specialist teaching staff of basic skills needed by physicians to manage and rehabilitate trauma patients at secondary level facilities.

- Assess adequacy of rehabilitation services available within tertiary centers, including accessability, competence, and appropriateness for local conditions of artificial limb fitting, fabrication, and maintenance.

(continued)

321

Table 15.2 Examples of research to be undertaken by the health sector—*Continued*

Research for improving basic supplies for health facilities

• Assess the extent to which tertiary facilities fulfill their potential to develop standardized protocols and supply lists for drugs and equipment to improve management of injuries at all levels of the health system.

Research for improving management decisions for allocation of resources for injury care

• For larger and wealthier developing countries, estimate the potential benefits and costs of establishing specialized regional trauma units and rehabilitation centers at the tertiary level, including any adverse impact on secondary facilities.

• For more wealthy countries, careful preliminary study of the appropriateness, cost-effectiveness, opportunity costs, maintenance costs, and availability of qualified technicians, repair personnel, and replacement parts for any planned purchases of expensive items such as computerized (CAT) scanners.

CONCLUSION

As for initial prevention of injuries, treatment and rehabilitation to control the harmful effects of injuries require a comprehensive program with policy interventions in different sectors. Intersectoral coordination of such efforts by policymakers is highly desirable.

Appropriate research at various levels is needed to guide policymakers in their decision-making, planning, and allocation of resources, and as a basis for training. The often insatiable demands for financing treatment systems should be weighed against the importance of primary and secondary prevention. For many injuries, death may seldom be prevented by improved treatment systems, but rather by preventing the injury provoking event; however, morbidity, and for certain injuries, mortality, may often be reduced or eliminated by more timely and better treatment and rehabilitation.

Basic epidemiologic studies of levels of mortality and morbidity from specific injuries in different locations may help in balancing the conflicting demands for resources for long-term primary and secondary prevention versus immediate needs for treatment and rehabilitation. For fatal injuries, the duration of the interval between the incident and death should be assessed. For certain types of injuries, this interval may be so short that it is obvious that primary or secondary prevention is essential. In view of previous neglect of training the public to deal with trauma, the capacity of families and individuals to recognize and respond to the effects of injuries needs special attention in remote areas.

Local self-reliance is particularly appropriate where regular treatment systems are already overloaded or are deteriorating as a result of inadequate resources for increasing numbers of victims. Rising treatment loads can result from the combined effect of factors such as rapid population growth, more patient referrals due to improved transport networks, deterioration in peripheral facilities, and rapid increases in the number of motor vehicles.

chapter 16

Conclusion

Attitudes towards injuries are changing. This should lead to a new era when scientific studies help guide decision makers toward effective leadership in the prevention of morbidity and mortality from injuries. We hope the material in this book has provided an introduction for the reader interested in preventing injuries, especially in neglected areas of developing countries or in indigenous, remote, and other underserved communities in industrialized countries. It should be obvious by now that relatively little injury surveillance and research has been done in such locations, especially for non-traffic injuries. This situation is changing as researchers and senior officials become aware of recent developments in injury control, acquire expertise in injury surveillance, improve local data sources, and begin to apply various interventions in their own countries.

There is abundant opportunity for both routine injury surveillance and creative research in developing countries and indigenous communities, including identification and study of local hazards, some of which are relatively unknown in major population centers in developed countries. There is also a need to develop effective and practical interventions adapted to local conditions. It is essential, however, that adequate funds be made available for research and evaluation locally, regionally, nationally and internationally. Routine descriptive injury research requires no expensive laboratories or experimental animals, but it does demand practical minds with basic epidemiological skills.

As an example of the lack of resources for injury control in many developing countries, it was reported that the total allocation for injury prevention programs in the 1990–91 World Health Organization Budget was only $5,000 for the 34 countries of the Western Pacific region, an average of $147 per country (Dietrich, 1990). More is expended during an average evening in many a local bar than is to be found in such shamefully low national injury research budgets.

The situation for research funding is generally better in some of the indigenous communities in developed countries. Information sharing between developing countries and indigenous communities in industrialized countries could be particularly beneficial regarding

When we watch a child trying to walk, we see its countless failures; its successes are but few. If we had time to limit our observation within a narrow space of time, the sight would be cruel. But we find that in spite of its repeated failures, there is an impetus of joy in the child which sustains it in its seemingly impossible task. We see it does not think of its falls so much as of its power to keep its balance, though for only a moment.

—Rabindranath Tagore,
Sādhanā: The Realisation of Life, *1913*

323

measures that can be taken to deal with the impact of rapid development on unintentional and intentional injuries. This could include interventions that have proven useful for dealing with injuries resulting from psychosocial stress due to loss of traditional lifestyles and social structures, physical hazards from introduction of new equipment, and personal risks due to aggressive marketing of alcohol and tobacco.

Public health professionals have been able to conduct many successful campaigns within the health sector to prevent infectious diseases, without needing multisectoral collaboration. Immunization campaigns provide dramatic examples of such successes. However, prevention and control of injuries are often more complex programs and tend to require multisectoral coalitions. Appropriate national and local organizations or networks must be created or strengthened to coordinate intersectoral collaboration to survey and control different types of injuries, including traffic injuries, drownings, fires, suicide, homicide, occupational injuries, and disasters.

The multifactoral etiology of different types of injuries provides scope for creative activity by professionals in various disciplines who share an interest in protecting the public from sudden death or disability by injury (Romer and Manciaux, 1986). Public health professionals, political leaders and legislators, policy makers, economists, business executives, union leaders, police, traffic engineers, firefighters, non-profit and other private organizations must collaborate to define the health and economic impact of specific injuries and their major determinants and to develop and evaluate interventions.

The World Health Organization's Ottawa Charter for Health Promotion provides a structured approach for considering possible interventions to prevent injuries and for integrating healthy public policies and legislation with other prevention activities by community organizations, health services, and individuals (WHO, 1986a). Health promotion should include the following:

- Building healthy public policy;
- Creating supportive environments;
- Strengthening community action;
- Developing personal skills;
- Reorienting health services.

These actions provide a starting point for a comprehensive approach to injury prevention. Advocacy for healthy public policy can be used to ensure that legislation and regulations at various levels serve to eliminate hazards. Environments must be not only supportive, but also user-friendly and protective of special vulnerable groups, such as toddlers. Community action to obtain safe environments must be backed by sound information and collaboration between organizations with shared goals. A link with the World Health Organization's Safe Community Programs and an awareness of the "Manifesto for Safe Communities" of the First World Conference on Injury Prevention in Stockholm could be useful in this context (WHO, 1989).

The health sector is faced with many of the consequences of uncontrolled injuries. Health services must be reoriented from only providing treatment for injuries to collaborating and participating in preventive activities, such as community surveillance for environmental hazards. Health professionals, including epidemiologists, carry out regular surveillance of the health impact of injuries and other health conditions using routine health data sources. On the basis of their extensive experience with the use of various indicators of mortality and morbidity, health professionals should be able to establish priorities that can be used to select specific injuries for prevention and control. This process can be strengthened by collaboration with demographers and economists.

Public health staff can share their epidemiological expertise to help others collect and analyze supplemental data to define the circumstances of important injuries of mutual interest. This collaborative information gathering may include standardized surveys of environmental, equipment, and personal risk factors for a specific category of injury at the level of mutual interest, be it community, regional, national, or international. Once the major circumstances of a specific injury have been ascertained, possible interventions can be developed jointly and selected on the basis of potential efficacy, feasibility, acceptability, and cost.

Political support is essential to develop effective legislation and regulations mandating changes in environmental, equipment, or personal factors at the appropriate level, and to obtain adequate funding for routine injury surveillance and special research. Carefully prepared epidemiological data on injuries helps to ensure the necessary support at all levels. Without effective enforcement, legislation may be ineffective. Thus, the collaboration of organizations with enforcement powers is needed, including groups such as police and industrial safety inspectors.

The Haddon matrix for injury prevention (Robertson, 1992) provides another means of structuring different injury prevention activities for control of personal, environmental, and equipment factors during pre-event, event, and postevent phases. The use of broad and comprehensive approaches to prevention, such as the Ottawa Charter for Health Promotion and the Haddon matrix, encourage lateral thinking, which is important to avoid becoming prematurely locked into a single strategy that might ultimately prove ineffective (de Bono, 1967, 1994).

Well-organized programs for injury surveillance identify personal, equipment, and environmental risk factors and hazardous activities for the specific injuries that are of greatest importance to the community, region, or nation. Injury surveillance also allows delineation of high-risk subgroups in the population. Planners must then consider whether to focus on protection of high risk subgroups, on the entire population, or on both (Rose, 1992).

The merits of population-based approaches versus a focus on high-risk individuals have been considered less for injuries than for many common diseases. Combinations of the two approaches may be effective depending upon the characteristics of the local population. Different approaches may complement each other or serve as backups if one fails.

It would appear that for certain general personal risk factors or determinants, such as alcohol abuse and cigarette smoking, shifts in national norms towards reduced or no consumption could benefit both the general population and high-risk groups as normative changes across the population cause downward shifts in consumption in both low and high-risk groups. Normative reductions in overall levels of consumption of alcohol and tobacco would benefit many other health and social conditions that are associated with these drugs, and provide additional justification for seeking to bring about such changes.

Environmental and equipment changes can often be implemented on a population-wide basis. While such interventions protect the population at large, they will provide the greatest protective effect or risk reduction for high-risk individuals. The introduction of enclosed stoves to replace open fires and kerosene stoves with open flames protect the general population against burns and housefires. However, the potential benefit in reduced risk of death or injury by burns is several times greater for certain high-risk individuals, such as persons with epilepsy, small girls and women with flammable dresses, and slow-moving elderly persons, than for the general population. The additional bonus of protection against smoke-induced respiratory damage is another strong incentive for replacement of open fires by enclosed stoves.

In industrialized countries, most of the population is regularly exposed to the risk of a crash while riding inside an automobile. Thus, to control traffic injuries, considerable effort and expense have been expended on occupant protection. Changes include special safety equipment, such as airbags and interior padding and reinforcement. These modifications have to be applied to all automobiles at the time of manufacture, since automobiles of the persons at highest risk of fatal crashes, such as alcoholics or young binge drinkers, cannot be selectively modified. Such high-risk individuals have the most to gain by the population-wide introduction of safety equipment that provides automatic passive protection.

Since a substantial proportion of all traffic fatalities occur among high-risk individuals, protection of such persons by standard population-wide equipment or environmental measures carries substantial benefits for society as a whole. Airbags and other built-in passive measures provide automatic protection in automobile crashes, since even intoxicated drivers or people who do not attach their safety belts receive considerable protection. Members of the general public who carefully fasten their seat belts receive a double dose of protection if a crash occurs, although their level of risk for crashes is lower.

As such engineering innovations are introduced, however, low-risk individuals, who need the extra protection less, may have it first, because they are better able to afford new cars equipped with all of the safety equipment. Appropriate taxation of private automobiles can help to reduce such inequalities if the revenues are used to finance alternative public transportation systems.

In many developing countries, a population approach to traffic injuries would focus on measures to protect pedestrians, cyclists, and passengers in the rear of pick-up trucks, rather than occupants of automobiles. In northern indigenous communities, many inhabitants are exposed to boat and snowmobile travel over icy waters, and prevention of transport-related deaths needs to include interventions to prevent drowning and hypothermia. A great challenge for injury control is to develop effective and feasible interventions to provide automatic protection for such populations.

The introduction of new technologies, such as tools, machines, motor vehicles, and chemicals, is often accompanied by serious hazards. It is better to anticipate and actively engineer away such hazards at the outset, rather than passively wait for damage to occur and then react. Similarly, the introduction of rapid change in traditional lifestyles and social structures can disrupt communities and lead to suicides and assaults, as well as a host of other health problems. The prevention and control of such damage to communities should be an essential component of any development project.

While specific preventive efforts should bear rich fruit, it must not be forgotten that for injuries, as for many diseases, poverty is often an underlying determinant. Social, educational, and economic equity and the concomitant safer living conditions greatly reduce the risk of many unintentional and intentional injuries and must be vigorously pursued, in conjunction with control programs directed towards specific injuries.

Violence is arguably the most serious public health problem of our era, and one of the greatest challenges in injury control is the prevention of intentional injuries. Violence prevention must occur at home, community, national, and international levels. This requires a new emphasis by industrialized countries on non-violent methods of resolving international conflicts, and alternatives for the firearms and defense industries to stimulate their economies. In developing countries, considerable rethinking is required to establish more equitable and harmonious relationships between men and women.

Shortage of renewable resources, such as forests, as a result of environmental degradation leads not only to environmental disasters, but also to mass migration and violence (Homer-Dixon et al., 1993). Thus, prevention of intentional injuries on a large scale may involve seemingly unrelated interventions, such as protection and restoration of forests, redistribution of land and wealth, population policy, and restraints on foreign companies that encourage rapid depletion of renewable resources or the production of export crops on land needed for local food production.

References

Aboutanos M, Baker SP. Wartime civilian injuries: epidemiology and intervention strategies. *J Trauma* 1997;43:719–726.

Acha PN, Aguilar FG. Studies on cysticercosis in Central America. *Am J Trop Med Hyg* 1964; 13:48–53.

Acha PN, Arambulo PV. Rabies in the tropics—history and current status. In: Kuwert E, Merieux C, Koprowski H, Bogel K, eds. *Rabies in the Tropics.* Berlin: Springer-Verlag, 1985:343–359.

Achutti A, Duncan BB, Schmidt MI. Factores de risco para doencas cronicas/nao-transmissiveis. Unpublished manuscript, Universidade Federal do Rio Grande do Sul, Porto Alegre, 1988. Cited in: World Bank. *Adult Health in Brazil: Adjusting to New Challenges.* Brazil Development Report No. 7807–BR. 1989:1–133.

Adala HS. Ocular injuries in Africa. *Soc Sci Med* 1983;17:1729–1753.

Adams JGU. Evaluating the effectiveness of road safety measures. *Traffic Engineering and Control* 1988;29(6):344–352.

Adrian M, Ferguson BS. The influence of income on the consumption of alcohol in Ontario—a cross-sectional study. In: Carmi A, Schneider S, eds. *Drugs and Alcohol,* Volume 6, Berlin: Springer-Verlag, 1986:151–157.

Adrian M, Ferguson BS. Pricing policies—their impact on impaired driving (Abstract). In: *North American Conference on Alcohol and Traffic Safety: Implications for Public Policy* (Oct 17–20), Quebec, QC: Conference Abstracts, 1993:17–18.

Adrian M, Ferguson BS, Her M. Can economic policies be used to reduce substance abuse problems? In: M Rosenberg, ed. *Health and Behaviour,* Kingston, ON: Queen's University Press, 1994:5–45.

Aggarwal MK. Ill-designed road junctions threat to traffic road safety (Abstract). *J Traffic Med* 1990;18(4):309.

Agran PF, Castillo DF, Winn DG. Limitations of data compiled from police reports on pedestrian and bicycle motor vehicle events. *Accid Anal Prev* 1990;22:361–370.

Akhtar R, Izhar N. The spatial distribution of health resources within countries and communities: examples from India and Zambia. *Soc Sci Med* 1986;22:1115–1129.

Alakija W. Poor visual acuity of taxi drivers as a possible cause of traffic accidents in Bendel State, Nigeria. *J Soc Occup Med* 1981;31: 167–170.

Alary M, Joly JR. Risk factors for contamination of domestic hot water systems by Legionellae. *Appl Environ Microbiol* 1991;57:2360–2367.

Alemayehu W, Cherinet A. Eye diseases and blindness. In: Kloos H, Zein ZA, eds. *The Ecology of Health and Disease in Ethiopia.* Boulder: Westview Press, 1993, 237–249.

Alexander DE. Death and injury in earthquakes. *Disasters* 1985;9:57–60.

Ali J, Naraynsingh V. Potential impact of advanced trauma life support (ATLS) program in a third world country. *Int Surg* 1987; 72(3): 179–184.

Al-Zahrani A, Bener A. An application of multiple regression model to road traffic accidents in

Riyadh, Saudi Arabia. *J Traffic Med* 1990; 18(4): 248.

American College of Surgeons. *Advanced Trauma Life Support Course*. Chicago: Committee on Trauma, American College of Surgeons. 1989: 1–298.

Anderson K. Overview of the problem of antipersonnel mines. In: *International Committee of the Red Cross. Symposium on Antipersonnel Mines*. Montreux, 21–23 April, 1993. Geneva: International Committee of the Red Cross, Report, 1993, 13–17.

Anderson MB. Which costs more: prevention or recovery? In: Kreimer A, Munasinghe M, eds. *Managing Natural Disasters and the Environment*. Washington, DC: Environmental Policy and Research Division, Environment Department, The World Bank, 1991:17–27.

Andreassen D. Population and registered vehicle data vs. road deaths. *Accid Anal Prev* 1991; 23(5):343–351.

Angell M, Kassirer JP. Alcohol and other drugs—Toward a more rational and consistent policy (Editorial). *N Engl J Med* 1994; 331:537–539.

Anywar WK, Brown S, Katz M, O'Carroll PW, Rosenberg ML. Injury and violence in developing countries. Background paper on Problems of Injuries in Developing Countries. In: *Risks Old and New: A Global Consultation on Health*. Atlanta: Emory University. April 27–May 1, 1986.

Appel H, Otte D, Wüstemann J. Epidemiologie von unfällen motorisierter Zweiradfahrer in der Bundesrepublik Deutsche Sicherheitsaspekte. In: Koch H, ed. *Der Motorradunfall: Beschreibung, Analyse, Prävention*. Bremerhaven, West Germany. Wirtschaftsverlag 1986:48–92. Cited in: Hancock PA, Wulf G, Thom D, Fossnacht. Driver workload during differing driving manoeuvers. *Accid Anal Prev* 1990;22: 281–290.

Armenian HK. Perceptions from epidemiologic research in an endemic war. *Soc Sci Med* 1989; 28(7):643–647.

Armitage P, Berry G. *Statistical Methods in Medical Research*. Oxford: Blackwell, 1987: 400–401, 403–405.

Arya AS. *Protection of Educational Buildings Against Earthquakes*. Bangkok: UNESCO. Educational Building Report 13. 1978:1–67.

Araya M, Aboud FE. Mental illness. In: Kloos H, Zein ZA, eds. *The Ecology of Health and Disease in Ethiopia*. Boulder: Westview Press, 1993, 493–505.

Ascherio A, Biellik R, Epstein A, Snetro G, Gloyd S, Ayotte B, Epstein PR. Deaths and injuries caused by land mines in Mozambique. *Lancet* 1995;346:721–724.

Ashtakala T, Barss P. Human and economic burden of disability from land mine injuries: possible legal approaches for a public health problem (Abstract). *Third International Conference on Injury Prevention and Control*, Melbourne, Australia. Adelaide, SA: National Injury Surveillance Unit, Australian Institute of Health and Welfare, 1996, 43.

Asian Disaster Preparedness Center. *Activity Report: 1986–1989*. Bangkok: Asian Institute of Technology. 1990:1–36.

Asogwa SE. The crash helmet legislation in Nigeria: a before-and-after study. *Accid Anal Prev* 1980a;12:213–216.

Asogwa SE. A review of coal-mining accidents in Nigeria over a 10-year period. *J Soc Occup Med* 1980b;30:(2)69–73.

Asogwa SE. Some characteristics of drivers and riders involved in road traffic accidents in Nigeria. *East African Med J* 1980c;57:399–404.

Asogwa SE. The health benefits of mechanization at the Nigerian Coal Corporation. *Accid Anal Prev* 1988;20:103–108.

Asogwa SE. Road traffic accidents in Nigeria: A review and a reappraisal. *Accid Anal Prev* 1992; 24(2):149–155.

Auchincloss JM, Grave GF. The problem of burns in Central Africa. *Tropical Doctor* 1976; 6:114–117.

Auerbach PS. Marine envenomations. *N Engl J Med* 1991;325:486–493.

Ayanru JO. Blindness in the Midwestern state of Nigeria. *Trop Geogr Med* 1974;26:325–332.

Ayati E. The cost-effectiveness of safety projects in Iran. *J Traffic Med* 1990;18(4):246.

Backstein R, Peters W, Neligan P. Burns in the disabled. *Burns* 1993;19(3):192–7.

Bagley C. Changing profiles of a typology of youth suicide in Canada. *Can J Public Health* 1992a;83(2):169–170.

Bagley C. The urban setting of juvenile pedestrian injuries: a study of behavioral ecology and social disadvantage. *Accid Anal Prev* 1992b; 24(6):673–678.

Bagley C, Jacobson S. Ecological variation of three types of suicide. *Psychol Med* 1976;6: 423–427.

Bagley C, Jacobson S, Rehin A. Completed suicide: a taxonomic analysis of clinical and social data. *Psychol Med* 1976;6:429–438.

Baker SP. Pedestrian deaths in Rio de Janeiro

and Baltimore. *Accid Anal Prev* 1977;9: 113–118.

Baker SP, Li G, Fowler C, Dannenberg AL. *Injuries to Bicyclists: A National Perspective*. Baltimore, MD: The Johns Hopkins Injury Prevention Center, 1993, 1–87.

Baker SP, O'Neill B, Ginsburg MJ, Li G. *The Injury Fact Book*. New York: Oxford University Press, 1992.

Baker SP, O'Neill B, Haddon W Jr, Long WB. The Injury Severity Score: a method for describing patients with multiple injuries and evaluating emergency care. *J Trauma* 1974; 14:187–196.

Baker SP, Fingerhut L, Higgins L, Chen L, Braver ER. *Injury to Children and Teenagers: State-by-State Mortality Facts*. Baltimore, MD: The Johns Hopkins Center for Injury Research and Policy, 1996.

Baker SP, Whitfield RA, O'Neill B. Geographic variations in mortality from motor vehicles. *N Engl J Med* 1987;316:1384–1387.

Baker T, MacKinney T. Changes in potential productive years of life lost through motor vehicle fatalities in Taiwan. Conference Presentation at: Symposium on Health, Environment, and Social Change—Emerging Health Problems in Rapid Socioeconomic Development. Taipei: Institute of Public Health, National Taiwan University. Unpublished paper. Department of International Health, The Johns Hopkins University. 1990.

Baldachin BJ, Malmud RN. Clinical and therapeutic aspects of kerosene poisoning: a series of 200 cases. *Br Med J* 1964;2:28–30.

Ballard JE, Koepsell TD, Rivara F. Association of smoking and alcohol drinking with residential fire injuries. *Am J Epidemiol* 1992; 135:26–34.

Balogun JA, Abereoje OK. Pattern of road traffic accident cases in a Nigerian University teaching hospital between 1987 and 1990. *J Trop Med Hyg* 1992;95:23–29.

Banerjee P, Bhattachariya S. Changing pattern of poisoning in children in a developing country. *Trop Ped Env Child Health* 1978: 136–139.

Bang A, Bang R. India: Action against sale of alcohol. *Lancet* 1992;340:720.

Bangdiwala SI, Anzola-Pérez E. Traffic accidents as a serious health problem in selected developing countries of the Americas. *Bull PAHO* 1987;21(1):38–47.

Bangdiwala SI, Anzola-Pérez E. The incidence of injuries in young people: II Log-linear multivariable models for risk factors in a collaborative study in Brazil, Chile, Cuba and Venezuela. *Int J Epidemiol* 1990;19: 125–132.

Bangdiwala SI, Anzola-Perez E, Glizer M. Statistical considerations for the interpretation of community utilized road traffic accident indicators: Implications for developing countries. *Accid Anal Prev* 1985;17:419–427.

Bangdiwala SI, Anzola-Pérez E, Glizer M, Romer C, Holder Y. Structured epidemiological approach for evaluation and intervention for traffic accidents: Experience in Latin American and Caribbean (Abstract). *J Traffic Med* 1990a;18(4):291.

Bangdiwala SI, Anzola-Pérez E, Romer C, Schmidt B, Valdez-Lazo F, Toro J, D'Suze C. The incidence of injuries in young people: I. Methodology and results of a collaborative study in Brazil, Chile, Cuba and Venezuela. *Int J Epidemiol* 1990b;19:115–124.

Barancik JI, Fife D. Discrepancies in vehicular crash injury reporting: Northeastern Ohio Trauma Study IV. *Accid Anal Prev* 1985;17: 147–154.

Barbaree JM, Breiman RF, Dufour AP, eds. *Legionella: Current Status and Emerging Perspectives*. Washington, DC: American Society for Microbiology, 1993, 1–311.

Barlow B, Nicmirska M, Gandhi RP, Leblanc W. Ten years of experience with falls from a height in children. *J Pediatr Surg* 1983; 18: 509–511.

Barnum H. Evaluating healthy days of life gained from health projects. *Soc Sci Med* 1987;24: 833–841.

Barss P. Injuries caused by garfish in Papua New Guinea. *Br Med J* 1982;284:77–79.

Barss P. Injuries due to falling coconuts. *J Trauma* 1984a;24:990–991.

Barss P. Wound necrosis caused by the venom of stingrays: pathological findings and surgical management. *Med J Aust* 1984b; 141: 854–855.

Barss P. Penetrating wounds caused by needlefish in Oceania. *Med J Aust* 1985a:143: 617–622.

Barss P. Inhalation hazards of "tropical peashooters". *Papua New Guinea Med J* 1985b; 28:45–46.

Barss P. Fractured hips in Melanesians: a nonepidemic. *Trop Geog Med* 1985c;37(2): 156–159.

Barss P. Renal failure and death after multiple stings in Papua New Guinea: ecology, prevention, and management of attacks by vespid wasps. *Med J Aust* 1989;151:659–653.

Barss P. *Health Impact of Injuries in the Highlands of Papua New Guinea: A Verbal Autopsy Study* (Dissertation). Baltimore, MD: The Johns Hopkins School of Hygiene and Public Health, 1991.

Barss P. Epidemic field investigation as applied to allegations of chemical, biological, or toxin warfare. *Politics and the Life Sciences* 1992; 11(1):5–22; 33–34.

Barss P. *Suicide and Parasuicide Among the Cree of Eastern James Bay Canada.* Montreal: Public Health Module for the Cree Region of James Bay, 1998a, 1–33.

Barss P. Drownings, near drownings, and other water-related injuries. In: *For the Safety of Canadian Children and Youth: From Data to Preventive Measures.* Ottawa, ON: Health Canada, 1998b.

Barss P, Blackford C. Medical emergency flights in remote areas: experience in Milne Bay Province, Papua New Guinea. *Papua New Guinea Med J* 1983;26:198–202.

Barss P, Dakulala P, Doolan M. Falls from trees and tree associated injuries in rural Melanesians. *Br Med J* 1984;289(6460):1717–1720.

Barss P, Ennis S. Injuries due to pigs in Papua New Guinea. *Med J Aust* 1988;149:649–656.

Barss P, Lehmann D, Hagen C, Hanley J, Kuate Defo B, Nishioka S. Epidemiologic, demographic, and biostatistical methods: assessing numbers, rates, causes, and determinants of mortality and morbidity in developing areas. In: JL Pickering, ed. *Health Research for Development: a Manual.* Ottawa, ON: Canadian University Consortium for Health in Development, 1997:48–100. (Available from: International Health Office, Dept. of Epidemiology, Biostatistics, and Occupational Health, McGill University, 1020 Pine Av. West, Montreal, QC, Canada H3A 1A2).

Barss P, Masson I. Failure by physicians to include external cause, contributing factors, and intent of injury in admission and discharge diagnoses: impact on validity of coding for external cause of injury and alcohol intoxication by hospital coders (Abstract). *Proceedings of the Third International Conference on Injury Prevention and Control, Melbourne, Australia.* Adelaide, SA: National Injury Surveillance Unit, Australian Institute of Health and Welfare, 1996, 43–44.

Barss P, Wallace K. Grass skirt burns in Papua New Guinea. *Lancet* 1983;1(8327): 733–734.

Batista-da-Costa M, Bonito RF, Nishioka SA. An outbreak of vampire bat bite in a Brazilian village. *Trop Med Parasitol* 1993;44:219–220.

Battle RM, Pathak D, Humble CG, et al. Factors influencing discrepancies between premortem and postmortem diagnoses. *JAMA* 1987;258: 339–344.

Bayoumi A. The epidemiology of fatal motor vehicle accidents in Kuwait. *Accid Anal Prev* 1981;13:339–348.

Beardsley T. Johns Hopkins leads the field in university military research. *Nature* 1987; 325:101.

Belotto AJ. Organization for mass vaccination for dog rabies in Brazil. In: Baer GM et al., eds. Research towards rabies prevention: a symposium. Washington DC. November 3–5, 1986. Chicago: University of Chicago. *Rev Inf Dis 1988;10(Suppl 4)*:S693.

Belsey MA. Child abuse: measuring a global problem. *World Health Statistics Quarterly* 1993;46: 69–77.

Bennett JD, Passmere DL. Correlates of coal mine accidents and injuries: a literature review. *Accid Anal Prev* 1984;16:37–45.

Bentham G. Proximity to hospital and mortality from motor vehicle traffic accidents. *Soc Sci Med* 1986;23:1021–1026.

Berg O, Adler-Nissen J. Housing and sickness in South Greenland: a sociomedical investigation. In: Shephard RJ, Itoh S, eds. *Proceedings III International Symposium Circumpolar Health.* Toronto: University of Toronto Press, 1976: 627–635.

Berger CJ, Tobeluk HA. Community-based suicide prevention programs in rural Alaska: Self determination as a new approach. In: Postl BD et al., eds. *Circumpolar Health 90 Proceedings of the 8th International Congress on Circumpolar Health,* Whitehorse, Yukon, May 20–25, 1990. Winnipeg, MA: University of Manitoba Press for Canadian Society for International Health, 1991;291–293.

Berger LR. Suicides and pesticides in Sri Lanka. *Am J Public Health* 1988;78:826–828.

Berger LR, Kalishman S, Rivara P. Injuries from fireworks. *Pediatrics* 1985;75:877–882.

Berhe D, Howe RC, Tedla T, Frommel D. Leprosy. In: Kloos H, Zein ZA, eds. *The Ecology of Health and Disease in Ethiopia.* Boulder: Westview Press, 1993, 251–264.

Bertazzi PA. Industrial disaster and epidemiology: a review of recent experiences. *Scand J Work Environ Health* 1989;15:85–100.

Bertelsen A. Grønlandsk Medicinsk Statistik og Nosografi. Grønlands befolkning statistik 190130 (Populations Statistics of Greenland 1901–30—In Danish) *Middr Grønland* 1935; 117:1–83. Cited in: Bjerregaard P. Fatal accidents in Greenland. *Arct Med Res* 1990a;49: 132–141.

Beverly MC, Rider TA, Evans MJ, Smith R. Local bone mineral response to brief exercise that stresses the skeleton. *Br Med J* 1989:299; 233–235.

Bezzaoucha A, Dekkar N, Ladjali M. Lives and limbs—the other price of modern road transport. *World Health Forum* 1988;9:84–87.

Bhatnagar MK, Smith GS. Trauma in the Afghan guerilla war: effect of lack of access to care. *Surgery* 1989;105:699–705.

Bijur PE, Golding J, Kurzon M. Childhood accidents, family size and birth order. *Soc Sci Med* 1988;26(8):839–843.

Binns CW. A deadly cure for lice: a case of paraquat poisoning. *Papua New Guinea Med J* 1976;19:105–107.

Bissell HH, Pilkington GB, Mason JM, Woods DL. Roadway cross section and alignment. In: *Synthesis of Safety Research Related to Traffic Control and Roadway Elements, Vol. 1.* Washington, DC: US Federal Highway Administration. 1982.

Bjärås G. *The Role of Community Development in Accident Prevention Program for a Large Urban Area: Experiences from the Stockholm County Accident Prevention Program* (Thesis). Sundbyberg, Sweden: Department of Social Medicine, Karolinska Institute, 1991.

Bjärås G. The potential of community diagnosis as a tool in planning an intervention programme aimed at preventing injuries. *Accid Anal Prev* 1993;25(1):3–10.

Bjerregaard P. Fatal accidents in Greenland. *Arct Med Res* 1990a;49:132–141.

Bjerregaard P. Geographic variation of mortality in Greenland: economic and demographic correlations. *Arct Med Res* 1990b; 49:16–24.

Bjerregaard P. Disease pattern in Greenland: Studies on morbidity in Upernavik 1979–1980 and mortality in Greenland 1968–1985. *Arct Med Res* 1991;50: Suppl. 4:1–62.

Bjerregaard P. Fatal non-intentional injuries in Greenland. *Arct Med Res* 1992;51: Suppl. 7: 22–26.

Bjerregaard P, Bjerregaard B. Disease pattern in Upernavik in relation to housing conditions and social group. *Meddr Grønland, Man and Soc* 1985;8:1–18.

Bjerregaard P, Juel K. Avoidable deaths in Greenland 1968–1985: Variations by region and period. *Arct Med Res* 1990;49:119–127.

Blanc PD, Maizlish N, Hiatt P, Olson KR, Rempel D. Occupational illness and poison control centers: referral patterns and service needs. *West J Med* 1990;152(2):181–4.

Bly PH. Vehicle engineering to protect vulnerable road users. *J Traffic Med* 1990;18(4):244 (Abstract).

Bogel K, Motschwiller E. Incidence of rabies and post-exposure treatment in developing countries. *Bull WHO* 1986;64:883–887.

Boldt M. A systematic and integrated interagency model for providing coordinated and comprehensive suicide prevention services. *Crisis* 1985;6(2):106–118.

Boldt M. Defining suicide: Implications for suicide behavior and for suicide prevention. *Crisis* 1987;8(1):3–13.

Boldt M. The meaning of suicide: Implications for research. *Crisis* 1988;9(2):93–108.

Borman B, Leiatua S. A general mortality atlas of New Zealand. Wellington, New Zealand: Department of Health, 1984. Cited in: Langley JD, McLoughlin E. Injury mortality and morbidity in New Zealand. *Accid Anal Prev* 1989; 21:243–254.

Bowers L, Thompson D, eds. *Where Our Children Play: Community Park Playground Equipment.* Reston, VA: American Alliance for Health, Physical Education, Recreation and Dance, 1989.

Boyce W, Khanlou N, Lysack C, Mulay S, Zakus D. Evaluating community participation. In: *JL Pickering, ed. Health Research for Development: A Manual.* Ottawa ON: Canadian University Consortium for Health Development, 1997: 132–162. (Available from International Health Office, Dept. of Epidemiology, Biostatistics and Occupational Health, McGill University, 1020 Pine Avenue, West, Montreal, QC, Canada H3A 1A2.)

Boyd JH. The increasing rate of suicide by firearms. *New Engl J Med* 1983;308:872–874.

Boyer R, Dufour R, Préville M, Bujold-Brown L. State of mental health. In: Jetté M, ed. *A Health Profile of the Inuit: Report of the Santé*

Québec Health Survey Among the Inuit of Nunavik, 1992. Montréal, QC: Ministère de la Santé et des Services Sociaux, Gouvernement du Québec, 1994a, 117–144.

Boyer R, Préville M, Légaré G. Mental health (Available in French and English). In: C Daveluy, C Lavallée, M Clarkson, E Robinson, eds. *Santé Québec: a health profile of the James Bay Cree.* Québec, Québec: Gouvernement du Québec, Santé Québec, 1994b, 161–173.

Bracker A. Drowning deaths: A cross-analysis of external cause and nature of injury codes. Ottawa, ON: Canadian Centre for Health Information, Statistics Canada, *Health Reports* 1989; 1(2):225–228).

Bradbury MD. Driving under the influence of drugs: A law-enforcement perspective (Abstract). *J Traffic Med* 1990;18(4):281.

Bradley SC. Attitudes and practices relating to marital violence among the Tolai of East New Britain. In: Toft S, ed. *Domestic Violence in Papua New Guinea.* Port Moresby: Papua New Guinea Law Reform Commission, Monograph No. 3, 1985, 32–71.

Brandão EO, Bastos HC, Nishioka SA, Silveira PVP. Lance-headed viper (Bothrops moojeni) bite wounding the eye. *Rev Inst Med Trop São Paulo* 1993;35:381–383.

Braver ER, Ferguson SA, Greene MA, Lund AK. Reductions in deaths in frontal crashes among right front passengers in vehicles equipped with passenger air bags. *JAMA* 1997; 178(17):1437–1439

Breinholdt F. Interpersonal violence among Greenlandic Inuit: Causes and remedies. In: Kern P, Cordtz T, eds. *NUNA MED '91—en Grønlandsmedicinsk Konference.* Nuuk, Greenland: Nuuk Offset, 1991:77–89.

Brennan ME, Lancashire R. Association of childhood mortality with housing status and unemployment. *J Epidemiol Community Health* 1978; 32:28–33.

Bresnitz EA. Poison Control Center follow-up of occupational disease. *Am J Public Health* 1990a; 80(6):711–2.

Bresnitz EA. A model system for occupational disease surveillance activities applying Centers for Disease Control guidelines to poison control centers. *J Occup Med* 1990b; 32(3): 255–9.

Brookhuis K, Van Schagen I, Rothengatter T. How to judge the safety of cyclists' behavior, observing and scaling traffic participation (Abstract). *J Traffic Med* 1990;18(4):262.

Brookoff D, Cook CS, Williams C, Mann CS. Testing reckless drivers for cocaine and marijuana. *N Engl J Med* 1994;331:518–522.

Brown B, Farley C, Forgues M. Identification of dangerous highway locations: Results of a community health department study in Québec (Unpublished paper). St-Lambert, Québec, Canada: Community Health Department, Charles LeMoyne Hospital, 1991:1–15.

Buchanan RC. The causes and prevention of burns in Malawi. *Cent Afr J Med* 1972; 18(3):55–56.

Buchner DM, Beresford SAA, Larson EB, LaCroix AZ, Wagner EH. Effects of physical activity on health status in older adults II: Intervention studies. *Annual Rev Publ Health* 1992; 13:469–488.

Budnick, LD, Ross DA. Bathtub-related drownings in the United States, 1971–81. *Am J Public Health* 1985;630–633.

Bull D. *A Growing Problem: Pesticides and the Third World Poor.* London: Oxford, 1982.

Bull JP. Disabilities caused by road traffic accidents and their relation to severity scores. *Accid Anal Prev* 1985;17(5):387–397.

Bureau of Labor Statistics. Workplace injuries and illnesses in 1992. Washington, DC: United States Department of Labor. *News,* 1993, Dec 15, 1–13.

Burns M. Prescription drugs and risk for the road user: Three studies of antihistamines (Abstract). *J Traffic Med* 1990;18(4):230.

Buzik SC, Hindmarsh KW. An alternative to the poison control system in Saskatchewan. *Vet Hum Toxicol* 1987;29(2):157–159.

Bwibo NO. Accidental poisoning in Uganda. *Br Med J* 1969;4:601–602.

Canadian Public Health Association. Ottawa Charter for Health Promotion. *Can J Public Health* 1986:425–427.

Canadian Red Cross Society. *Drowning Among 1 to 4–Year Old Children in Canada: a High-risk Group for Water Related Fatalities.* Ottawa, ON: Special Research Report, 1994a, 1–32 (also available in French).

Canadian Red Cross Society. *Drowning Among Boaters in Canada: a Problem of Adult Males in Small Powerboats and Canoes.* Ottawa, ON: Special Research Report, 1994b, 1–66 (also available in French).

Canadian Red Cross Society. *National Drowning Report: Annual Surveillance Report for 1994: Analysis of Water-Related Fatalities in Canada for 1992.* Ottawa, ON: 1994c, 1–108 (also available in French).

Canadian Red Cross Society. *Drownings of Swimmers in Canada: Circumstances and Prevention.* Ottawa, ON: Special Research Report, 1996a, 1–71 (also available in French).

Canadian Red Cross Society. *National Drowning Report: Analysis of Water-Related Fatalities in Canada for 1993.* Comprehensive Surveillance Report. Ottawa, ON, 1996b, 1–180 (also available in French).

Canadian Red Cross Society. *National Drowning Report: Analysis of Water-Related Fatalities in Canada for 1994 and 1995.* Concise Visual Surveillance Report. Ottawa, ON, 1997, 1–122.

Canadian Red Cross Society, *Drownings and Other Injury Fatalities during Boating: National Report.* Ottawa, ON, 1997b, 1–62.

Cardim MS, et al. Epidemiologia descriptiva de alcoolismo em grupos populacionais do Brazil. *Cadernos de Saude Publica (Rio de Janeiro)* 1986;2:191–211. Cited in: World Bank. Adult Health in Brazil: Adjusting to New Challenges. *Brazil Development Report No. 7907-BR.* 1989:1–133.

Carmo JC, Costa DF, Santos UP, Settimi, MM. Occupational accident prevention: A public health experience. In: *Preprints: Accident Prevention in Developing Countries. International Conference on Strategies for Occupational Accident Prevention.* Stockholm, Sweden, September 21–22, 1989. Solna, Sweden: Publication Service, National Board of Occupational Safety and Health, 1989:1–11.

Carter D, Heath GW, Hovmork G, Sax H. Space applications for disaster mitigation and management. *Acta Astronautica* 1989;19(3): 229–240.

Cavin SH, Pierce JP. Low-cost cigarettes and smoking behavior in California, 1990–1993. *Am J Prev Med* 1996;12:17–21.

Celis A. Asfixia por inmersión en Jalisco: 1983–89. *Salud Pública de México* 1991;33: 585–589.

Centers for Disease Control. Occupational mortality in the oil industry—Louisiana. *MMWR* 1980;29:230–231.

Centers for Disease Control. Premature mortality due to sudden infant death syndrome. *MMWR/JAMA* 1986;255:1992–1993.

Centerwall BS. Television and violence—The scale of the problem and where to go from here. *JAMA* 1992;267(22);3059–3063.

Central Road Research Institute. Road user cost study in India. New Delhi: *Central Road Research Institute.* 1982.

Ccsari D. Pedestrian protection and car design (Abstract). *J Traffic Med* 1990;18(4):268.

Chabasse P. The proliferation of anti-personnel landmines in developing countries: considerable damage in human terms and a dramatically insufficient medico-social response. In: International Committee of the Red Cross. *Symposium on Antipersonnel Mines.* Montreux, 21–23 April, 1993. Geneva: International Committee of the Red Cross, Report, 1993, 85–95.

Chalmers DJ, Marshall SW, Langley JD, et al. Height and surfacing as risk favors for injury in falls from playground equipment: a case-control study. *Injury Prevention* 1996;2: 98–104.

Chamie M. Survey design strategies for the study of disability. *World Health Statistics Quarterly* 1989;42(3):122–140.

Chandramohan D, Maude GH, Rodrigues LC, Hayes RJ. Verbal autopsies for adult deaths: Issues in their development and validation. *Int J Epidemiol* 1994;23:213–222.

Chao TC. Deaths from poisons in Singapore, 1960–1969. *Med Sci Law* 1971;11:41–45.

Chari SR, Nath KMB. Accident causative factors under mixed traffic conditions—a case study of Hyderabad City (Abstract). *J Traffic Med* 1990;18(4):249.

Chen LE, Huq E, D'Souza. Sex bias in the family allocation of food and health care in rural Bangladesh. *Population and Development Review,* 1981;7:55–70.

Chesnais J-Cl. *Histoire de la Violence.* Ed. Robert Laffont, Paris, 1981.

Chesnais JC. The prevention of deaths from violence. In: Vallin J, Lopez AD (Eds.). *Health Policy, Social Policy and Mortality Prospects.* Institut National d'Etudes Demographiques (INED) and International Union for the Scientific Study of Population (IUSSP), Ordina Editions 1985:261–279.

Chiang Y. A national head and spinal injury program in Taiwan, Republic of China. Paper presented at National Programmes on Accident and Injury Prevention. National Board of Health and Welfare, Stockholm 1989. Division of Health Education, Department of Health, Taiwan, 1989.

Choinière R, Robitaille Y, Dorval D, Sauvageau Y. *Profil des Traumatismes au Québec: Disparités Régionales et Tendances de la Mortalité (1976 à 1990) et des Hospitalisations (1981 à 1991).* Quebec, Québec: Gouvernement du Québec, Ministère de la Santé et des Services sociaux, 1993.

Chomsky N. *The Culture of Terrorism.* New York: Black Rose, 1988.

Chomsky N. *Pirates and Emperors.* Montréal: Black Rose, 1991.

Choudhry VP, Jalali AJ, Haider G, Qureshi MA. Spectrum of accidental poisonings among children in Afghanistan. *Ann Trop Pediatrics* 1987;7:278–81.

Christiani DC, Xue-qi G. Occupational health in selected developing countries: The People's Republic of China. In: *Occupational Health: Recognizing and Preventing Work-Related Disease.* Levy BS, Wegman DH, eds. Boston: Little, Brown, 1988:560–568.

Ciborowski A. Some aspects of physical development planning for human settlements in earthquake-prone regions. In: *The Assessment and Mitigation of Earthquake Risk.* Paris: UNESCO. 1978:274–284.

Cifuentes EE. Program for the elimination of urban rabies in Latin America. *Rev Inf Dis* 1988;10(Suppl 4):S689.

Clark JR. Coastal zone management. In: Kreimer A, Munasinghe M, eds. *Managing Natural Disasters and the Environment.* Washington, DC: Environmental Policy and Research Division, Environment Department, The World Bank, 1991:115–119.

Clarke RV, Lester D. Toxicity of car exhausts and opportunity for suicide: Comparison between Britain and the United States. *J Epidemiol Community Health* 1987;41:114–120.

Claymore BJ. A public health approach to suicide attempts on a Sioux reservation. *American Indian and Alaska Native Mental Health Research* 1988;1(3):19–24.

Coburn AW, Pomonis A, Sakai S. Assessing strategies to reduce fatalities in earthquakes. In: Jones N, Noji E, Smith G, Krimgold F, eds. *International Workshop on Earthquake Injury Epidemiology for Mitigation and Response.* Baltimore: The Johns Hopkins University, 1989:107–132.

Cock J. Hidden consequences of state violence: spinal cord injuries in Soweto, South Africa. *Soc Sci Med* 1989;29(10):1147–1155.

Cohen R. Rio's murder wave takes on the aura of a class struggle. Poor start to view killings as acts of social justice; bodies along a highway. *Wall Street J* 1989 May 9(A):1,15.

Cole DC, McConnell R, Murray DL, et al. Pesticide illness surveillance: The Nicaraguan experience. *Bull PAHO* 1988;22:119–132.

Colodey D, Griew AR. Surveying for disability in the developing world: Suggestions for a methodology. *Int J Rehab Research* 1982;5(3):317–325.

Collis ML. Survival behaviour in cold water immersion. In: *Proceedings of the Cold Water Symposium, Toronto, 1976.* Toronto, ON: The Royal Life Saving Society Canada, 1976, 25–27.

Committee on Accident and Poison Prevention. *Injury Control for Children and Youth.* Elk Grove Village, IL: American Academy of Pediatrics, 1987.

Committee on Injury Scaling. *The Abbreviated Injury Scale, 1990 Revision.* Des Plaines IL: Association for the Advancement of Automotive Medicine, 1990.

Committee on Trauma Research, Commission on Life Sciences, National Research Council and the Institute of Medicine. *Injury in America: a Continuing Public Health Problem.* Washington D.C.: National Academy Press, 1985.

Conway S. Are accidents at work being exported to developing countries? Some indications from the Philippines. *J R Soc Health* 1984; 104/5:177–179.

Corbin DOC, Fraser HS. A review of 98 cases of near-drowning at the Queen Elizabeth Hospital, Barbados. *West Indian Med J* 1981;30:22–9.

Cormier L. Trainer manual for integrated pesticide safety; development of training curriculum for integrated project; List of Project Handouts to be Used in the Training Curriculum; list of curriculum training objectives for each session. Colombo, Sri Lanka: *Care International,* 1993.

Courtright P, Haile D, Kohls E. The epidemiology of burns in rural Ethiopia. *J Epidemiol Community Health* 1993;47:19–22.

Coye MJ, Fenske R. Agricultural workers. In: *Occupational Health: Recognizing and Preventing Work-Related Disease.* Levy BS, Wegman DH, eds. Boston: Little, Brown, 1988:511–521.

Crome P. Paraquat poisoning 1986. *Lancet* 1986; 1:333–334.

Crum RM, Bucholz KK, Helzer JE, Anthony JC. The risk of alcohol abuse and dependence in adulthood: The association with educational level. *Am J Epidemiol* 1992;135(9):989–999.

Cuellar A. Occupational health and safety in the smelting and foundry industries in Mexico. *Am J Indust Med* 1980;1:261–3.

Cummings SR, Kelsey JL, Nevitt MC, O'Dowd KJ. Epidemiology of osteoporosis and osteoporotic fractures. *Epidemiol Rev* 1985;7: 178–208.

Cummins D. Foot trauma due to rodents in Sierra Leone. *Tropical Doctor* 1988;18: 189–190.

Dab W, Abenhaim LL. Connaissance scientifique et action en santé publique: l'utilité de la recherche dans l'élaboration d'un programme de santé. *Can J Public Health* 1984; 75:388–392.

Dalton LM, Hanns CT. Nelson EA, Hughs T. Public health aspects of stray dogs in Barrow, Alaska. *Arct Med Res* 1988;47: Suppl. 1:83–89.

Damestoy N. *Injury Mortality Among the Cree of Northern Québec 1982–91* (MSc thesis). Montréal, Québec: McGill University, Department of Epidemiology and Biostatistics, 1994.

Damestoy N, Barss P. Acceptability and usefulness of verbal autopsies for determining the circumstances of fatal injuries in remote indigenous communities in northern Canada (Abstract). *Third International Conference on Injury Prevention and Control*, Melbourne, Australia. Adelaide, SA: National Injury Surveillance Unit, Australian Institute of Health and Welfare, 1996, 17–18.

Datey S, Murthy NS, Taskar AD. A study of burn injury cases from three hospitals. *Indian J Public Health* 1981;15(3):117–24.

Dave PK, Rastogi S. Accident profile of vulnerable road users (Abstract). *J Traffic Med* 1990; 18(4):272.

Davies JE, Freed VH, Whittemore FW, eds. *An Agromedical Approach to Pesticide Management: Some Health and Environmental Considerations.* Miami, FL: Consortium for International Crop Protection/University of Miami Printing (576 B), 1982.

Davis S, Smith LS. Alcohol and drowning in Cape Town: a preliminary report. *S Afr Med J* 1982; 62:931–3.

de Bono E. *The Use of Lateral Thinking.* London: Penguin, 1967, 1–141.

de Bono E. *Parallel Thinking: from Socratic Thinking to de Bono Thinking.* London, UK: Viking, Penguin Books Ltd., 1994.

DeBruycker M, Greco D, Lechat MF. The 1980 earthquake in southern Italy: morbidity and mortality. *Int J Epidemiol* 1985;14:113–117.

DeBruyn LM, Lujan CC, May PA. A comparative study of abused and neglected American Indian children in the southwest. *Soc Sci Med* 1992;35(3):305–315.

DeCock KM, Barrere B, Diaby L, LaFontaine MF, Gnaore E, Porter A, Pantobe D, Lafontant GC, Dago-Akribi A, Ette M, Odehouri K, Heyward WL. AIDS—the leading cause of adult death in the West African city of Abidjan, Ivory Coast. *Science* 1990;249: 793–796.

DeCodes J, Baker TD, Schumann D. The hidden costs of illness in developing countries. *Research in Human Capital Development* 1988; 5:127–45.

DeGuevara L. Alcohol abuse and traffic sinestrability in Madrid, Spain (Abstract). *J Traffic Med* 1990;18(4):231.

Demamu S. *Community-based Study of Childhood Injuries in Adamitulu District, Ethiopia* (Thesis). Addis Abbaba University, Department of Community Health, 1991.

Demissie K. *The Occurrence and Determinants of Accidents: a Case Control Study Among Workers in the Assab Port* (Thesis). Addis Ababa University, Department of Community Health, 1988. Cited in: Larson CP, Dessie T. Unintentional and intentional injuries. In: Kloos H, Zein ZA, eds. *The Ecology of Health and Disease in Ethiopia.* Boulder: Westview Press, 1993, 473–482.

Dempsey M. Decline in tuberculosis: the death rate fails to tell the whole story. *Am Rev Tuberculosis* 1947;56:157–164.

Dennis PJ. Potable Water Systems: Insights into Control. In: Barbaree JM, Breiman RF, Dufour AP, eds. Legionella: *Current Status and Emerging Perspectives.* Washington, DC: American Society for Microbiology, 1993: 223–225.

Dennis PJ, Brenner DJ, Thacker WL, Wait R, Vesey G, Steigerwalt AG, Benson RF. Five new Legionella species isolated from water. *Int J Syst Bacteriol* 1993;43(2):329–37.

de Preux J. Quoted in: Monod J-M. *Mines and Humanitarian Activities.* In: International Committee of the Red Cross. *Symposium on Antipersonnel Mines.* Montreux, 21–23 April, 1993. Geneva: International Committee of the Red Cross, Report, 1993, 3–6.

Deputy Commissioner of Traffic Police, Delhi. Report on road accidents in Delhi 1988. *Delhi: Traffic Police,* 1989:7.

Desai NB, Chawda SK, Shad JD, Bhatt HK. Road users' involvement spectrum for road accident—Case study (Abstract). *J Traffic Med* 1990b;18(4):307.

Desai NB, Shad JD, Chawda SK, Shad JD. Road users' safety —some studies (Abstract). *J Traffic Med* 1990a;18(4):307.

DeSouza LJ. The pattern of trauma at Mulago Hospital, Kampala. *East Afr Med J* 1968;45: 523–31.

Dessie T, Larson CP. The occurrence and driver characteristics associated with motor vehicle injuries in Addis Ababa, Ethiopia. *J Trop Med Hyg* 1991;94:395–400.

Dhara S. A brief history of public interest action for greater occupational safety in India. In: *Preprints: Accident Prevention in Developing Countries. International Conference on Strategies for Occupational Accident Prevention.* Stockholm, Sweden: National Board of Occupational Safety and Health, 1989.

Diekema DS, Quan L, Holt VL. Epilepsy as a risk factor for submersion injury in children. *Pediatrics* 1993;91:612–616.

Diekstra RFW, Gulbinat W. The epidemiology of suicidal behaviour: a review of three continents. *Wld Hlth Statis Quart* 1993;46:52–68.

Dietrich P. WHO's to blame: fixing world health aid. *Wall Street Journal* 1990 May 11:12 (col 4–6).

Doege TC. An injury is no accident. *N Engl J Med* 1978;298(9):509–510.

Dougherty G, Pless IB, Wilkins R. Social class and the occurrence of traffic injuries and deaths in urban children. *Canadian J Public Health* 1990;81:204–209.

Downing A. Traffic injury column, Holder Y, ed. *Carec Surveillance Report* 1990;16(9):3–4.

Downing AJ. Road safety in developing countries. Crowthorne, Berkshire, UK: Overseas Unit, *Transport and Road Research Laboratory,* 1992: 1–15

Downing AJ, Baguley CJ, Hills BL. Road safety in developing countries: an overview. In: PTRC. *Nineteenth Transport, Highways, and Planning Summer Annual Meeting. Proceedings of Seminar C. University of Sussex 9–13 September 1991.* 1991: 1–26.

Duhl LJ. The healthy city: Its function and its future. *Health Promotion* 1986;1(1):55–60.

Durrani KM. The epidemiology of burn injuries. *Report of the Burns Research Project at Civil Hospital,* Karachi, Dow Medical College, 1974.

Durrani KM, Raza SK. Studies on flammability of clothing of burn victims, changes therein, and their wearability after a borax rinse. *J Pakistan Med Assoc* 1975;25(5):99–102.

Dwyer T, Ponsonby A. Sudden infant death syndrome—insights from epidemiological research. *J Epidemiol Community Health* 1992;46: 98–102.

Dykes EH, Spence LJ, Chipman M, Bohn DJ, Wesson DE. Fatal bicycle accidents in children: a plea for safety education (Abstract). *First World Conference on Accident and Injury Prevention (Stockholm, Sweden): Abstract Guide.* Sundyberg: Karolinska Institute, September 17–20, 1989.

Eastwood R. Suicide and parasuicide. In: Last J, ed. *Public Health and Preventive Medicine.* New York: Appleton-Century Crofts, 1980: 1359–1371.

Ebong WW. Falls from trees. *Trop Geogr Med* 1978;30:63–67.

Economist. Ban the land mine and cut the casualties. *Globe and Mail (Toronto)* 1994 Jan 14:A17(col 1–4).

Edwards G. Drinking problems: putting the third world on the map. *Lancet* 1979;2: 402–404.

Eibl-Eibesfeldt I. *The Biology of Peace and War: Men, Animals, and Aggression.* London: Thames and Hudson, 1979:1–294.

Eid AM. Road traffic accidents in Qatar. The size of the problem. *Accid Anal Prev* 1980;12: 287–298.

Elias T. *Incidence of Injuries and Their Determinants in Akaki Textile Factory* (Thesis). Addis Ababa University, Department of Community Health, 1991. Cited in: Larson CP, Dessie T. Unintentional and intentional injuries. In: Kloos H, Zein ZA, eds. *The Ecology of Health and Disease in Ethiopia.* Boulder: Westview Press, 1993, 473–482.

Enders J, Dodd RS. Airport safety: a survey of accidents and available approach and landing aids. Flight Safety Foundation. *Flight Safety Digest,* March 1996, p. 9.

EQE Engineering. The December 7, 1988 Armenia, USSR earthquake: an EQE summary report. San Francisco: *EQE Engineering.* 1989.

Ergun G. Condition of vehicles in Saudi Arabia. *Accid Anal Prev* 1987;19(5):343–358.

Eriksson A, Björnstig U. Fatal snowmobile accidents in northern Sweden. *J Trauma* 1982;22: 977–982.

Eun CH, Kim KC, Cha CW. Occupational burns. *Contact Dermatitis* 1984;10:20–22

European Conference of Ministers of Transport. *Statistical Report on Road Accidents in 1981.* Paris: ECMT, 1984.

Evans L. The fraction of traffic fatalities attributable to alcohol. *Accid Anal Prev* 1990;22: 587–602.

Evans L. *Traffic Safety and the Driver.* New York, NY: Van Nostrand Reinhold, 1991, 1–405.

Evans L, Frick MC. Alcohol's effect on fatality

risk from a physical insult. *J Stud Alcohol* 1993;54: 441–449.

Evans WA, Courtney AJ. An analysis of accident data for franchised public buses in Hong Kong. *Accid Anal Prev* 1985;17:355–366.

Ewert D, Alleyne D. Risk of exposure to outdoor advertising of cigarettes and alcohol (Letter). *Am J Public Health* 1992;82(6): 895–896

Fallon WF, Robertson LM, Alexander RH. Seizure disorders and trauma. *South Med J* 1989;82(9):1093–1095.

Fang YY. On the role of worker's behavior and accomplishment in prevention of accidents and injuries. In: Preprints: *Accident Prevention in Developing Countries.* International Conference on Strategies for Occupational Accident Prevention. Stockholm, Sweden: National Board of Occupational Safety and Health, 1989:1–6.

Fauveau U, Blanchet T. Deaths from injuries and induced abortion among rural Bangladeshi women. *Soc Sci Med* 1989;29: 1121–1127.

Feachem RGA, Kjellstrom T, Murray CJL, Over M, Phillips MA, eds.. *The Health of Adults in the Developing World.* The World Bank. New York: Oxford University Press, 1992.

Feck G, Baptiste MS, Greenwald P. The incidence of hospitalized burn injuries in upstate New York. *Am J Public Health* 1977; 67:966–967.

Federal Office of Road Safety. *Towards Traffic Calming: a Practitioners' Manual on Implemented Local Area Traffic Management and Blackspot Devices.* CR 126, Australian Government Publishing Service, Canberra, Australia, 1994.

Ferguson SA. Update on Airbag Performance in the United States: Benefits and Problems. Washington DC: Insurance Institute for Highway Safety, 1996.

Fernando LVR. Towards the development of effective occupational health services in Ceylon. *Ceylon Med J* 1970;15:88–95.

Ferrante AM, Rosman DL, Knuiman MW. The construction of a road injury database. *Accid Anal Prev* 1993;25:659–665.

Ferreira FF, Mendes R. Alguns aspectos epidemiologicos dos accidentes de trabalho fatais ocorridos em Campinas, SP (Brasil), 1972–78. *Rev Saude Publica* 1981;15:251–262.

Fife D. Injuries and deaths among elderly persons. *Am J Epidemiol* 1987;126:936–941.

Fife D, Davis J, Tate L, Wells JK, Mohan D, Williams AF. Fatal injuries to bicyclists: the experience of Dade County, Florida. *J Trauma* 1983;23:745–55.

Fife D, Rappaport E. What role do injuries play in the deaths of old people? *Accid Anal Prev* 1987;19:225–230.

Fisher R. *Improving Compliance with International Law.* Charlottesville: University Press of Virginia. 1981.

Fisher R, Brown S. *Getting Together: Building a Relationship That Gets to Yes.* Boston: Houghton Mifflin. 1988.

Fisher R, Ury W. *Getting to Yes: Negotiation Agreement Without Giving In.* New York: Penguin, 1991.

Foege WH. Violence and public health. In: U.S. Department of Health and Human Services. *Surgeon General's Workshop on Violence and Public Health.* DHHS Publication No. HRS–D–MC 86–1, 1986:19–34.

Ford AB. Reducing the threat of hip fracture. *Am J Public Health* 1989;79:269–270.

Forjuoh SN, Guyer B, Smith GS. The epidemiology and home-based treatment of childhood burns in Ghana. Baltimore MD: Department of Maternal and Child Health, *The Johns Hopkins Bulletin of Hygiene and Public Health,* 1994.

Forjuoh SN, Guyer B, Strobino DM. Determinants of modern health care use by families after a childhood burn in Ghana. *Injury Prevention* 1995;1:31–34.

Forjuoh SN, Gyebi-Ofosu. Injury surveillance: Should it be a concern to developing countries? *J Public Health Policy* 1993;14:355–359.

Foster HMcA, Webb SJ. Skin cancer in the North Solomons. *Aust NZ J Surg* 1988;58: 129–133.

Fouracre PR, Jacobs GD. Comparative accident costs in developing countries. TRRL Report SR 206 UC. Crowthorne: *Transport and Road Research Laboratory.* 1976.

French JG, Holt KW. Floods. In: Gregg MB, ed. *The Public Health Consequences of Disasters 1989.* Atlanta: US Dept of Health and Human Services, Centers for Disease Control, 1989.

Frenk J, Bobadilla JL, Sepulveda J, Cervantes ML. Health transition in middle-income countries: new challenges for health care. *Health Policy Planning* 1989;4:29–39.

Friederici H. Reflections on the postmortem audit. *JAMA* 1988;260:3461–3465.

Friesen B. Haddon's strategy for prevention: application to Native house fires. *Circumpolar*

Health, Seattle, WA: U. of Washington Press, 1985;84:105–109.

Frimodt-Møller B, Bay-Nielsen H. Classification of accidents in the Arctic. A suggestion for adaptation of the Nordic classification for accident monitoring. *Arct Med Res* 1992;51: Suppl. 7:15–21.

Fulle A. *Injuries in Urban Factories of Ketena One* (Thesis). Addis Ababa University, Department of Community Health, 1988. Cited in: Larson CP, Dessie T. Unintentional and intentional injuries. In: Kloos H, Zein ZA, eds. *The Ecology of Health and Disease in Ethiopia.* Boulder: Westview Press, 1993, 473–482.

Gadjusek DC. Introduction of Taenia solium into West New Guinea with a note on an epidemic of burns from cysticercosis epilepsy in the Ekari people of the Wissel Lakes area. *Papua New Guinea Med J* 1978;21:321–342.

Gaind BN, Mohan M, Ghosh S. Changing pattern of poisoning in children. *Indian Pediatr* 1977; 14(4):295–301.

Gallaher MM, Fleming DW, Berger LR, Sewell CM. Pedestrian and hypothermia deaths among Native Americans in New Mexico. Between bar and home. *JAMA* 1992;267(10): 1345–1348.

Garenne M, Fontaine O. Assessing probable causes of death using a standardized questionnaire: A study in rural Senegal. In: Vallin J, D'Souza S, Palloni A, eds. *Measurement and Analysis of Mortality: New Approaches.* International Studies in Demography, International Union for the Scientific Study of Population. Oxford: Clarendon Press, Oxford University Press, 1990:123–142.

Garfield RM. War-related changes in health and health services in Nicaragua. *Soc Sci Med* 1989; 28(7):669–676.

Gee RWK, Sinha SN. The epidemiology of spinal cord injuries in Papua New Guinea. *Papua New Guinea Med J* 1982;25:97–99.

Geissler E. *Biological and Toxin Weapons Today.* Oxford: Oxford Press. (Stockholm International Peace Research Institute). 1986.

Gekonge N. Traffic accidents and their economic implications in Kenya (Abstract). *J Traffic Med* 1990;18(4):265.

Gielen AC. Health education and injury control: Integrating approaches. *Health Education Quarterly* 1992;19(2):203–218.

Gittlesohn AM. On the distribution of underlying causes of death. *Am J Public Health* 1982;72: 133–140.

Glass RI, Craven RB, Bregman DJ, et al. Injuries from the Wichita Falls tornado: implications for prevention. *Science* 1980;207: 734–738.

Glass RI, Urrutia JJ, Sibony S. Earthquake injuries related to housing in a Guatemalan village. *Science* 1977;197:638–43.

Golden FSTC, Rivers JF. The immersion incident. *Anaesthesia* 1975;30:364–373.

Gordon JE. The epidemiology of accidents. *Am J Public Health* 1940;39:504–515.

Gordon JE. Epidemiology—Old and New. In: *The Challenge of Epidemiology: Issues and Selected Readings.* Buck C, Llopis A, Nájera E, Terris M, eds. Washington, DC: Pan American Health Organization, 1988, 135–141. (From: J Michigan State Med Soc 1950;49:194–199—Presented at 84th annual session of the Michigan State Medical Society at Grand Rapids, September 24, 1949).

Gordon JE, Gulati PV, Wyon J. Traumatic accidents in rural tropical regions: An epidemiological field study in Punjab, India. *Am J Med Sci* 1962;243(3):158–178.

Gosselin P, Chapdelaine A, Johnson PM. Les institutions: le rôle de l'intersectorialité. In: Beaulne G, ed. *Traumatismes au Québec—Comprendre pour Prévenir.* Québec, Québec: Les Publications du Québec. 1991:299–316.

Govinda LA. The importance of ritual. In: *Buddhist Reflections.* York Beach, Maine: Samuel Weiser, Inc., 1991, 69–73.

Graham I. Castlemilk, Glasgow: Application to become a member of the Safe Community Network. KI White Report 276. Sundbyberg, Sweden: WHO Collaborating Centre on Community Safety Promotion, Department of Social Medicine, Karolinska Institute, 1992.

Graitcer PL. Injury surveillance in developing countries. *MMWR* 1992;41(No.SS–1):15–20.

Gray RH. The integration of demographic and epidemiologic approaches to studies of health in developing countries. In: Ruzicka L, Wunsch G, Kane P, eds. *Differential Mortality: Methodological Issues and Biosocial Factors.* International Studies in Demography, International Union for the Scientific Study of Population. Oxford: Clarendon Press, Oxford University Press, 1989:36–63.

Gray RH. Epidemiologic methods and case-control studies of mortality and morbidity. In: Vallin J, D'Souza S, Palloni A, eds. *Measurement and Analysis of Mortality: New Approaches.* International Studies in Demography, International Union for the Scientific Study of Population. Oxford: Clarendon Press, Oxford University Press, 1990:65–83.

Gray RH, Smith GS, Barss PG. The use of verbal autopsies to determine selected causes of death in children. IIP Occasional Paper No.10. Baltimore: The Johns Hopkins Institute for International Programs, 1990:1–46. (Also available as: *The Use of Verbal Autopsy Methods to Determine Selected Causes of Death in Children.* Liège, Belgium: International Union for the Scientific Study of Population, IUSSP Paper no. 30, 1990.

Gregg MB, ed. *The Public Health Consequences of Disasters 1989.* Atlanta: US Dept of Health and Human Services, Centers for Disease Control, 1989.

Grieshop JI, Winter DM. Agricultural pesticide accidents and prevention in Ecuador. *Accid Anal Prev* 1989;21:394–398.

Griew AR, Colodey D. The prevalence of major disability in urban and rural coastal Papua New Guinea—Results of a pilot survey. *Papua New Guinea J Education* 1982.

Grossman DC, Milligan BC, Deyo RA. Risk factors for suicide attempts among Navajo adolescents. *Am J Public Health* 1991;81(7) 870–874.

Grubb GS, Fortney JA, Saleh S, et al. A comparison of two cause-of-death classification systems for deaths among women of reproductive age in Menoufia, Egypt. *Int J Epidemiol* 1988;17: 385–391.

Guidotti TL, Clough VM. Occupational health concerns of firefighting. *Annual Rev Publ Health* 1992;13:151–171.

Gupta JL. Epidemiology of burns in children. In: Rukhean PP, Hecker WC, Prevot, eds. *Pediatric Surgery in Tropical Countries.* Prog Pediat Surg 1982;15:255–270.

Gupta RC, Bhasin SK, Khanka BS. Drive-belt or patta injuries. *Injury* 1982;13(6):495–499.

Gupta RG. Safety measures for a super metropolitan city— Delhi (Abstract). *J Traffic Med* 1990;18(4):248.

Guptill KS, Hargarten SW, Baker TD. American travel deaths in Mexico: Causes and prevention strategies. *West J Med,* 1991; 154: 169–171.

Guria JC. The expected loss of life quality from traffic injuries requiring hospitalization. *Accid Anal Prev* 1993;25:765–772.

Guthrie R. Prevention of lead poisoning in children: an issue for both developing and industrialized countries. *Pediatrics* 1988;83: 524–525.

Haberal M. Electrical burns: a five-year experience. 1985 Evans Lecture. *J Trauma* 1986;26: 103–109.

Haddon W, Jr. The changing approach to the epidemiology, prevention, and amelioration of trauma: the transition to approaches etiologically rather than descriptively based. *Am J Public Health* 1968;58:1431–1438.

Haddon W, Jr. On the escape of tigers: an ecologic note. *Am J Public Health* 1970;60: 2229–2234.

Haddon W, Jr. A logical framework for categorizing highway safety phenomena and activity. *J Trauma* 1972;12:193–207.

Haddon W, Jr. Energy damage and the ten countermeasure strategies. *J Trauma* 1973; 13(4): 321–331.

Haddon W, Jr. Advances in the epidemiology of injuries as a basis for public policy. *Public Health Rep* 1980a;95:411–421.

Haddon W, Jr. The basic strategies for reducing damage from hazards of all kinds. *Hazard Prevention* 1980b;16:8–12.

Haddon W, Jr. Options for prevention of motor vehicle injury. *Israel J Med Sci* 1980c;16:45–65.

Haddon W, Jr. Reducing damage from hazards of all kinds. *Foresight, The Journal of Risk Management* 1981;6(8):16–22.

Haddon W, Jr., Valien P, McCarroll JR, Umberger CJ. A controlled investigation of the characteristics of adult pedestrians fatally injured by motor vehicles in Manhattan. *J Chronic Dis* 1961;14:655–678.

Haight, FA. Traffic safety in developing countries (Editorial). *J Safety Res* 1980; 12:50–58.

Haight, FA. Traffic safety in developing countries: Part 2. *J Safety Res* 1983;14:1–12.

Haimanot RT, Kidane Y, Wuhib E, Kassina A, Endeshaw Y, Alemu T, Spencer PS. The epidemiology of lathyrism in north and central Ethiopia. *Ethiop Med J* 1993;31:15–24.

Halabi S, Zurayk H, Awaida R, Darwish M, Saab B. Reliability and validity of self and proxy reporting of morbidity data: A case study from Beirut, Lebanon. *Int J Epidemiol* 1992;21(3): 607–612.

Hamdy CR, Dhir A, Cameron B, Jones H, Fitzgerald GWN. Snowmobile injuries in northern Newfoundland and Labrador: an 18–year review. *J Trauma* 1988;28:1232–1237.

Hammoudeh M, Snounou H. Methanol poisoning from cologne ingestion. *Saudi Med J* 1988:9:412–415.

Hamour BA. Epidemiology of road accidents. In: Sebai ZA, ed. *Community Health in Saudi Arabia.* London: Macmillan. 1982:45–50.

Hampton KK, Peatfield RC, Pullar T, Bodansky HJ, Walton C, Feely M. Burns because of epilepsy. *Br Med J* 1988;296:1659–1660.

Hancock PA, Wulf G, Thom D, Fassnacht P. Driver workload during different driving maneuvers. *Accid Anal Prev* 1990;22:281–290.

Haponik EF, Crapo RO, Herndon DN, Traber DL, Hudson L, Moylan J. Smoke inhalation. *Am Rev Respir Dis* 1988;138:1060–1063.

Hargarten SW. Availability of safety devices in rental cars: An international survey. *Trav Med Int* 1992;109–110.

Hargarten SW. Injury prevention: A crucial aspect of travel medicine. *J Travel Med* 1994; 1(1):48–50.

Hargarten S, Baker S. Fatalities in the Peace Corps. *JAMA* 1985;254(10):1326–1329.

Hargarten SW, Baker TD, Guptill K. Overseas fatalities of United States citizen travelers: An analysis of deaths related to international travel. *Ann Emer Med* 1991;20(6):622–626.

Hargarten S, Bouc G. Emergency air medical transport of U.S. citizen tourists: 1988–1990. *Air Med J* 1993:398–402.

Harris JR, Kobayashi JM, Frost F. Injuries from fireworks. *JAMA* 1983;249:2460.

Harris S. The real number of road traffic accident casualties in the Netherlands. A yearlong survey. *Accid Anal Prev* 1990;22: 371–378.

Hassan HM, Luscombe W. Remote sensing and disaster technology in developing countries. In: Kreimer A, Munasinghe M, eds. *Managing Natural Disasters and the Environment.* Washington, DC: Environmental Policy and Research Division, Environment Department, The World Bank, 1991:141–144.

Hatakka M, Keskinen E, Katila A, Laapotti S. New drivers versus light traffic (Abstract). Supplement: International Conference on Traffic Safety, New Delhi, India, 1991. *J Traffic Med* 1990;18(4):290.

Hatfield EM. Eye injuries due to fireworks: results of a 1969 survey. *Sight Sav Rev* 1970; 40:93–99.

Havanonda S, Mohan D, Svanström L, Moller J. *Report of the Second Travelling Seminar on Safe Communities.* Sundbyberg, Sweden: Depart-

ment of Social Medicine, Karolinska Institute, 1991.

Havanonda S, Romer C, Svanström L, Moller J. Formulating guidelines for safe communities. *WHO Travelling Seminar.* Sundbyberg, Sweden: Department of Social Medicine, Karolinska Institute, 1989.

Hayes MV, Willms SM. Healthy community indicators: The perils of the search and the paucity of the find. *Health Promotion Int* 1990;5(2): 161–166.

Hayes WJ. Factors limiting injury from pesticides. *J Environ Sci Heath* 1980;B15(6): 1005–1021.

Hayward L, Zubrick SR, Silburn S. Blood alcohol levels in suicide cases. *J Epidemiol Community Health* 1992;46:256–260.

Health Canada. *Trends in first nations mortality 1979–93,* 1996, p 1–82.

Health Canada. *Drowning Among First Nations and Inuit Peoples of Canada: Circumstances and Prevention.* Ottawa, ON: Special Research Report. In collaboration with: Régie Régionale de la Santé et des Services Sociaux de Montréal-Centre, The Canadian Red Cross Society, Lifesaving Society, 1998.

Health Situation and Trend Assessment Program, PAHO. Surveillance of living conditions and the health situation. *Epidemiol Bull PAHO* 1991;12(3):7–10.

Healthy Cities Symposium. Summary Report: Fourth Annual Healthy Cities Symposium. *Health Promotion Int* 1990;5(3):245–248.

Heise L. Violence against women: the hidden health burden. *World Health Statistics Quarterly* 1993;46:78–85.

Herman ES, Chomsky N. *Manufacturing Consent: the Political Economy of the Mass Media.* New York: Pantheon, 1988:1–413.

Híjar-Medina MC, Tapia-Yáñez JR, Lozano-Ascencio R, López-López MV. Accidentes en el hogar en niños menores de 10 años. Causas y consecuencias. *Salud Pública de México* 1992;34: 615–625.

Hills PJ, Jones-Lee MW. The role of safety highway investment appraisal for developing countries. *Accid Anal Prev* 1983;15:355–370.

Himmelstein J. Low back pain syndrome. In: Weeks JL, Levy BS, Wagner GR, eds. *Preventing Occupational Disease and Injury.* Washington, DC: American Public Health Association, 1991:396–404.

Hipp LL, Taylor JS. Industrial dermatoses. In:

Plog BA, ed. *Fundamentals of Industrial Hygiene.* Chicago: National Safety Council. 1988: 145–161.

Hislop GT, Threlfall WJ, Gallagher RP, Band PR. Accidental and intentional violent deaths among British Columbia Native Indians. *Can J Public Health* 1987;78:271–274.

Hobart CW. Socioeconomic correlates of mortality and morbidity among Inuit infants. In: Shephard RJ, Itoh S, eds. *Proc III Int Symp Circumpolar Health.* Toronto: University of Toronto Press, 1976:452–461.

Hobcraft JN, McDonald JW, Rutstein SO. Socioeconomic factors in infant and child mortality: a cross-national comparison. *Population Studies* 1984;38:192–223.

Hollenbach KA, Barrett-Conner E, Edelstein SL, Holbrook T. Cigarette smoking and bone mineral density in older men and women. *Am J Public Health* 1993;83:1265–1270.

Holman RG, Olszewski A, Maier RV. The epidemiology of logging injuries in the northwest. *J Trauma* 1987;27:1044–1050.

Homer-Dixon TF, Boutwell JH, Rathjens GW. Environmental change and violent conflict. *Scientific American* 1993;Feb:38–45.

Honkanen R, Ertama L, Kuosmanen P, Linnoila M, Alha A, Visuri T. The role of alcohol in accidental falls. *J Stud Alcohol* 1983;44(2) 231–245.

Hoque MM. An analysis of fatal bicycle accidents in Victoria (Australia) with a special reference to nighttime accidents. *Accid Anal Prev* 1990;22:1–11.

Howard-Pitney B, LaFromboise TD, Basil M, September B, Johnson M. Psychological and social indicators of suicide ideation and suicide attempts in Zuni adolescents. *J Consult Clin Psychol* 1992;60(3):473–476.

Hu X, Wesson D, Venney B. Home injuries to children. *Can J Public Health* 1993;84: 155–158.

Hudgens RW. Preventing suicide (Editorial). *N Engl J Med* 1983;308:897–898.

Hutchinson TP. *Road accident statistics.* Adelaide Australia: Rumsby Scientific Publishing, 1987.

IAFF. 1980 *Annual death and injury survey.* Washington DC: International Association of Fire Fighters, 1980.

Igbedioh SO. Effects of agricultural pesticides on humans, animals, and higher plants in developing countries. *Archiv Environ Health* 1991; 46(4):218–224.

Ilsar M, Chirambo M, Belkin M. Ocular injuries in Malawi. *Br J Ophthalmol* 1982;66:145–148.

Insurance Institute for Highway Safety. Discounts for automatic restraints. *IIHS Status Report.* 1990a:25:5.

Insurance Institute for Highway Safety. Texas Law triggers a dramatic jump in helmet use. *IIHS Status Report.* 1990b:25:1.

Insurance Institute for Highway Safety. Relationship found between motorcycle crashes and operator licensure. *IIHS Status Report.* 1990c: 25:3.

Insurance Institute for Highway Safety. Airbags. *IIHS Status Report.* 1997;9:1–7.

International Committee of the Red Cross. *Mines: a Perverse Use of Technology.* Geneva: International Committee of the Red Cross, 1992, 1–17.

International Committee of the Red Cross. *Symposium on Antipersonnel Mines,* Montreux, 21–23 April, 1993. Geneva: International Committee of the Red Cross, Report, 1993, 1–321.

International Conference on Traffic Safety. The vulnerable road user. *J Traffic Med* 1990; 18(4):220–324

Irwin KL, Mannino S, Daling J. Sudden infant death syndrome in Washington State: Why are Native American infants at greater risk than white infants? *J Pediatr* 1992;121: 242–247.

Ityavyar DA, Ogba LO. Violence, conflict and health in Africa. *Soc Sci Med* 1989;28(7): 649–657.

Iwegbu CG. Traumatic paraplegia in Zaria, Nigeria: The case for a centre for injuries of the spine. *Paraplegia* 1983;21:81–85.

Jacobs GD, Bardsley MN. Research on road accidents in developing countries. *Traffic Engineering and Control* 1977;18(4):1–5.

Jacobs GD, Downing AJ. *A Study of Bus Safety in Delhi.* Crowthorne, Berkshire, UK: Transport and Road Research Laboratory, Supplementary Report 758, 1982.

Jacobs GD, Sayer I. Road accidents in developing countries. *Accid Anal Prev* 1983;15: 337–353.

Jacobson S, Bagley C, Rehin A. Clinical and social variables which differentiate suicide, open and accident verdicts. *Psychol Med* 1976;6:417–421.

Jadaan KS. Traffic accidents in Kuwait: An economic dimension. *Accid Anal Prev* 1990;22: 399–401.

Jadamba Z. Accident and injury prevention in South-East Asia. In: *Proceedings National Programmes on Accident and Injury Prevention.* Stockholm, Sweden: Swedish National Board of Health and Welfare, 1991:31–33.

Jar QF, Fan YS, Huang HK. Research on explosion prevention in pneumatic conveyance and dust removal system. In: Preprints: *Accident Prevention in Developing Countries.* International Conference on Strategies for Occupational Accident Prevention. Stockholm, Sweden: National Board of Occupational Safety and Health, 1989.

Jarvis GK, Boldt M. Death styles among Canada's Indians. *Soc Sci Med* 1982;16:1345–1352.

Jarvis GK, Boldt M, Butt J. Medical examiners and manner of death. *Suicide and Life-Threatening Behavior* 1991;21(2):115–113.

Jeanneret O, Sand EA. Intentional violence among adolescents and young adults: an epidemiological perspective. *World Health Statistics Quarterly* 1993;46:34–51.

Jensen LR, Williams SD, Thurman DJ, Keller PA. Submersion injuries in children younger than 5 years in urban Utah. *West J Med* 1992;57:641–644.

Jeyaratam J, de Alwis, Senevirante RS, Copplestone JF. Survey of pesticide poisonings in Sri Lanka. *Bull WHO* 1982;60(4):615–619.

Jeyaratam J, Lun KC, Poon WO. Survey of acute pesticide poisonings among agricultural workers in four Asian countries. *Bull WHO* 1987; 65:521–527.

Jinadu MK. Pattern of disease and injury among road construction workers in Plateau and Bauchi areas, northern Nigeria. *Ann Trop Med Parasitol* 1980;74:577–435.

Johnson MS, Moore MA, Kennedy RD. Injuries in the Alaskan Arctic. *Arct Med Res* 1992;51: Suppl. 7:45–55.

Joly M, Foggin P, Pless B. A case-control study of traffic accidents among child pedestrians (Abstract). *J Traffic Med* 1990;18(4): 286.

Jones NE, Pieper CF, Robertson LS. The effect of legal drinking age on fatal injuries of adolescents and young adults. *Am J Public Health* 1992;82:112–115.

Jorge MHPM. Accidentes e outras causas violentas de morte: epidemiologia e programas. Paper commissioned by the World Bank, 1988, 1–31. Cited in *Adult Health in Brazil: Adjusting to New Challenges.* Brazil Development Report 7807-BR. Washington DC: World Bank, 1989: 1-133.

Jørgensen NO. Urban speed management, the state of the art. *Accid Anal Prev* 1992; 24(1): 1–2.

Joscelyn KB, Maickel RP. *Report on an International Symposium on Drugs and Driving.* Report No. DOT-HS-4–00994–75–1. Springfield, VA: National Technical Information Service, 1975.

Joshi V. Depressed in India turn to 10–cent tablet to bring them death. *The Gazette (Montréal, Canada)* 1991 Oct 11:B8 (Col 1–6).

Joubert PH. Toxicology units in developing countries: Different priorities? *J Toxicol Clin Toxicol* 1982;19(5):509–16.

Kadiyali LR, Bhaskaran P, Geetha. Analysis of historical trend of road accident data in India and some inferences (Abstract). *J Traffic Med* 1990;18(4):243.

Kahane CJ. *An Evaluation of Head Restraints: Federal Motor Vehicle Safety Standard 202.* Washington, DC: National Highway Traffic Safety Administration, US Dept. of Transport. 1982.

Kale OO. Epidemiology and treatment of dog bites in Ibadan: A 12–year retrospective study of cases seen at the University College Hospital Ibadan (1962–1973). *Afr J Med Sci* 1977;6(3): 133–140.

Kalter HD, Gray RH, Black RE. Validation of a port-mortem interview method to ascertain selected causes of death in children in the Philippines. *Int J Epidemiol* 1989.

Kandela P. Road accidents in Jordon (News). *Lancet* 1993;342:426.

Katcher ML. Scald burns from hot tap water. *JAMA* 1981;246:1219–1222.

Katcher ML, Shapiro MM. Lower extremity burns related to sensory loss in diabetes mellitus. *Journal of Family Practice* 1987;24: 149–151.

Keatinge WR. Death after shipwreck. *Brit Med J* 1965;2:1537–1540.

Kellermann AL, Reay DT. Protection or peril? An analysis of firearm-related deaths in the home. *N Engl J Med* 1986;314:1557–1560.

Kelsey JL, Hochberg MC. Musculoskeletal disorders. In: Last JM, Wallace RB, eds. *Maxcy-Rosenau-Last, Public Health and Preventive Medicine.* Norwalk, Conn.: Appleton and Lange, 1992, 913–928.

Kelsey JL, Thompson WD, Evans AS. *Methods in*

Observational Epidemiology. New York: Oxford University Press, 1986:187–211.

Khatter K. Drowning Among Native Indians (Unpublished manuscript). Montréal, Québec: Injury Prevention Program, Department of Community Health, Montreal General Hospital, 1990;1–9.

Kimati VP. Childhood accidents in Dar Es Salaam. *Trop Geogr Med* 1977;29:91–94.

Kirkwood B. An experimental driver education programme in New Zealand (Abstract). *J Traffic Med* 1990;18(4):247.

Klang M, Andersson, Lindqvist K, eds. *Safe Communities: the Application to Industrialized Countries*. Linköping, Sweden: Universitet i Linköping, Linköping Collaborating Centre Occasional Papers 5, 1992.

Kleevens JW. Accidents in Hong Kong. *Public Health* 1982;96(5):297–304.

Kling GW, Clark MA, Compton HR, et al. The 1986 Lake Nyos gas disaster in Cameroon, West Africa. *Science* 1987;236:169–175.

Kloos H. Health impacts of war. In: Kloos H, Zein ZA, eds. *The Ecology of Health and Disease in Ethiopia*. Boulder: Westview Press, 1993, 121–132.

Kloos H, Zein ZA. Other diseases. In: Kloos H, Zein ZA, eds. *The Ecology of Health and Disease in Ethiopia*. Boulder: Westview Press, 1993, 507–515.

Kobori N, Yamaki T, Nagagawa Y. The mortality rate in motorcycle accidents cannot be reduced simply by wearing helmets (Abstract). *J Traffic Med* 1990;18(4):261.

Kotulak R. The biology of violence: How a chemical in the brain can curb or unleash violence. *Gazette (Montreal)* 1993 Dec 26:A1(col 2–3,A6(col 1–4).

Kraus JF. Fatal and non-fatal injuries in occupational settings: a review. *Ann Rev Public Health* 1985;6:403–418.

Kraus JF. Homicide and assault. In: Weeks JL, Levy BS, Wagner GR, eds. *Preventing Occupational Disease and Injury*. Washington, DC: American Public Health Association, 1991:317–320.

Kraus RF, Buffler PA. Sociocultural stress and the American Native in Alaska: An analysis of changing patterns of psychiatric illness and alcohol abuse among Alaska Natives. *Culture, Medicine, and Psychiatry* 1979;3:111–151.

Kreimer A, Munasinghe M. Managing environmental degradation and natural disasters: an overview. In: Kreimer A, Munasinghe M, eds. *Managing Natural Disasters and the Environment*. Washington, DC: Environmental Policy and Research Division, Environment Department, The World Bank, 1991a:3–6.

Kreitman N, Platt S. Suicide, unemployment, and natural gas detoxification in Britain. *J Epidemiol Comm Hlth* 1984;38:1–6.

Krishnarajah V. Falls from trees. *Ceylon Med J* 1978;3(2–3):76–78.

Kroeger A. Health interview surveys in developing countries: a review of the methods and results. *Int J Epidemiol* 1983;12:465–481.

Krugman R. Child abuse and neglect. *World Health* 1993;46th year(1):22–23.

Laditan AAO. Accidental scalds and burns in infancy and childhood. *J Trop Pediatr* 1987; 33:199–202.

Lancet Editorial. Community approach to psychiatric illness. *Lancet* 1992a;340:703.

Lancet Editorial. Depression and suicide: are they preventable? *Lancet* 1992b;340:700–701.

Lancet Editorial. Discounting health care: Only a matter of timing. *Lancet* 1992c;340: 148–149.

Lancet Editorial. Indoor air pollution and acute respiratory infections in children. *Lancet* 1992d;339:396–398.

Lancet Editorial. Reel violence. *Lancet* 1994; 343: 127–128.

Lancet Editorial. Antipersonnel mines, the all too–conventional weapon. *Lancet* 1995;346: 715.

Lancet Editorial. In the shadow of epilepsy. *Lancet* 1997;349:1851.

Langley J. Fencing of private swimming pools in New Zealand. *Community Health Studies* 1983;7(3):285–289.

Langley J. The need to discontinue the use of the term "accident" when referring to unintentional injury events. *Accid Anal Prev* 1988;20: 1–8.

Langley J, McLoughlin E. *A Review of Research on Unintentional Injury: a Report to the Medical Research Council of New Zealand*. Auckland: Medical Research Council of New Zealand, Special Report Series No. 10, 1987.

Lao Tzu. War. In: *The Sayings of Lao Tzu* (Translated from the Chinese). London: John Murray, 1905, 45–46.

Larson CP, Dessie T. Unintentional and intentional injuries. In: Kloos H, Zein ZA, eds. *The Ecology of Health and Disease in Ethiopia*. Boulder: Westview Press, 1993, 473–482.

Last JM, ed. *A Dictionary of Epidemiology*. International Epidemiological Association. New York: Oxford University Press, 1990.

Last JM. War and the demographic trap (Commentary). *Lancet* 1993;342:508–509.

Lau EMC, Cooper C. Wickham C, et al. Hip fracture in Hong Kong and Britain. *Int J Epidemiol* 1990;19:1119–1120.

Laue JH, ed. Using mediation to shape public policy. *Mediation Quarterly*, 1988 (Vol 20 Summer).

Laurell A. Mortality and working conditions in agriculture in underdeveloped countries. *Int J Health Serv* 1981;11:3–20.

Lawson SD, Edwards PJ. The involvement of ethnic minorities in road accidents: Data from three studies of young pedestrian casualties. *Traffic Engineering and Control* 1991; 32(1): 12–19.

Laxminarayan, Dhanbad. Ocular injuries in coal mines. *J All-India Ophthal Soc* 1968;16: 186–191.

Leach EH, Peters RA, Rossiter RJ. Experimental thermal burns, especially the moderate temperature burn. *Quart J Exper Physiol* 1943–44;32:67–86.

Learmonth AM. Domestic child burn and scald accidents. *J Ind Med Assoc* 1979;73(2):43–47.

LeBras J, Semenor M, Gate C. Importance, repartition et causes principales des accidents observés en 1980 dans deux formations sanitaires rurales de Côte d'Ivoir: étude comparative. *Medicine Tropicale* (Mars) 1982;42(2):129–144.

Lechat MF. Disasters and public health. *Bull WHO* 1979;57:11–17.

Lechat MF. The International Decade for Natural Disaster Reduction: Background and Objectives. *Disasters* 1990a;14(1):1–6.

Lechat MF. The epidemiology of health effects of disasters. *Epidemiol Rev* 1990b;12:192–198.

Lee KN, Choi YO, Kim CH, Yun DR. An epidemiological study on the incidence of carbon monoxide poisoning in Korea. *J Korea Prev Med Soc* 1971;4:95–106.

Lee ST. Two decades of specialized burns care in Singapore. *Ann Acad Med Singapore* 1982; 11(3):358–365.

Lees B, Molleson T, Arnett TR, Stevenson JC. Differences in proximal femur bone density over two centuries. *Lancet* 1993;341:673–675.

Lehmann D. Tari Research unit: *Final Report for the Southern Highlands Rural Development Project*. Mendi, Southern Highlands Province: Media Unit, Provincial Government 1984: 1–304.

Lester D, Abe K. The effects of the switch from coal gas to natural gas on the accidental death rate: A study of the United States and Japan. *Accid Anal Prev* 1992;24(2):157–160.

Levav I, Lima B, Somosa-Lenon M, Kramer M, González R. Salud mental para todos en América latina y el Caribe. Bases epidemiológicas para la acción. Boletin de la Oficina Sanitaria Panamericana 1989;107(3):196–219. Cited in: Pan American Health Organization. *Health Conditions in the Americas, 1990 Edition. Volume I*. Washington, DC, Pan American Health Organization Scientific Publication No. 524, 1990:109.

Leung PC, Ng TKW. A preliminary look into the causative factors of occupational hand injury in Hong Kong. Bull Hong Kong Med Assoc 1978;30:37–42. Cited by Ong SG in: *Proceedings of 10th Asian Conference on Occupational Health* 1982.

Levy BS, Widess E. Pesticide poisoning. In: Weeks JL, Levy BS, Wagner GR, eds. *Preventing Occupational Disease and Injury*. Washington, DC: American Public Health Association, 1991: 462–482.

Lewis DO. From abuse to violence: Psychophysiological consequences of maltreatment. *J Am Academy Child and Adolescent Psychiatry* 1991;31: 383–391.

Lewis LM, Naunheim R, Standeven J, Naunheim KS. Quantitation of impact attenuation of different playground surfaces under various environmental conditions using a tri-axial accelerometer. *J Trauma* 1993;35(6): 932–935.

Lewis ND. Disease and development: ciguatera fish poisoning. *Soc Sci Med* 1986;10:983–393.

Li G, Baker SP. A comparison of injury death rates in China and the United States, 1986. *Am J Public Health* 1991;81:605–609.

Li G, Baker SP. Alcohol in fatally injured bicyclists. *Accid Anal Prev* 1994;26:543–548.

Li G, Baker SP. Injuries to bicyclists in Wuhan, The People's Republic of China. *Am J Public Health* 1997;87:1049–1052.

Lillibridge SR. Industrial disasters. In: Noji EK, ed. *The Public Health Consequences of Disasters*. New York: Oxford University Press, 1997.

Lines CJ. Urban safety management in the UK (Abstract). *J Traffic Med* 1990;18(4):283

Lingam TSK. 70 muertos por envenenamiento en celebración de fin de año. *El Nuevo Pais*

(Caracas, Venezuela) 1992: No. 1035 Jan 2: 23(Col 1 and 2).

Linwood ME. Accidents in the community. *Recent Advances in Nursing* 1988;22:49–61.

List W. Under the gun about safety. *Globe and Mail (Toronto)* 1994 Jan 4:B14(col 1–3).

Litovitz TL; Schmitz BF; Bailey KM. 1989 annual report of the American Association of Poison Control Centers. National Data Collection System. Data Collection Committee, American Association of Poison Control Centers, Washington, DC. *Am J Emerg Med* 1990;8(5): 394– 442.

Litovitz TL, White JD. Occupational and environmental illness and the poison center. National Capital Poison Center, Georgetown University Medical Center, Washington, DC. *West J Med* 1990;152(2):178–80.

Lloyd EL. Hypothermia and cold. *Sci Prog Oxf* 1989;73:101–116.

Locklear GL. A retrospective case-control study of porch step falls occurring on the Fort Apache Indian Reservation—1987 to 1989. Phoenix, Arizona: Environmental Health Services Branch, Phoenix Area Office, Public Health Service, 1991, 1–20.

Loevinsohn ME. Insecticide use and increased mortality in rural central Luzon, Philippines. *Lancet* 1987;1:359–362.

Logue JN, Melick ME, Hansen H. Research issues and directions in the epidemiology of health effects of disasters. *Epidemiol Reviews* 1981;3: 140–162.

Loh RCK, Ramanathan TK. Occupational eye diseases and injuries in Singapore. *Singapore Med J* 1968;9:245–248.

Loomes G, McKenzie L. The use of QALY's in health care decision making. *Soc Sci Med* 1989; 28:299–308.

Lopez AR, Miranda PP, Tejada EV, Fishbein DB. Outbreak of human rabies in the Peruvian jungle. *Lancet* 1992;339:408–412.

Lowe MD. *The Bicycle: Vehicle for a Small Planet.* Washington, DC: Worldwatch Institute, Worldwatch Paper 90, 1989:1–62.

Lowenfels AB, Miller TT. Alcohol and trauma. *Ann Emerg Med* 1984;13:1056–1060.

Lowenfels AB, Wynn PS. One less for the road: International trends in alcohol consumption and vehicular fatalities. *Ann Epi* 1992;2: 249–256.

Lujan CC. Alcohol-related deaths of American Indians: Stereotypes and strategies. *JAMA* 1992a; 267(10):1384.

Lujan CC. An emphasis on solutions rather than problems. *American Indian and Alaska Native Mental Health Research* 1992b;4(3): 101–104.

Lundgren RI, Lang R. `There is no sea, only fish': Effects of United States policy on the health of the displaced in El Salvador. *Soc Sci Med* 1989;28(7):697–706.

Machumu WB. Safety and health conditions at construction sites in Tanzania. In: Preprints: *Accident Prevention in Developing Countries.* International Conference on Strategies for Occupational Accident Prevention. Stockholm, Sweden: National Board of Occupational Safety and Health, 1989.

Mackay M, Petrucelli E. Strategies for the reduction of traffic injuries internationally (Abstract). *First World Conference on Accident and Injury Prevention (Stockholm, Sweden)*: Abstract Guide. Sundyberg: Karolinska Institute, September 17–20, 1989.

Mackay M, Petrucelli E. Strategies for reducing traffic injury (Abstract). *J Traffic Med* 1990; 18(4):233

Maddy KT, Edmiston S, Richmond D. Illness, injuries, and deaths from pesticide exposures in California 1949–1988. California Department of Food and Agriculture, Sacramento. *Rev Environ Contam Toxicol* 1990; 114:57–123

Maher MJ, Mountain LJ. The identification of accident blackspots: a comparison of current methods. *Accident Anal Prev* 1988;20(2): 143–151.

Makky A. Effects of rapid increase in motorization levels on road fatality rates in some rich developing countries. *Accid Anal Prev* 1985; 17:101–109.

Makonnen F. Rabies in Ethiopia. *Am J Trop Med Hyg* 1982;115:266–273.

Malek M, Guyer B, Lescohier I. The epidemiology and prevention of child pedestrian injury. *Accid Anal Prev* 1990;22:301–313.

Malini M. Road safety education: the missing link in the education chain (Abstract). *J Traffic Med* 1990;18(4):274.

Malini E, Victor DJ. Measures to improve pedestrian safety; lessons from experience in Madras (Abstract). *J Traffic Med* 1990;18(4): 266.

Manciaux M. Violent youth. *World Health* 1993;46th year(1):24–25.

Manson-Bahr PEC, Bell DR. Tropical ulcer. In: Manson-Bahr PEC, Bell DR, eds. *Manson's*

Tropical Diseases. London: Baillière Tindall Publishers, 1987:725–728.

Mao T, Morrison H, Semenciw R, Wigle D. Mortality on Canadian Indian reserves 1977–1982. *Can J Public Health* 1986;77: 263–268.

Marcusson H, Oehmisch RW. Accident mortality in childhood in selected countries of different continents. *WHO Statistical Report* 1977;30(1): 57–92.

Marcusson HW, Oehmisch W, Pechmann W. Der Unfall im Kindes-und Jugendalter. 1. Mortalität und prophylaxe. Eine sozial-hygienische Studie. Berlin. 1970. Cited in: Marcusson H, Oehmisch W. Accident mortality in childhood in selected countries of different continents. *WHO Stat Report* 1977;30(1): 57–92.

Marshall DL, Soule S. Accidental deaths and suicides in Southwest Alaska: Actual versus official numbers. *Alaska Med* 1988;30(2): 45–52.

Marzuk PM, Leon AC, Tardiff K, Morgan EB, Stajic M, Mann J. The effect of access to lethal methods of injury on suicide rates. *Arch Gen Psychiatry* 1992;49:451–458.

Masalawala KS. Experiences with traumatic paraplegia patients in India. *Paraplegia* 1975; 13: 29–35.

Mathews RN, Radakrishnan T. First aid for burns (letter). *Lancet* 1987;1:1371.

Mathieu-Nolf M, Furon D. Answering calls from the general public: A necessity for poison centers? *Vet Hum Toxicol* 1990;32(1): 32–34.

May PA. Alcohol and drug misuse prevention programs for American Indians: Needs and opportunities. *J Stud Alcohol* 1986;47(3): 187–195.

May PA. Suicide and self-destruction among American Indian youths. *Am Indian Alaska Native Mental Health Research* 1987;1(1): 57–74.

May PA. *Suicide and Suicide Attempts Among American Indians and Alaska Natives.* An annotated bibliography (Revised edition). Albuquerque, NM: University of New Mexico, 1991.

May PA. Alcohol policy considerations for Indian reservations and bordertown communities. *American Indian and Alaska Native Mental Health Research* 1992;4(3):5–59.

Maynard A. Economic aspects of addiction policy. *Health Promotion* 1986;1(1):61–71.

McCarthy TJ. Human depredation by vampire bats (Desmodus rotundus) following a hog cholera campaign. *Am J Trop Med Hyg* 1989; 40:320–322.

McDonald RS. Accidental poisoning in children in Capetown with special reference to kerosene and salicylates. *S Afr Med J* 1961; 35:21–25.

McGrath R. The reality of the present use of mines by military forces. In: *International Committee of the Red Cross. Symposium on Antipersonnel Mines.* Montreux, 21–23 April, 1993. Geneva: International Committee of the Red Cross, Report, 1993a, 7–12.

McGrath R. Trading in death: anti-personnel mines. *Lancet* 1993b;342;628–629.

McLean AJ, Chen Paul CY, Wong TW, Ukai T. Motorcyclist licensing requirements and subsequent injury experience in four countries (Abstract). *J Traffic Med* 1990;18(4):289.

McShane WR, Roess RP. *Traffic Engineering.* Englewood Cliffs, New Jersey: Prentice Hall, 1990;20:147–165.

Meade MS. Potential years of life lost in countries of Southeast Asia. *Soc Sci Med* 1980;14D: 277–281.

Mekky A. Effects of rapid increase in motorization levels on road fatality rates in rich developing countries. *Accid Anal Prev* 1985;17: 101–109.

Melius J, Binder S. Industrial disasters. In: Gregg MB, ed. *The Public Health Consequences of Disasters 1989.* Atlanta: US Dept of Health and Human Services, Centers for Disease Control. 1989:97–102.

Mello-Jorge MH, Marques MB. Violent childhood deaths in Brazil. *Bull PAHO* 1985;19: 288–299.

Mendes R. *Importancia das Pequenas Empresas Industriais No Problema de Accidentes do Trabalho em São Paulo.* (Master's thesis). São Paulo, Brazil, 1975. Cited in: Occupational health in Latin America and the Caribbean: consideration of some problems, alternatives, trends, and challenges for its promotion. Washington, DC: PAHO, 1982: 32.

Merani NS. The International Decade for Natural Disaster Reduction. In: Kreimer A, Munasinghe M, eds. *Managing Natural Disasters and the Environment.* Washington, DC: Environmental Policy and Research Division, Environment Department, The World Bank, 1991: 36–39.

Michaels D, Mendes R. Occupational health in selected developing countries: Latin America. In: *Occupational Health: Recognizing and Preventing Work-Related Disease*. Levy BS, Wegman DH, eds. Boston: Little, Brown, 1988: 553–560.

Middaugh J. Epidemiology of injuries in Northern areas. *Arct Med Res* 1992;51: Suppl. 7: 5–14.

Middaugh J, Miller J, Dunaway CE, et al. *Causes of Death in Alaska: an Analysis of the Causes of Death, Years of Potential Life Lost, and Life Expectancy*. Anchorage, AK: Section of Epidemiology, Division of Public Health, Dept. of Health and Social Services, State of Alaska, 1991:1–266.

Middelhauve V, Appel H. Safety measures on trucks for the protection of pedestrians and cyclists (Abstract). *J Traffic Med* 1990;18(4): 320.

Mierley MC, Baker SP. Fatal housefires in an urban population. *JAMA* 1983;249:1466–1468.

Milio N. Healthy Cities: the new public health and supportive research. *Health Promotion Int* 1990;5(4):291–297.

Millar WJ, Adams OB. Socio-demographic correlates of personal risk, Canada 1988 (Abstract). *First World Conference on Accident and Injury Prevention (Stockholm, Sweden)*: Abstract Guide. Sundyberg: Karolinska Institute, September 17–20, 1989.

Miller TR, Luchter S, Brinkman CP. Crash costs and safety investment. *Accid Anal Prev* 1989; 21(4):303–315.

Milliner N, Pearn J, Guard R. Will fenced pools save lives? A 10-year study from Mulgrave Shire, Queensland. *Med J Aust* 1980;2: 510–511.

Ministry of Health, Mozambique. Mantakassa: an epidemic of spastic paraparesis associated with chronic cyanide intoxication in a cassava staple area of Mozambique. I. Epidemiology and clinical and laboratory findings in patients. *Bull WHO* 1984;62:477–484.

Mintsis G, Pitsiava-Latinopoulou. Traffic accidents with fixed roadside obstacles: a study of the Greek rural road network. *Traffic Engineering and Control* 1990;31(5):306–311.

Mirza S, Mirza M, Chotani H, Luby S. Observation of the behavior of bus commuters and bus drivers predisposing them to the risk of traffic accidents in Karachi, Pakistan. *Accid Anal Prev*, in press.

Misfeldt J, Senderovitz F. Suicide in Greenland. *Arct Med Res* 1989;48:122–123.

Mishra BK, Banerji AK, Mohan D. Two-wheeler injuries in Delhi, India: A study of crash vic-

tims hospitalized in a neurosurgery ward. *Accid Anal Prev* 1984;16(5/6):407–416.

Mitchell RG. Antecedents of handicap. *Lancet* 1981;i:86–87.

Mittal BN, Indrayan A, Sengupta RK, Bagchi SC. Epidemiological triad in domestic accidents. *Indian J Med Res* 1975;63(9): 1344–1352.

Mittleman MA, Maldonado G, Gerberich SG, Smith GS, Sorock GS. Alternative approaches to analytical designs in occupational injury epidemiology. *Am J Indust Med* 1997;32(2):129–141.

MMWR. Guidelines for investigating clusters of health events. *MMWR* 1990;39(RR–11):1–23.

MMWR. April through June 1991 Table reporting alcohol involvement in fatal motor-vehicle crashes. *JAMA* 1992;268(8):970.

Mock CN, Adzotor KE, Conklin E, Denno DM, Jurkovich GJ. Trauma outcomes in the rural developing world: comparison with an urban level I trauma center. *J Trauma* 1993;35: 518–523.

Mohan D. Accidental death and disability in India: a stocktaking. *Accid Anal Prev* 1984;16 (4): 279–288.

Mohan D. Childhood Injuries in India: extent of the problem and strategies for control. *Indian J Pediatr* 1986a;53:607–615.

Mohan D. A report on amputees in India. *Orthotics and Prosthetics* 1986b;40(1):16–32.

Mohan D. Road Traffic Injuries in Delhi: Technology Assessment, Agenda for Control. Fifth Annual State Bank Lecture. New Delhi: *Indian Institute of Technology, Centre for Biomedical Engineering* 1986c:1–33.

Mohan D. Food vs limbs: Pesticides and physical disability in India. *Economic and Political Weekly* 1987a; XXII:13,A–23–A–29.

Mohan D. Lessons from Bhopal. *Business India* 1987b;254:76–85.

Mohan D. Injuries and the 'poor' worker. *Ergonomics* 1987c;30:373–377.

Mohan D. A safer world for the vulnerable road user. *J Traffic Med* 1990a;18(4):225.

Mohan D. The vulnerable road user (Editorial). *J Traffic Med* 1990b;18:153–155.

Mohan D. Vulnerable road users: an era of neglect. *J Traffic Med* 1992;20:121–128.

Mohan D. Avoidable dangers on the farm. *World Health* 1993;1:12–13.

Mohan D, Bawa PS. An analysis of road traffic fatalities in Delhi, India. *Accid Anal Prev* 1985;17(1):33–45.

Mohan D, Kajzer J, Bawa Bhalla LS, Chawla A. Impact modeling studies for a three-wheeled scooter taxi. *Accid Anal Prev* 1997;29(2): 161–170.

Mohan D, Kumar M. Road traffic fatalities in Delhi India: lessons for low income countries (Abstract). *First World Conference on Accident and Injury Prevention (Stockholm, Sweden)*: Abstract Guide. Sundyberg: Karolinska Institute, September 17–20, 1989.

Mohan D, Kumar S, Kothiya KP, et al. *Firework Injuries During Diwali: a Study of Patients Brought to Two Hospitals in Delhi.* New Delhi, India. Centre for Biomedical Engineering, Indian Institute of Technology, 1984.

Mohan D, Kumar A, Patel R, Qadeer I. Injuries in agricultural activities. *Indian J Rural Development* 1989;1(1):71–80.

Mohan D, Qadeer I. Injuries sustained by women and children in agricultural activities in India. *Proc. XII Asian Conference on Occupational Health*, Bombay, 1988.

Mohan D, Varghese M. Fireworks cast a shadow on India's festival of lights. *World Health Forum* 1990;11:323–326.

Moharty S, Rao CJ, Kumar A. Problems with penetrating injuries of the head in rural India. *J Indian Med Assoc* 1980;74:107–108.

Monk M. Epidemiology of suicide. *Epidemiological Review* 1987;9:51–69

Moore CW. *The Mediation Process: Practical Strategies for Resolving Conflict.* San Francisco: Jossey–Bass, 1986.

Morgan G. Satellite remote sensing applications for natural hazard preparedness and emergency response planning. In: Kreimer A, Zador M, eds. *Colloquium on Disasters, Sustainability and Development: a Look to the 1990's.* Washington, DC: Environment Department, World Bank. Environment Working Paper No. 23. 1989.

Moritz AR, Henriques FC. Studies of thermal injury. II. The relative importance of time and surface temperature in the causation of cutaneous burns. *Am J Pathol* 1947;23: 695–720.

Morrisson W, Rice C, Roberts H. Corkerhill, Glasgow: Application to become a member of the Safe Community Network. *KI White Report 275.* Sundbyberg, Sweden: WHO Collaborating Centre on Community Safety Promotion, Department of Social Medicine, Karolinska Institute, 1992.

Moscicki EK, O'Carroll PW, Rae DS, Roy AG,

Locke BZ, Regier DA. Suicidal ideation and attempts: The epidemiologic catchment area study. In: *Alcohol, Drug Abuse, and Mental Health Administration. Report of the Secretary's Task Force on Youth Suicide.* Volume 4: Strategies for the prevention of youth suicide. DHHS Pub. No. (ADM) 89–1624. Washington, DC: US Government Printing Office, 1989: 115–128.

Moses M. Pesticides. In: Last JM and Wallace RB, eds, *Maxcy-Rosenau-Last, Public Health and Preventive Medicine.* Norwalk, CN: Appleton and Lange 1992:479–489.

Moskowitz H, ed. Special issue on drugs and driving. *Accid Anal Prev* 1976;8:1.

Moskowitz H, ed. Marihuana and driving. *Accid Anal Prev* 1985;17(4):323–345.

Moulder J. Alcohol and drug impairment in crash–involved commercial drivers in North America (Abstract). *J Traffic Med* 1990;18(4): 297.

Mountain L, Fawaz B. The accuracy of estimates of expected accident frequencies obtained using an Empirical Bayes approach. *Traffic Engineering and Control* 1991;32(5): 246–251.

Mowbrey DL. Pesticide poisoning in Papua New Guinea and the South Pacific. *Papua New Guinea Med J* 1986;29:131–141.

Moyer LA, Boyle CA, Pollock DA. Validity of death certificates for injury-related causes of death. *Am J Epidemiol* 1989;130:1024–1032.

Mufti MH. Medico-legal aspects of seat belt legislation in Saudi Arabia. *Saudi Med J* 1986; 7(1):84–90.

Muir BL. *Health Status of Canadian Indians and Inuit—1990.* Ottawa, Canada: Indian and Northern Health Services, Medical Services Branch, Health and Welfare Canada, 1991: 1–58.

Muller A. An evaluation of the effectiveness of motorcycle headlight use laws. *Am J Public Health* 1982;72:1136–1141.

Murray CJL, Lopez AD, eds. *The Global Burden of Disease, Volume I.* World Health Organization, Harvard University Press, 1996, 1–990.

Murray CJL, Yang G, Qiao X. Adult Mortality: Levels, Patterns, and Causes. In: Feachem RGA, Kjellstrom T, Murray CJL, Over M, Phillips MA, eds. *The Health of Adults in the Developing World.* The World Bank. New York: Oxford University Press, 1992:23–112.

Myntti C, Said A, Aqlan G, Al-Rubayh S. Using

post-mortem interviews at the community level: an example from Yemen. *Health Policy and Planning* 1991;6(3):282–290.

Nader R. *Unsafe at Any Speed: the Designed In Dangers of the American Automobile.* New York: Knightsbridge Publishing, 1991:1–368.

Naraqi S. Treatment of acute methyl alcohol intoxication in developing countries. *Med J Aust* 1979;2:194–199.

Naraynsingh V. Potential impact of the advanced trauma life support (ATLS) program in a third world country. *Int Surg* 1987;72 (3):179–184.

Nash N. Bankrupt system takes glitter off golden years: Argentina/A series of suicides has called national attention to the economic plight of retirees. *Globe and Mail* 1992 Nov 17, A6 col 1–4.

Natarajan M. Accident and emergency medical services: a project for Tamil Nadu State. Madras: Tamil Nadu State Planning Commission 1978:1–35.

Nathani MB. Status of occupational safety in Pakistan. In: Preprints: *Accident Prevention in Developing Countries.* International Conference on Strategies for Occupational Accident Prevention. Stockholm, Sweden: National Board of Occupational Safety and Health, 1989: 1–12.

Nation's Health. EPA urged to add secondhand smoke to most toxic list. American Public Health Association, December, 1992:1.

National Center for Health Statistics. (Collins JG). Persons injured and disability days due to injuries, United States, 1980–81. *Vital and Health Statistics.* Series 10, No. 149, DHHS Pub. No. (PHS) 85–1577. Public Health Service. Washington: U.S. Government Printing Office, March 1985.

National Center for Health Statistics. *Prevention profile. Health, United States, 1989.* Hyattsville, Maryland: Public Health Service 1990; 139–140.

National Center for Health Statistics. 1993 *National Mortality Followback Survey: Followback for the Future.* Hyattsville, Maryland: Division of Vital Statistics. National Center for Health Statistics, Centers for Disease Control, 1992.

National Committee for Injury Prevention and Control. *Injury Prevention: Meeting the Challenge.* New York: Oxford, American J Preventive Medicine 1989;5(Suppl):115–144, 296–299.

National Epidemiology Board of Thailand. *Review of the Health Situation of Thailand: Priority Ranking of Diseases.* Sukon K, ed. Bangkok: National Epidemiology Board of Thailand. 1987.

National Highway Traffic Safety Administration (NHTSA). *Facts of Alcohol and Highway Safety.* Washington: U.S. Department of Transportation Office of Alcohol Countermeasures, 1984.

National Highway Traffic Safety Administration (NHTSA). *Fatal Accident Reporting System,* 1987. Washington: U.S. Department of Transportation, 1988.

National Safety Council of Singapore. *21st Annual Report for the Year 1986/87.* 1988.

National Safety Council. *Accident Facts.* Chicago: National Safety Council, 1994.

Natsios AS. Economic incentives and disaster mitigation. In: Kreimer A, Munasinghe M, eds. *Managing Natural Disasters and the Environment.* Washington, DC: Environmental Policy and Research Division, Environment Department, The World Bank, 1991: 111–114.

Nelson DC, Strueber JV. Measuring road safety using a relative safety index (Abstract). *J Traffic Med* 1990;18(4):249.

Nelson DC, Strueber JV. The effect of open-back vehicles on casualty rates: The case of Papua New Guinea. *Accid Anal Prev* 1991; 23:109–117.

Newberger EH. Child abuse. In: Last JM and Wallace RB, eds, *Maxcy-Rosenau-Last, Public Health and Preventive Medicine.* Norwalk, CN: Appleton and Lange, 1992:1046–1048.

Ng SC, Chao TC, How J. Deaths by accidental drowning in Singapore, 1973–76. *Singapore Med J* 1978;19:14–19.

Nicholson AJ. The variability of accident costs. *Accid Anal Prev* 1985;17(1):47–56.

Niiranen M. Perforating eye injuries. *Acta Ophthalmologica (Kbh)* 1978;135(Suppl):1–87.

Nikander P, Seppala T, Kilonzo GP, et al. Ingredients and contaminants of traditional alcoholic beverages in Tanzania. *Trans R Soc Trop Med Hyg* 1991;85:412–415.

Nishioka SA, Handa ST, Nunes RS. Pig bite in Brazil: a case series from a teaching hospital. *Revista da Sociedade Brasileira de Medicina Tropical* 1994;27(1):15–18.

Nishioka SA, Silveira PVP. Bacteriology of abscesses complicating bites of lance-headed vipers. *Annals Trop Med Parasitol* 1992a;86: 89–91.

Nishioka SA, Silveira PVP. Clinical and epidemiologic study of 292 cases of lance-headed viper bite in a Brazilian teaching hospital. *Am J Trop Med Hyg* 1992b;47:805–810.

Nishioka SA, Silveira PVP, Menezes LB. Coral snake bite and severe local pain. *Ann Trop Med Parasitol* 1993a;87:429–431.

Nishioka SA, Silveira PVP, Pereira CAD. Scorpion sting on the penis. *J Urology* 1993b; 150:1501.

Nishioka SA, Silveira PV, Ugrinovich R, De Oliviera RC. Scorpion sting with cranial nerve involvement (letter). *Toxicon* 1992;30: 685–686.

Nixon JW, Pearn JH. An investigation of sociodemographic factors surrounding childhood drowning accidents. *Soc Sci Med* 1978; 12: 387–390.

Nixon JW, Pearn JH, Dugdale AE. Swimming ability of children: a survey of 4,000 Queensland children in a high drowning region. *Med J Aust* 1979;6(4):271–272.

Nkwi P. The Lake Nyos gas explosion: different perceptions of the phenomenon. Nairobi: Academy Science Publishers. *Discovery and Innovation* 1990;2(2):7–19.

Noji EK. *The Nature of Disasters.* In: Noji EK, ed. *The Public Health Consequences of Disasters.* New York: Oxford University Press, 1997.

Nordic Medico-Statistical Committee. *Classification for Accident Monitoring.* Copenhagen: NOMESCO, Nordic Statistical Secretariat, 1990.

Nordic Medico-Statistical Committee. *Classification of External Causes of Injuries in the Arctic.* Copenhagen: NOMESCO, Nordic Statistical Secretariat, 1993, 1–106.

Nur IM. Disaster preparedness and response in Africa. In: *Colloquium on the Environment and Natural Disaster Management.* Washington, DC: Environment Department, World Bank. 1990.

Nur IM. Writing an action plan for disaster preparedness in Africa. In: Kreimer A, Munasinghe M, eds. *Managing Natural Disasters and the Environment.* Washington, DC: Environmental Policy and Research Division, Environment Department, The World Bank, 1991:191–196.

Obembe A, Fagbayi A. Road traffic accidents in Kaduna metropolis: a 3–month survey. *East African Med J* 1988;65:572–577.

O'Brien SJ, Vertinsky PA. Unfit survivors: Exercise as a resource for aging women. *Gerontologist* 1991;31(3):347–357.

O'Carroll PW. Suicide. In: Last JM and Wallace RB, eds, *Maxcy-Rosenau-Last, Public Health and Preventive Medicine.* Norwalk, CN: Appleton and Lange, 1992:1054–1062.

O'Carroll PW, Mercy JA, Steward JA. CDC recommendations for a community plan for the prevention and containment of suicide clusters. *MMWR* 1988;37(S–6):1–12.

O'Carroll PW, Rosenberg ML, Mercy JA. Suicide. In: Rosenberg ML, Fenley MA, eds. *Violence in America: a Public Health Approach.* New York: Oxford University Press, 1991:184–196.

Odero W, Garner P, Zwi A. Road traffic injuries in developing countries: A comprehensive review of epidemiological studies. *Trop Med Int Health* 1997;2:445–460.

Office of Technology Assessment, U.S. Congress. Hierarchy of Controls. In: *Preventing Illness and Injury in the Workplace.* Washington: OTA–H–257. 1985:175–185.

Ogden KW. *An Aid to Road Safety Engineering.* Sydney, Avebury Technical, 1996.

Okonkwo CA. Spinal cord injuries in Enugu, Nigeria— preventable accidents. *Paraplegia* 1988;26(1):12–18.

Olkkonen S. Alcohol-involved bicycle fatalities in Finland. J Traffic Med 1993;21:29–37. Abstracted in: *ICADTS Reporter* 1993;4:3.

Olkkonen S, Honkanen R. The role of alcohol in nonfatal bicycle injuries. *Accid Anal Prev* 1990;22:89–96.

Olurin O. Ocular injuries in Nigeria. *Am J Ophthalmol* 1971;72:159–166.

Oluwasanmi AJ. Road accident trends in Nigeria. *Accid Anal and Prev* 1993;25:485–487.

O'Neill B. The uses and limitations of motor vehicle insurance in prevention (Abstract). *J Traffic Med* 1990;18(4):226.

Onuba O. Pattern of burn injury in Nigerian children. *Trop Doct* 1988;18:106–108.

Onyoyo HA. Abstract on chemical accidents and disaster in Kenya. In: Preprints: *Accident Prevention in Developing Countries.* International Conference on Strategies for Occupational Accident Prevention. Stockholm, Sweden: National Board of Occupational Safety and Health, 1989.

Orer M. Heavy vehicle shaker (Abstract). *J Traffic Med* 1990;18(4):275.

Organisation for Economic Co-operation and Development. *Participatory Development and Good Governance.* Paris; Development Cooperation Guidelines Series 1995:1–30. (Bilingual English-French publication, French 36 pp).

Osler T, Baker SP, Long W. A modification of the Injury Severity Score that both improves accuracy and simplifies scoring. *J Trauma* 1997;43(6):922-926.

Orski CK. Can management of transportation demand help solve our growing traffic congestion and air pollution problems? *Transportation Quarterly* 1990;44(4):483–498.

Östrom M, Huelke DF, Waller PF, Eriksson, Blow F. Some biases in the alcohol investigative process in traffic fatalities. *Accid Anal Prev* 1992;24(5):539–545.

O'Toole BI. Intelligence and behavior and motor vehicle accident mortality. *Accid Anal Prev* 1990;22:211–221.

Otte D. Injury mechanisms in pedestrian accidents and the possibility of injury reduction by vehicle geometrics (Abstract). *J Traffic Med* 1990;18(4):269.

Overseas Development Council. Foreign aid: The Reagan legacy. *Policy Focus* 1988;2:1–10.

Pacqué-Margolis S, Pacqué M, Dukuly Z, Boateng J, Taylor HR. Application of the verbal autopsy during a clinical trial. *Soc Sci Med* 1990;31: 585–591.

Paixao MLT DA, Dewar RD, Cossar JH, et al. What do Scots die of when abroad? *Scot Med J* 1991;36:114–116.

Pakkala L. The flammability of different textiles and its influence on the severity of skin burns. *Ann Chir Gynaecol* 1980;69(5): 240–243.

Palca J. Cameroon lake gas disaster: a lesson for the future. *Nature* 1987;325:475.

Pan American Health Organization. *A Guide to Emergency Health Management After Natural Disasters.* Washington, D.C.: Pan American Health Organization Scientific Publication No. 407, 1981.

Pan American Health Organization. Fatal occupational accidents. *Epidemiol Bull PAHO* 1984; 5(3):9–11.

Pan American Health Organization. *Health Conditions in the Americas, 1981–1984.* Volume I. Washington, DC, Pan American Health Organization Scientific Publication No. 500, 1986.

Pan American Health Organization. Health profiles, Brazil, 1984. *PAHO Epidemiological Bull* 1988;9(2):6–12.

Pan American Health Organization. *Health Conditions in the Americas, 1990 Edition.* Volume I. Washington, DC, Pan American Health Organization Scientific Publication No. 524, 1990: 1–504.

Pan American Health Organization. *Consideraciones Sobre la Prevención, el Control y la Vigilancia Epidemiológica de la Rabia Humana Transmitida por Vampiros en las Americas.* Reunion de consulta sobre la atención a personas expuestas a la rabia transmitida por vampiros. Washington, D.C., 1991.

Pantelic J. The link between reconstruction and development. In: Kreimer A, Munasinghe M, eds. *Managing Natural Disasters and the Environment.* Washington, DC: Environmental Policy and Research Division, Environment Department, The World Bank, 1991:90–96.

Parikh DJ, Vyas JB, Patel VG, Kashyap SK. Studies on occupational accidents in small scale industries. In: Preprints: *Accident Prevention in Developing Countries.* International Conference on Strategies for Occupational Accident Prevention. Stockholm, Sweden, Sept 21–22, 1989. Solna, Sweden, Publication Service, National Board of Occupational Safety and Health, 1989.

Patel NS, Bhagwatt GP. Road traffic accidents in Lusaka and blood alcohol. *Med J Zambia* 1977; 11(2):46–49.

Patel R, Mohan D. Epidemiologic studies and design of agricultural implements (Abstract). *First World Conference on Accident and Injury Prevention* (Stockholm, Sweden): Abstract Guide. Sundyberg: Karolinska Institute, September 17–20, 1989.

Patel R, Mohan D. Human factors approach for improving designing of motorcycle helmets in India (Abstract). *J Traffic Med* 1990a; 18 (4):296.

Patel R, Mohan D. Design of shopping bag as a safety vest for two wheeler rider (Abstract). *J Traffic Med* 1990b;18(4):276.

Patel R, Mohan D, Kumar A, Shah SJ, Kumar H. Epidemiological studies and design of agricultural implements. In: *Preprints: Accident Prevention in Developing Countries.* International Conference on Strategies for Occupational Accident Prevention. Stockholm, Sweden: National Board of Occupational Safety and Health, 1989:1–7.

Paux P, Bahuaud J. Injuries caused by garfish in New Caledonia and its dependencies. *Med Trop* (Mars) 1989;49(3): 289–292.

A Paz é Possivel em Timor Leste. *Timor Oriental Santa Cruz: L'Armée Indonésienne Tire Sur La Foule.* Lisbon, Portugal: A Paz é Possivel em Timor Leste, 1992, 1–17.

Pearce NE, Davis PB, Smith AH, Foster FH. Mortality and social class in New Zealand II: Male mortality by major disease groupings. *NZ Med J* 1983;96:711–716.

Pearce NE, Davis PB, Smith AH, Foster FH. Mortality and social class in New Zealand III: Male mortality by ethnic group. *NZ Med J* 1984; 97:31–35.

Pearn JH. Drowning and near-drowning in the Australian Capital Territory: a five-year total population study of immersion accidents. *Med J Aust* 1977;1:130–133.

Pearn JH. Survival rates after serious immersion accidents in childhood. *Resuscitation* 1978;6(4): 271–278.

Pearn JH, Bart R, Yamaoka R. Drowning risks to epileptic children: a study from Hawaii. *Br Med J* 1978;2:1284–1285.

Pearn JH, Brown J, Hsia EY. Swimming pool drownings and near drownings involving children: a total population study from Hawaii. *Military Medicine* 1980;15–18.

Pearn JH, Brown JB, Wong R, et al. Bathtub drownings: report of seven cases. *Pediatrics* 1979a;64:68–70.

Pearn JH, Nixon J, Wilkey I. Freshwater drowning and near drowning accidents involving children: a five-year total population study. *Med J Aust* 1976;2:942–946.

Pearn JH, Wong RYK, Brown J III, Ching YC, Bart R Jr, Hammar S. Drowning and near-drowning involving children: a five-year total population study from the city and county of Honolulu. *Am J Public Health* 1979b;69: 450–454.

Perneger T, Smith GS. The driver's role in fatal two-car crashes: a paired "case-control" study. *Am J Epidemiol* 1991;134:1138–1145.

Petawabano BH, Gourdeau É, Jourdain F, Palliser–Tulugak, Cossette J. *Mental Health and Aboriginal People of Quebec*. Québec, QC: La Comité de la santé mentale du Québec, 1994, 1–124.

Petricciani JC. Ongoing tragedy of rabies. *Lancet* 1993;342:1067–1068.

Petrucelli E. The evolution of injury scaling since 1970 (Abstract). *J Traffic Med* 1990;18 (4):251.

Phelps CE. Death and taxes: an opportunity for substitution. *J Health Econ* 1988;7:1–24.

Pineault R, Daveluy C. *La Planification de la Santé: Concepts, Méthodes, Stratégies*. Montréal: Agence d'ARC Inc. (les éditions), 1986.

Pless IB. National childhood injury prevention conference. *Can J Public Health* 1989; 80:427–430.

Pleuckhahn VD. Alcohol and accidental drowning: a 25–year study. *Med J Aust* 1984; 141:22–25.

Poe GS, McLaughlin JK, Powell-Griner E, Parsons CR, Robinson K. The time interval between deaths and next-of-kin contact and its effects on response rates and data quality. *Am J Epidemiol* 1991;134:1454–62.

Pooley AC, Hines T, Shield J. Attacks on humans. In: Ed. CA Ross. *Crocodiles and Alligators*. New York: Facts on File, Inc., 1989, pp. 172–187.

Popkin C. Cited in: Women at risk. *Prevention File: Alcohol, Tobacco and Other Drugs*. University of California, San Diego 1992;7(5): 19–20.

Posanau C. *A Study of the Relationship of Alcohol and Road Traffic Accidents in the National Capital District of Papua New Guinea* (Thesis). Port Moresby: Department of Community Medicine, University of Papua New Guinea, 1990.

Price J, Karim I. Suicide in Fiji: a two-year survey. *Acta Psychiatr Scand* 1975;52:153–159.

Prince RL, Smith M, Dick IM, Price RI, Garcia Webb P, Henderson NK, Harris MM. Prevention of postmenopausal osteoporosis. A comparative study of exercise, calcium supplementation, and hormone replacement therapy. *N Engl J Med* 1991;325:1189–1195.

Pugh RNH, Theakston RDG. Incidence and mortality of snakebite in Savanna Nigeria. *Lancet* 1980;2:1181–1183.

Punnet L. Carpal tunnel syndrome. In: Weeks JL, Levy BS, Wagner GR, eds. *Preventing Occupational Disease and Injury*. Washington, DC: American Public Health Association, 1991a: 194–203.

Punnet L. Peripheral nerve entrapment syndromes. In: Weeks JL, Levy BS, Wagner GR, eds. *Preventing Occupational Disease and Injury*. Washington, DC: American Public Health Association, 1991b:445–453.

Punnet L. Tendinitis, tenosynovitis. In: Weeks JL, Levy BS, Wagner GR, eds. *Preventing Occupational Disease and Injury*. Washington, DC: American Public Health Association, 1991c: 553–562.

Qadeer I, Mohan D. Occupational injuries in agriculture: an epidemiological study in Northern India. In: *Proceedings of the International Conference on Ergonomics, Occupational*

Safety and Health and the Environment, Beijing, China 1988:2:1072–1080.

Qadeer I, Mohan D. Man, machine, and morbidity: a study of injuries in a green revolution district of India (Abstract). *First World Conference on Accident and Injury Prevention* (Stockholm, Sweden): *Abstract Guide.* Sundyberg: Karolinska Institute, September 17–20, 1989:343.

Qi-chun XU, Fend-chong, L. Study on ergonomics and its use in the harvesting system. In: *Preprints: Accident Prevention in Developing Countries.* International Conference on Strategies for Occupational Accident Prevention. Stockholm, Sweden: National Board of Occupational Safety and Health, 1989:1–9.

Quan L, Gore EJ, Wentz K, Allen J, Novack AH. Ten-year study of pediatric drownings and near-drownings in King County, Washington: Lessons on injury prevention. *Pediatrics* 1989; 83:1035–1040.

Radjak HA, Agustiono E. Successful helmetization program in Indonesia. Jakarta: Ministry of Health. Paper presented at *National Programmes on Accident and Injury Prevention.* National Board of Health and Welfare. Stockholm, Sweden, 1989.

Rainey DY, Runyan CW. Newspapers: a source for injury surveillance? *Am J Public Health* 1992; 82(5):745–746.

Ramsay R, Bagley C. The prevalence of suicidal behaviors, attitudes and associated social experiences in an urban population. *Suicide and Life-Threatening Behavior* 1985; 15(3):151–167.

Ranganathan N, Sharma AK, Gupta S, Raju MP. Spatial and temporal characteristics of traffic accidents in a metropolitan city (Abstract). *J Traffic Med* 1990;18(4):308.

Rankin JG, Ashley MJ. Alcohol-related health problems. In: Last JM, Wallace RB, eds. *Maxcy-Rosenau-Last, Public Health and Preventive Medicine.* Norwalk, Conn.: Appleton and Lange, 1992, 741–767.

Rao BS. Burns in childhood and early adolescence: an epidemiologic study of hospitalized cases. *J Indian Med Assoc* 1966;46(1): 23–27.

Rao DP, Venkataram BM. Urban road users traffic safety knowledge: A case study of Visakhapatnam City, India (Abstract). *J Traffic Med* 1990;18(4):238.

Rausch A, Wong J, Kirkpatrick M. A field test of two single center, high-mounted brake light systems. *Accid Anal Prev* 1982;14:287–291

Ravenholt RJ. Addiction mortality in the United States, 1980: tobacco, alcohol, and other substances. *Population and Development Review* 1984;10:697–724. Cited in: Secretary of Health and Human Services. *Sixth Special Report to the U.S. Congress on Alcohol and Health.* Washington, DC: Alcohol, Drug Abuse, and Mental Health Administration, DHSS publication no. (ADM) 87–1519. 1987.

Razouki SS. Abnormality of speed spectra as a phenomenon of roads with high accident potential (Abstract). *J Traffic Med* 1990;18 (4):254.

Recker RR, Davies KM, Hinders SM, Heaney RP, Stegman MR, Kimmel DB. Bone gain in young women. *JAMA* 1992;268:2403–2408.

Reilly MSJ. Have "formal investigations" into fishing vessel losses ceased? *Br J Indust Med* 1987a; 28:27–35.

Reilly MSJ. Safety at sea is a forgotten frontier (Editorial). *Br J Indust Med* 1987b;44:1–6.

Replogle MA. Sustainable transportation strategies for Third-World development. Washington, DC: Transportation Research Board, National Research Council. *Transportation Research Record* 1991;No. 1294:1–8.

Retting R, Schwartz SI, Kuliwecz M, Buhrmeister D. Queens Boulevard pedestrian safety project. Injury Control. *MMWR* 1989;38(5), reprinted in Injury Control MMWR Reprints, Compilation #6, October 1988–December 1989, 1990:12–14.

Reuters. Panel convinced of TV-violence link. *Globe and Mail* (Toronto) 1993 Aug 11:A13 (col 5–6).

Rhoades ER, Brenneman G, Lyle J, Handler A. Mortality of American Indian and Alaska Native infants. *Annual Rev Publ Health* 1992;13: 269–285.

Ribeiro LA, Jorge MT, Piesco RV, Nishioka SA. Wolf spider bites in São Paulo, Brazil: A clinical and epidemiological study of 515 cases. *Toxicon* 1990;28:715–717.

Rice DP, MacKenzie EJ, and Associates (Jones AS, Kaufman SR, De Lissovoy GV, Max W, McLoughlin E, Miller TR, Robertson LS, Salkever DS, Smith GS). *Cost of Injury in the United States: a Report to Congress.* San Francisco: Institute for Health and Aging, University of California and Injury Prevention Center, The Johns Hopkins University, 1989.

Riley ID, Lehmann D, Alpers MP, Marshall TFD, Gratten H, Smith D. Pneumococcal vaccine prevents death from acute lower respiratory tract infections in Papua New Guinean children. *Lancet* 1986;ii:877–881.

Ritson EB. Community response to alcohol-related problems: Review of an international study. Geneva: *World Health Organization Public Health Papers No. 81*, 1985:1–58.

Rivara FP, Dicker BG, Bergman AB, Dacey R, Herman C. The public cost of motorcycle trauma. *JAMA* 1988;260:221–223.

Roberts I. Differential recall in a case-control study of child pedestrian injuries. *Epidemiology* 1994;5:473–475.

Roberts I. What does a decline in child pedestrian injury rates mean? (letter) *Am J Public Health* 1995;85:268–269.

Roberts I, Lee-Joe T. Effect of exposure measurement error in a case-control study of child pedestrian injuries. *Epidemiology* 1993;4:477–479.

Roberts I, Marshall R, Lee-Joe T. The urban traffic environment and the risk of child pedestrian injury: a case-crossover approach. *Epidemiology* 1995a;6:169–171.

Roberts I, Norton R, Jackson R. Driveway-related child pedestrian injuries: a case-control study. *Pediatrics* 1995b;95:405–408.

Robertson, LS. Crash involvement of teenaged drivers when driver education is eliminated from high school. *Am J Public Health* 1980;70:599–603.

Robertson LS. Report of the twelfth Ross roundtable on critical approaches to common pediatric problems. In: Bergman AB, ed. *Prevention of Childhood Injuries.* Columbus, OH: Ross Laboratories, 1982.

Robertson LS. *Injuries: Causes, Control Strategies, and Public Policy.* Lexington, MA: Lexington Books, 1983.

Robertson LS. Motor vehicle injuries. In: Weeks JL, Levy BS, Wagner GR, eds. *Preventing Occupational Disease and Injury.* Washington, DC: American Public Health Association, 1991: 425–429.

Robertson LS. *Injury Epidemiology.* New York: Oxford, 1992.

Robertson LS, Kelley AB, O'Neill B, et al. A controlled study of the effect of television messages on safety belt use. *Am J Public Health* 1974;64:1071–1080.

Robertson LS, Zador PL. Driver education and crash involvement of teenaged drivers. *Am J Public Health* 1978;68:959–965.

Robine JM. Estimating disability-free life expectancy (DFLE) in the Western countries in the last decade—how can this new indicator of health status be used? (Summary). *World Health Stat Q* 1989;42(3):147.

Robitaille Y, Barss P. Traumatismes et facteurs de risque (Available in French and English as Santé Québec: A Health Profile of the Cree). In: Daveluy C, Lavallée C, Clarkson M, Robinson E, eds. *Santé Québec: a health profile of the James Bay Cree.* Québec, Québec: Gouvernement du Québec, Santé Québec, 1994, 145–160.

Rodgers DD. Community crisis intervention in suicide epidemics. In: Postl BD et al., eds. *Circumpolar Health 90 Proceedings of the 8th International Congress on Circumpolar Health,* Whitehorse, Yukon, May 20–25, 1990. Winnipeg, MA: University of Manitoba Press for Canadian Society for International Health, 1991:276–280.

Rogers J, Dennis PJ, Lee JV, Keevil. Effects of water chemistry and temperature on the survival and growth of *Legionella pneumophila* in potable water systems. In: *Legionella: Current Status and Emerging Perspectives.* Barbaree JM, Breiman RF, Dufour AP, eds. Washington, DC: American Society for Microbiology, 1993, 248–250.

Romeder JM, McWhinnie JR: Potential years of life lost between ages 1 and 70: an indicator of premature mortality for health planning. *Int J Epidemiol* 1977;6:143–151.

Romer CJ. WHO Injury Prevention Program: How to implement the safe community concept worldwide. In: *Proceedings National Programmes on Accident and Injury Prevention.* Stockholm, Sweden: Swedish National Board of Health and Welfare, 1991:17–20.

Romer CJ, Manciaux M. Research and intersectoral cooperation in the field of accidents. *World Health Stat Q* 1986;39:281–284.

Rongfang S, Xiaomin M, Wei C. A preliminary study of strategic systems planning for disaster prevention and relief in Shanghai area. In: Preprints: *Accident Prevention in Developing Countries.* International Conference on Strategies for Occupational Accident Prevention. Stockholm, Sweden: National Board of Occupational Safety and Health, 1989:1–7.

Rose G. *The Strategy of Preventive Medicine.* Oxford: Oxford University Press, 1992:1–138.

Rosenberg ML, Fenley MA, eds. *Violence in America: a Public Health Approach.* New York: Oxford University Press, 1991:1–199.

Rosenberg ML, Gelles RJ, Holinger PC, Zahn MA, Stark E, Conn JM, Fajman NM, Karlson TA. Violence: homicide, assault, and suicide. In: Amler RW, Dull HVB, eds. *Closing the Gap: the Burden of Unnecessary Illness.* New York: Oxford University Press; *Am J Prev Med* 1987;3(Suppl 5):164–78.

Rosenberg ML, Mercy JA. Assaultive violence. In: Last JM and Wallace RB, eds, *Maxcy-Rosenau-Last, Public Health and Preventive Medicine.* Norwalk, CT: Appleton and Lange, 1992: 1035–1039.

Rosenthal CB. *A Study of Violent Death in the State of São Paulo, Brazil; Homicide, Suicide, and Motor Vehicle Accident Mortality from 1945 to 1990* (Dissertation). Baltimore, MD, Johns Hopkins School of Hygiene and Public Health, 1995.

Ross HL. *Confronting Drunk Driving. Social Policy for Saving Lives.* New Haven, CT: Yale University Press, 1992, 1–220.

Ross HL. Prevalence of alcohol-impaired driving: An international comparison. *Accid Anal Prev* 1993;25:777–779.

Rothman KJ. *Modern Epidemiology.* Boston: Little, Brown and Company. 1986:64–72; 311–326.

Rowe B, Bota G. Serious snowmobile trauma in a northern Ontario community: a case series. *Annals RCPSC* 1991;24:501–505.

Rubinstein DH. Epidemic suicide among Micronesian adolescents. *Soc Sci Med* 1983; 17(10):657–665.

Ruehsen MM, Abdul-Wahab AM. The epidemiology of trauma in an intensive care unit in Bahrain. *J Trauma* 1989;29:31–36.

Ruegg RT, Weber SF, Lippiatt BC, Fuller SK. *Improving the Fire Safety of Cigarettes: an Economic Impact Analysis.* Washington, DC: U.S. Consumer Product Safety Commission, 1987.

Runyan CW, Bangdiwala SI, Linzer MA, Sacks JJ, Butts J. Risk factors for fatal residential fires. *N Engl J Med* 1992;327(12):859–863.

Ryan CA, Dowling. Drowning deaths in people with epilepsy. *Can Med Assoc J* 1993;148: 781–784.

Ryan GA. *Prevention and Control of Road Traffic Accidents: Solomon Islands.* World Health Organization, Regional Office for the Western Pacific, Assignment Report, 1989a:1–24.

Ryan GA. *Prevention and Control of Road Traffic Accidents: Papua New Guinea.* World Health Organization, Regional Office for the Western Pacific, Assignment Report, 1989b:1–18.

Ryan GA. *Prevention and Control of Road Traffic Accidents: Papua New Guinea.* World Health Organization, Regional Office for the Western Pacific, Assignment Report, 1990:1–17.

Ryan GA, Ukai T. *Prevention and Control of Road Traffic Accidents: People's Republic of China.* World Health Organization, Regional Office for the Western Pacific, Assignment Report, 1988: 1–32.

Sahlu T, Larson C. The prevalence and environmental risk factors for moderate to severe trachoma in southern Ethiopia. *J Trop Med Hyg* 1992;95:36–41.

Sainsbury P. Validity and reliability of trends in suicide statistics. *World Health Stat Q* 1983; 3/4:339–348.

Saleh S, Gadalla S, Fortney JA, Rogers SM, Potts DM. Accidental burn deaths to Egyptian women of reproductive age. *Burns* 1986; 12:241–245.

Sambasivan M. Survey of the problems of head injuries in India. *Neurology India* 1977;25: 51–59.

Sande J, Thorson J. An evaluation of the official Swedish statistics on seriously injured in road traffic accidents. *Scand J Soc Med* 1975;3:5–11.

Sanfaçon G, Blais R. Les intoxications. In: Beaulne G, ed. *Les Traumatismes au Québec.* Québec, Québec: Gouvernement du Québec, Ministère de la Santé et des Services sociaux, 1991:177–190.

Saravanapavanthan. Injuries caused by homemade explosives. *Forensic Sci Int* 1978;12: 131–136.

Sarin SM, Sharfuddin, Dindayal, Sharma ML, Kaushal SC. Design and performance of speed breakers for better safety and conspicuity (Abstract). *J Traffic Med* 1990a;18 (4):309.

Sarin SM, Sharfuddin, Dindayal, Sharma ML, Kaushal SC. Characteristics of pedestrians and cyclists involved in road fatalities (Abstract). *J Traffic Med* 1990f;18(4):279.

Sarin SM, Shukla A, Suri BL, Chhabra S. Driver vision under dynamic road traffic conditions (Abstract). *J Traffic Med* 1990b;18(4):278.

Sarin SM, Suri BL, Bajpai RK, Luthra HR, Saxena A, Singh H. Road accidents in India and other South-east Asian countries (Abstract). *J Traffic Med* 1990c;18(4):316.

Sarin SM, Suri BL, Chhabra S, Kaushal SC. Knowledge of road traffic signs and road traffic rules among truck drivers in India (Abstract). *J Traffic Med* 1990d;18(4):247.

Sarin SM, Suri BL, Sharfuddin, Bajpai RK, Luthra HR, Singh H. A study of road accidents on a national highway in India and countermeasures (Abstract). *J Traffic Med* 1990e;18(4):316.

Sattin RW. Falls among older persons: A public health perspective. *Annual Rev Publ Health* 1992;13:489–508.

Saxena PS, Sharma SM, Singh M, Saxena M. Camel bite injuries. *J Indian Med Assoc* 1982; 79(5&6):65–68.

Sayer I, Hitchcock R. An analysis of police and medical road accident data: Sri Lanka 1977–81. Crowthorne, Berkshire, UK: Overseas Unit, Transport and Road Research Laboratory, *TRRL Supplementary Report* 834, 1984: 1–27.

Schelp L. *Community Intervention and Accidents: Epidemiology as a Basis for Evaluation of a Community Intervention Programme on Accidents* (Thesis). Sundbyberg, Sweden: Department of Social Medicine, Karolinska Institute, 1987.

Schelp L. The role of organizations in community participation—prevention of accidental injuries in a rural Swedish municipality. *Soc Sci Med* 1988;26:1087–1093.

Schilling RSF. Hazards of deep sea fishing. *Br J Indust Med* 1971;28:27–35.

Schnarch B. *Alcohol and Injuries from Fights and Motor Vehicles.* Data from: Kuujjuag, QC, Canada: Nunavik Regional Council of Health and Social Services, Internal report, 1994.

Schroeder G, Eidam J, Windus G, Bosch U. Injury patterns in relation to bumper design in simulated car/pedestrian collisions (Abstract). *J Traffic Med* 1990;18 (4):269.

Schuller E, Beier G, Ettemeyer M. The effects of vehicle frontal design on pedestrian injury in real accidents (Abstract). *J Traffic Med* 1990; 18(4):268.

Schulze-Robbecke R, Buchholtz K. Heat susceptibility of aquatic mycobacteria. *Appl Environ Microbiol* 1992;58(6):1869–73.

Schulze-Robbecke R, Janning B, Fischeder R. Occurrence of mycobacteria in biofilm samples. *Tuber Lung Dis* 1992;73(3):141–1.

Schwab L. Blindness from trauma in developing nations. *Int Ophthalmol Clin* 1990;30: 28–29.

Schweig KH. Pedestrian-related goals and innovations, step by step. *Transportation Quarterly* 1990;44(4):595–606.

Schweitzer A, Anderson E. In: E Anderson. *The Schweitzer Album.* 1965, 44, 65.

Scottolini AG, Weinstein SR. The autopsy in clinical quality control. *JAMA* 1983;250: 1192–1194.

Seah HC, Chao TC. Carbon monoxide poisoning in Singapore. *Singapore Med J* 1975;16(3): 174–176.

Secretary of Health and Human Services. *Sixth Special Report to the U.S. Congress on Alcohol and Health.* Washington: Alcohol, Drug Abuse, and Mental Health Administration, DHSS publication no. (ADM) 87–1519. 1987.

Secretary of Health and Human Services. *Seventh Special Report to the U.S. Congress on Alcohol and Health.* Washington: Alcohol, Drug Abuse, and Mental Health Administration, DHSS publication no. (ADM) 90–1656. 1990.

Seeman I, Poe G, Powell-Griner E. Development, methods and response characteristics: 1986 National Mortality Followback Survey. Rockville, MD. National Center for Health Statistics, *Vital and Health Statistics*, Series 2, 1993.

Sehgal S. Tollwut in Indien. *Die Gelben Helte* 1992;38:126–129.

Seiden RH. Suicide prevention: A public health-public policy approach. *OMEGA* 1977; 8(3): 267–276.

Selya RM. Deaths due to accidents in Taiwan: A possible indicator of development. *Soc Sci Med* 1980;14D:361–367.

Sen RN, Ghosal S. An ergonomic study on traffic accidents in Calcutta. (Abstract). *First World Conference on Accident and Injury Prevention (Stockholm, Sweden): Abstract Guide.* Sundyberg: Karolinska Institute, September 17–20, 1989:353.

Sengupta SK, Purohit RC, Buck AT. Chloroquine poisoning. *Papua New Guinea Med J* 1986; 29:143–147.

Shah AR, Chawda SK, Shah JD, Shah HJ. Economic analysis of road characteristics with rate of accidents in NH 8 in Gujarat (Abstract). *J Traffic Med* 1990; 18(4):264.

Sharma OP, Kumar R. Problems of minor injuries in general practice. *J Indian Med Assoc* 1974; 62:161–162.

Shinar D. Demographic and socioeconomic correlates of safety belt use. *Accid Anal Prev* 1993; 25:745–755.

Shorvon SD. Epidemiology, classification, natural history, and genetics of epilepsy. *Lancet* 1990; 336:93–96.

Shorvon SD, Farmer PJ. Epilepsy in developing countries: a review of epidemiological, sociocultural and treatment aspects. *Epilepsia* 1988; 29 (Suppl 1):36–53.

Shun ZG. The lesson from an explosion of a fuel depot. In: Preprints: *Accident Prevention in Developing Countries.* International Conference on Strategies for Occupational Accident Prevention. Stockholm, Sweden: National Board of Occupational Safety and Health, 1989:1–6.

Siddique AK, Eusof A. Cyclone deaths in Bangladesh, May 1985: Who was at risk? *Trop Geogr Med* 1987;39:3–8.

Siegel SR, Witham P. UNDP coordination of disaster and development planning. In: Kreimer A, Munasinghe M, eds. *Managing Natural Disasters and the Environment.* Washington, DC: Environmental Policy and Research Division, Environment Department, The World Bank, 1991: 163–171.

Silveira PVP, Nishioka SA. Non-venomous snake bite and snake bite without envenoming in a Brazilian teaching hospital. Analysis of 91 cases. *Rev Inst Med Trop São Paulo* 1992a;34: 499–503.

Silveira PVP, Nishioka SA. South American rattlesnake bite in a Brazilian teaching hospital. Clinical and epidemiological study of 87 cases, with analysis of factors predictive of renal failure. *Tran Roy Soc Trop Med Hyg* 1992b;86: 499–503.

Simpson SG, Reid R, Baker SP, Teret S. Injuries among the Hopi Indians: A population-based survey. *J Am Med Assoc* 1983;249: 1873–1876.

Singh K, Jain NR, Khullar BMP. A study of suicide in Delhi State. *J Indian Med Assoc* 1971;57: 412–419.

Sinha SN, Sengupta SK. Road traffic accident fatalities in Port Moresby: a ten-year survey. *Accid Anal Prev* 1989;21:297–301.

Sinha SN, Sengupta SK, Purohit RC. A five-year review of deaths following trauma. *Papua New Guinea Med J* 1981;24:222–228.

Sivard RL. *World Military and Social Expenditures.* Washington, DC: World Priorities, 1991.

SKEPHI and ORIGIN (Organization for the Control of Indigenous People Genocide in Indonesia). Systematic genocide and ethnocide on Papua Lands. PO Box 88 Jatra, Jati Rawamangun, Jakarta Timur, Indonesia. *Setiakawan* 1990;Jan–June No.4–5:9–54.

Sklar DP. Emergency medicine and the developing world. *Am J Emerg Med* 1988;6:390–393.

Sloan JH, Kellermann AL, Reay DT, Ferris JA, Koepsell T, Rivara FP, Rice C, Gray L, LoGerfo J. Handgun regulations, crime, assaults, and homicide—A tale of two cities. *N Engl J Med* 1988;319(19):1256–1262.

Smith D. Suicide in a remote preliterate society in the highlands of Papua New Guinea. *Papua New Guinea Med J* 1981;24:242–246.

Smith GS. Measuring the gap for unintentional injuries. The Carter Center Health Policy Project. *Public Health Rep* 1985;100:565–568.

Smith GS, Barss P. Unintentional injuries in developing countries: the epidemiology of a neglected problem. *Epidemiologic Reviews* 1991;13: 228–266.

Smith GS, Falk H. Unintentional injuries. *Am J Prev Med* 1987;(Suppl 5):143–163.

Smith GS, Kraus JF. Alcohol and residential, recreational and occupational injuries: a review of the epidemiologic evidence. *Ann Rev of Public Health* 1988;9:99–121.

Smith P. The occurrence of accidents in Greenland and their bearing on the death-rate. In: Sundhedstilstanden i Grønland (The State of Health in Greenland. Annual Report from the Chief Medical Officer in Greenland). Godthaab 1961:75–81. Cited in: Bjerregaard P. *Fatal Accidents in Greenland. Arct Med Res* 1990;49:132–141.

Smith SM, Middaugh JP. An assessment of potential injury surveillance data sources in Alaska using an emerging problem: All-terrain vehicle-associated injuries. *Public Health Reports* 1989;104(5):493–498.

Snow RW, Armstrong JF, Forster D, Winstanley MT, Marsh VM, Newton CRJC, et al. Childhood deaths in Africa: uses and limitations of verbal autopsies. *Lancet* 1992;340:351–355.

Snyder MB, Knoblaugh RL. *Pedestrian Safety: the Identification of Precipitating Factors and Possible Countermeasures.* Vol 2. FH–117312. Washington, DC. US Department of Transportation, National Highway Safety Administration, 1971.

Sonnen AEH. Epilepsy and swimming, No. 42. In: Epilepsy, Clinical and Experimental Research. *Monogr Neural Sci* 1980;5:265–270.

Sorensen S. Suicide among the elderly: Issues facing public health. *Am J Public Health* 1991; 81(9):1109–1110.

Sorensen TH, Vindenes H. Scalding injuries in children. *Tidsskr Nor Laegeforen* 1993;113(14): 1716–8.

Sposito MMM, Casalis MEP, Ferraretto I. Follow-up of paraplegic patients after comprehensive rehabilitation. *Paraplegia* 1984;22: 373–378.

Stackhouse J. Home truths ignored in India. *Globe and Mail* (Toronto) 1993 Dec 9:A1(col 2–4),A8(col 1–4).

Stackhouse J. Cloud of health problems still hangs over Bhopal. *Globe and Mail* (Toronto) 1994 Jan 25:A1(col 3–5),A2(col 5–6).

Steele JH. Rabies in the Americas and remarks on global aspects. In: Research towards rabies prevention: a symposium. Washington DC. November 3–5, 1986. GM Baer et al., eds. Chicago: University of Chicago. *Rev Inf Dis* 1988;10(Suppl 4):S585–597.

Steffen R, Lobel HO. The Epidemiologic Basis for the Practice of Travel Medicine. *J Wilderness Med* 1994; 5(1):156–166.

Stein H. Fleet Experience with Daytime Running Lights in the United States—Preliminary Results. Washington, DC: Insurance Institute for Highway Safety. 1985.

Stephens PW. Reliability of lay reporting of morbidity and cause-of-death data: an evaluation of reported cases and deaths from measles in rural Senegal. In: Vallin J, D'-Souza S, Palloni A, eds. *Measurement and Analysis of Mortality: New Approaches.* Oxford: Clarendon Press, Oxford University Press, 1990:142.

Stewart D, Chudworth CJ. A remedy for accidents at bends. *Traffic Engineering and Control* 1990; 31(2):88–93.

Stout JE, Yu VL, Muraia P, Joly J, Troup N, Tompkins LS. Potable water as a cause of sporadic cases of community acquired Legionnaires' disease. *N Engl J Med* 1992;326: 151–155.

Stutts JC, Williamson JE, Whitley J, Sheldon FC. Bicycle accidents and injuries: A pilot study comparing hospital- and police-reported data. *Accid Anal Prev* 1990;22:67–78.

Subianto DB, Tumada LR, Margono SS. Burns and epileptic fits associated with cysticercosis in mountain people of Irian Jaya. *Trop Geogr Med* 1978;30(3):275–278.

Subrahmanyam M. Bicycle injury pattern among children in rural India. *Trop Geogr Med* 1984; 36(3):243–247.

Subrahmanyam M, Date VN, Samant NA, Patil AJ, Arwade DJ. Bicycle injuries in children. *J Indian Med Assoc* 1980;75:220–221.

Suchman EA, Munoz RA. Accident occurrence and control among sugar-cane workers. *J Occ Med* 1967;9:407–414.

Sugarman JR, Warren CW, Oge L, Helgerson SD. Using the behavioral risk factor surveillance system to monitor year 2000 objectives among American Indians. *Public Health Reports* 1992; 107(4):449–456.

Sundarason R, Kim TC. A review of burns in Singapore. *Singapore Med J* 1969;10:98–102.

Supramanian V, VanBelle G, Sung JFC. Fatal motorcycle accidents in peninsular Malaysia. *Accid Anal Prev* 1984;16:157–162.

Susskind LE, Cruikshank J. *Breaking the Impasse: Consensual Approaches to Resolving Public Disputes.* New York: Basic Books, 1987.

Svanström L. Reduction of traffic injuries through community participation (Abstract). *J Traffic Med* 1990;18(4):246.

Svanström L. *Report 1989–1991 from The Karolinska Institute Department of Social Medicine Kronan Health Centre in its Capacity as a WHO Collaborating Centre on Community Safety Promotion.* Sundbyberg, Sweden: WHO Collaborating Centre on Community Safety Promotion, Department of Social Medicine, Karolinska Institute, 1991.

Svanström L, Schelp L, Skjönberg G. Sweden: The establishment of a National Safety Promotion Programme for prevention of accidents and injuries—the first Swedish "Health for All" programme implemented in practice. In: *Proceedings National Programmes on Accident and Injury Prevention.* Stockholm, Sweden: Swedish National Board of Health and Welfare, 1991: 201–208.

Svanström K, Svanström L. *A Safe Community— How to Prevent Accidents at the Local Level.* Prepared for WHO Travelling Seminar on Community Safety. Sweden-Thailand. Sundbyberg, Sweden: Department of Social Medicine, Karolinska Institute, 1989:1–211

Tagore R. *Sādhanā: the Realisation of Life.* New York: Macmillan, 1913, 50–51.

Tagore R. *Gitanjali.* London: Macmillan and Co. Ltd., 1921, 24–25

Tahzib F. Camel injuries. *Trop Doctor* 1984;14: 187–188.

Tamrat A. Accidents and poisoning in children (Abstract). *Ethiop Med J* 1981;24:39–40.

Tanga MR, Kawathekar P. Injury due to bull goring. *Int Surg* 1973;58(9):635 -636.

Tekle-Haimanot R. Neurological disorders. In: Kloos H, Zein ZA, eds. *The Ecology of Health and Disease in Ethiopia.* Boulder: Westview Press, 1993, 483–491.

Tekle-Haimanot R, Mekkonen Abebe L, Forsgren et al. Public attitude towards epilepsy in rural Ethiopia. *Soc Sci Med* 1991; 32:203–209.

Tekle Wold F. Accidents in childhood. *Ethiop Med J* 1973;11:41–46.

Teret SP, Jacobs M. Prevention and torts: the role of litigation in injury control. *Law, Medicine, and Health Care* 1989;17:17–22.

Terrill JR, Montgomery RR, Rehihardt CF. Toxic gases from fires. *Sueme* 1978;200:1343–1347.

Thapa NB. Injury prevention in Nepal. *Souvenir Napas J* 1984;3(1):136–139.

Thapa NB. *Report of Injury Survey in Bhumisthan Village Panchayat Dhadhing and in Bir Hospital Kathmandu*. Paper presented at: National Programmes on Accident and Injury Prevention. National Board of Health and Welfare, Stockholm, 1989.

Thapa NB. Accidents and injury in childhood. In: Wallace HM, Giri K, eds. *Health Care of Women and Children in Developing Countries*. Oakland, CA: Third Party Publishing Co., 1990;428–440.

Theakston RDG, Reid HA, Larrick JW, Kaplan J, Yost JA. Snake venom antibodies in Ecuadorian Indians. *J Trop Med Hyg* 1981;84:199–202.

Thomas C, Ferguson E, Feng D, DePriest J. *Policy Implications of Increasing Motorization on Non-motorized Transport in Developing Countries: the Case of Guangzhou, Peoples Republic of China*. Paper presented at the 71st annual meeting of the Transportation Research Board. Washington, DC: Transportation Research Board, National Research Council, Preprint Paper No. 920788, 1992:1–11.

Thomas V. Quoted in: World Bank changes approach. *Globe and Mail* (Toronto) 1991 July 8: A4(col 1–5).

Thompson RS, Rivara FP, Thompson DC. A case-control study of the effectiveness of bicycle safety helmets. *N Engl J Med* 1989;320:1361–1367.

Thorn JJ, Hansen PK. Incidence and etiology of jaw fractures in Greenland. In: *Circumpolar Health* 84, 1984:110–112.

Thorslund J. Inuit suicides in Greenland. *Arct Med Res* 1990;49:25–33.

Thorslund J, Misfeldt J. On suicide statistics. *Arct Med Res* 1989;48:124–130.

Toe T. Spinal injuries in Rangoon, Burma. *Paraplegia* 1978–79;16:118–120.

Tournier-Lasserve C, Veillard JM, Samouth M, Dischino M. Un aspect méconnu de la traumatologie tropicale: les plaies pénétrantes de l'abdomen por corne de buffle. À propos de 64 observations cambodgieènes. *Medicine Tropicale* (Mars) 1982;42(2):161–167.

Townsend J. Department of Health reports on tobacco advertising: A ban would significantly cut consumption (Editorial). *BMJ* 1992;305: 1110–1111.

Transport and Road Research Laboratory. *Information Note: Road Safety in Developing Countries*. Crowthorne, Berkshire, UK: Overseas Unit, Transport and Road Research Laboratory, 1986:1–86.

Transport and Road Research Laboratory. *Proposed Guideline Design of Police Booklet for Use in Developing Countries*. Crowthorne, Berkshire, UK: Overseas Unit, Transport and Road Research Laboratory, 1988:1–20.

Transport and Road Research Laboratory. *Towards Safer Roads in Developing Countries: A Guide for Planners and Engineers*. Crowthorne, Berkshire, UK: Overseas Unit, Transport and Road Research Laboratory, 1991.

Transport and Road Research Laboratory. *Costing Road Accidents in Developing Countries*. Crowthorne, Berkshire, UK: Overseas Unit, Transport and Road Research Laboratory, ORN 10, 1994.

Transport and Road Research Laboratory. *Microcomputer Accident Analysis Package* (information leaflet). Crowthorne, Berkshire, UK: Overseas Unit, Transport and Road Research Laboratory, nd.

Transportation Research Board. *Designing Safer roads: Practices for Resurfacing, Restoration, and Rehabilitation*. Washington: National Research Council, 1987.

Trinca GW, Johnson IR, Campbell BJ, Haight FA, Knight PR, Mackay GM, McLean AJ, Petrucelli E. *Reducing Traffic Injury—A Global Challenge*. Melbourne, Australia: Royal Australasian College of Surgeons, 1988:1–119.

Trovato F. Mortality differential in Canada: 1951–1971: French, British, and Indians. *Culture, Medicine, and Psychiatry* 1988;12: 459–477.

Tucker A, ed. *Safecomm—91: The First International Conference on Safe Communities*. Falköping, Sweden, 3–5 June 1991. Sundbyberg, Sweden: WHO Collaborating Centre on Community Safety Promotion, Department of Social Medicine, Karolinska Institute, nd.

Tursz A, Crost M, Lavaud J. Childhood traffic injuries in France: From epidemiology to preventive measures (Abstract). *J Traffic Med* 1990; 18(4):234.

Tylleskär T, Banea M, Bikangi N, Cooke RD, Poulter NH, Rosling H. Cassava cyanogens and konzo, an upper motoneuron disease found in Africa. *Lancet* 1992;339:208–211.

Udo ES. A case study of working conditions and accidents in the Nigerian logging industry. In: *Preprints: Accident Prevention in Developing Countries*. International Conference on Strategies for Occupational Accident Prevention. Stockholm, Sweden: National Board of Occupational Safety and Health, 1989.

Ugalde A, Vega RR. Review essay: State terrorism, torture, and health in the Southern Cone. *Soc Sci Med* 1989;28(7):759–767.

UNDRO (Office of the United Nations Disaster Relief Coordinator). *Report on International Relief Assistance for the Earthquake of 7 December 1988 in the Soviet Socialist Republic of Armenia*. Geneva: UNDRO. United Nations report no. UNDRO/89/6, February, 1989.

United Nations. *Low-cost Construction Resistant to Earthquakes and Hurricanes*. New York: Department of Economic and Social Affairs, United Nations. 1975:1–205.

United Nations. *Report of the Expert Group on Development of Statistics on Disabled Persons*. New York, Department of International Economic and Social Affairs, Statistical Office, ESA/STA/AC. 18/7, 1984.

United Nations. *United Nations Disability Statistics Data Base, 1975–1986—Technical Manual*. New York, Department of International Economic and Social Affairs, Statistical Office, ST/ESA/STAT/Ser.Y/3, 1988.

United Nations. *Disability Statistics Compendium*. New York, United Nations, ST/ESA/STAT/Ser. Y/4, 1990.

United Nations Centre for Human Settlements (Habitat). *Transportation Strategies for Human Settlements in Developing Countries*. Nairobi 1981.

United Nations Centre for Human Settlements (Habitat). *Human Settlements and Natural Disasters*. Nairobi: Habitat 1989:1–40.

Uradosa CG. Occupational hazards among granite workers in Ceylon. *J Trop Med Hyg* 1968; 71:267–270.

U.S. Consumer Product Safety Commission. *Handbook for Public Playground Safety*. Washington, DC, 1997.

U.S. Department of Transport. *General Estimates System 1989: a Review of Information on Police-reported Traffic Crashes in the United States*. National Highway Traffic Administration, 1990: 1–146.

Vahl HG, Giskes J. *Traffic Calming Through Integrated Urban Planning*. Paris, France, Editions Amarcande, 1990.

Vaidhya VG, Naik VG, Joshi JK, Hussaini SMR. Retrospective analysis into aetiology of industrial hand injuries. *Proceedings of 10th Asian Conference on Occupational Health*. 1982: 310–316.

Van Weperen W. Guidelines for the development of safety-related standards for consumer products. *Accid Anal Prev* 1993;25(1): 11–18.

Varghese M. Analysis of 198 medical-legal records of road traffic accident victims treated in a Delhi hospital (Abstract). *J Traffic Med* 1990; 18(4):280.

Varghese M, Mohan D. Occupational injuries among agricultural workers in rural Haryana, India. *J Occup Accid* 1990a;12: 237–244.

Varghese M, Mohan D. Transportation injuries in rural Haryana, North India (Abstract). *J Traffic Med* 1990b;18(4):242.

Verma S. Eye injuries. In: Weeks JL, Levy BS, Wagner GR, eds. *Preventing Occupational Disease and Injury*. Washington, DC: American Public Health Association, 1991:245–249.

Vess RW, Anderson RL, Carr JH, Bond WW, Favero MS. The colonization of solid PVC surfaces and the acquisition of resistance to germicides by water micro-organisms. *J Appl Bacteriol* 1993;74(2):215–21.

Vilanilam JV. A historical and socioeconomic analysis of occupational safety and health in India. *Int J Health Servs* 1980;10(2):233–249.

Villerme LR. A description of the physical and moral state of workers employed in cotton, wool, and silk mills. In: *The Challenge of Epidemiology: Issues and Selected Readings*. Buck C, Llopis A, Nájera E, Terris M, eds. Washington, DC: Pan American Health Organization, 1988, 33–36.

Vimpani G. The role of injury surveillance within the Australian Injury Prevention Program In: *Proceedings National Programmes on Accident and Injury Prevention*. Stockholm, Sweden: Swedish National Board of Health and Welfare, 1991: 39–47.

Vincent I. Colombia: Censors defy tradition to box in TV crime. *Globe and Mail* (Toronto) 1993 Aug 13:A1(col 5–6),A2(col2–5).

Viravan C, Looareesuwan S, Losakarn W, Wuthiekanun V, McCarthy CJ, Stimson AF, Bunnag D, Harinasuta T, Warrell DA. A national hospital-based survey of snakes responsible for bites in Thailand. *Trans R Soc Trop Med Hyg* 1992;86:100–106.

Voas RP. Development of a national impaired driving policy for commercial drivers (Abstract). *J Traffic Med* 1990;18(4):297.

Voltaire FA. Atomes. Questions sur l'Encyclopédie, deuxième partie, 1770. In: *Oeuvres Complètes de Voltaire: Dictionnaire Philosophique I*. Paris: Garnier Frères. 1848:479.

Vulcan P. Road trauma prevention. In: Ozanne-Smith J, Williams F (eds). *Injury Research and Prevention: a Text*. Melbourne, Monash University Accident Research Centre, 1995: 75–97.

Vural N, Saygi S. A survey of blood alcohol effect on drivers in Ankara. Paper presented at the International Workshop on Drugs and Driving, Padua, Italy, 1991. Cited in: Ross HL. Prevalence of alcohol-impaired driving: An international comparison. *Accid Anal Prev* 1993;25: 777–779.

Wacholder S, McLaughlin JK, Silverman DT, Mandel JS. Selection of controls in case-control studies. I. Principles. *Am J Epidemiol* 1992a; 135(9):1019–1028.

Wacholder S, Silverman DT, McLaughlin JK, Mandel JS. Selection of controls in case-control studies. II. Types of controls. *Am J Epidemiol* 1992b;135(9):1029–1041.

Wacholder S, Silverman DT, McLaughlin JK, Mandel JS. Selection of controls in case-control studies. III. Design options. *Am J Epidemiol* 1992c;135(9):1042–1050.

Wagenaar AC, Streff FM, Schultz RH. Effects of the 65 mph speed limit on injury morbidity and mortality. *Accid Anal Prev* 1990;22: 571–585.

Wagner EH, LaCroix AZ, Buchner DM, Larson EB. Effects of physical activity on health status in older adults I: Observational studies. *Annual Rev Publ Health* 1992;13:451–468.

Walker J. *Distress Signals: an Investigation of Global Television* (Video, film, 55 minutes). Ottawa: National Film Board of Canada, 1990.

Wallace CF. Opening remarks. In: *Research Towards Rabies Prevention: a Symposium*. Washington DC. November 3–5, 1986. Baer GM et al., eds. Chicago: University of Chicago. *Rev Infect Dis* 1988;10(Suppl 4):S579–580.

Waller JA. *Injury Control: A Guide to the Causes and Prevention of Trauma*. Lexington: Lexington Books, 1985:107.

Waller JA. Injury: conceptual shifts and preventive implications. *Ann Rev Public Health* 1987; 8: 21–49.

Waller P. Cited in: *Women at Risk*. Prevention file: alcohol, tobacco and other drugs. San Diego: University of California 1992;7(5):1 9–20.

Wallace WA. The increasing incidence of fractures of the proximal femur: an orthopaedic epidemic. *Lancet* 1983;1(8339):1413–1414.

Walsh SS, Jarvis SN. Measuring the frequency of "severe" accidental injury in childhood. *J Epidemiol Community Health* 1992;46:26–32.

Wandeler AI, Budde A, Capt S, Kappeler A, Matter H. Dog ecology and dog rabies control. In: *Research Towards Rabies Prevention: a Symposium*, Washington, DC, November 3–5, 1986. Baer GM et al., eds. Chicago: University of Chicago. *Rev Inf Dis* 1988;10(Suppl 4):S684–688.

Warrell DA. Animal poisons. In: Manson-Bahr PEC, Bell DR, eds. *Manson's Tropical Diseases*. London: Baillière Tindall Publishers, 1987: 855–898.

Warrell DA. *Venomous and Poisonous Animals*. In: Warren KS, Mahmoud AAF, eds. New York: McGraw-Hill, 1990:542–548.

Warrell DA, Warrell MJ. Human rabies and its prevention: an overview. In: Research towards rabies prevention: a symposium. Washington DC. November 3–5, 1986. Baer GM et al., eds. Chicago: University of Chicago. *Rev Inf Dis* 1988;10(Suppl 4):S726–731.

Watson GF, Zador PL, Wilks A. The repeal of helmet use laws and increased motorcyclist mortality in the United States, 1975–1978. *Am J Public Health* 1980;70:579–592.

Weddell JM, McDougall A. Road traffic injuries in Sharjah. *Int J Epidemiol* 1981;10:155–159.

Weeks JL. Injuries, fatal; Injuries, non-fatal. In: Weeks JL, Levy BS, Wagner GR, eds. *Preventing Occupational Disease and Injury*. Washington, DC: American Public Health Association, 1991:347–367.

Werner, D. *Where There is No Doctor*. Palo Alto, CA: Hesperian Foundation, 1977.

Werner D. *Disabled Village Children*. Palo Alto, CA: Hesperian Foundation, 1987.

West JG, Williams MJ, Trunkey DD. Trauma systems: current status—future challenges. *JAMA* 1988;259(24):3597–3600.

West-Oram F. Measuring danger on the road. *Traffic Engineering and Control* 1989;30(11): 529–532.

West-Oram F. Casualty reductions—whose problem? *Traffic Engineering and Control* 1990; 31(8/9):474–479.

West-Oram F. The one-third reduction target. *Traffic Engineering and Control* 1991;32(7/8): 359–363.

White JAM. Shark attack in Natal. *Injury* 1975;6(3):187–197.

White JR. *Terrorism: an Introduction.* Pacific Grove, CA: Brooks/Cole Publishing Company, 1991: 1–294.

WHO Collaborating Centre. *Criteria for the Safe Community Network.* Sundbyberg, Sweden: Department of Social Medicine, Karolinska Institute, 1992.

WHO Collaborating Centre. *Community Based Interventions— an Emerging Dimension of Injury Control Models.* Sundbyberg, Sweden: Department of Social Medicine, Karolinska Institute, nd.a.

WHO Collaborating Centre. *Research on Community Safety Promotion.* Sundbyberg, Sweden: Department of Social Medicine, Karolinska Institute, nd.b.

Wickham CAC, Walsh F, Cooper C, Barker DJP, Margetts BM, Morris J, Bruce SA. Dietary calcium, physical activity and risk of hip fracture: a prospective study. *Br Med J* 1989;299: 889–892.

Wilkins R, Adams O, Brancker A. Changes in mortality by income in urban Canada from 1971 to 1986. *Health Reports* 1989;1(2): 137–174.

Williams AF, Zador PL, Harris SF, et al. The effect of raising the legal minimum drinking age on involvement in fatal crashes. *J Legal Stud* 1983;12:169–79.

Wintemute GJ. Is motor vehicle-related mortality a disease of development? *Accid Anal Prev* 1985;17:223–237.

Wintemute GJ, Kraus JF, Teret SP, Wright M. Drowning in childhood and adolescence: A population-based study. *Am J Public Health* 1987;77:830–832.

Wintemute GJ, Teret SP, Kraus JF, Wright M. Alcohol and drowning: An analysis of contributing factors and a discussion of criteria for case selection. *Accid Anal Prev* 1990;22: 291–296.

Wong J. China's dogs. You can beat 'em or eat 'em, but you can't keep 'em. *Globe and Mail* (Toronto) 1994a Jan 26:A1(col 4–5), A8(col 1–3).

Wong J. Great leap into the driver's seat. *Globe and Mail* (Toronto) 1994b;Jan 14;A1(col 4–6), A2(col 2–4).

Wong TW, Lee J, Phoon WO, Yiu PC, Fung KP, McLean JA. Driving experience and the risk of traffic accident among motorcyclists. *Soc Sci Med* 1990;30:639–640.

Wood T, Milne P. Head injuries to pedal cyclists and the promotion of helmet use in Victoria, Australia. *Accid Anal Prev* 1988;20:177–185.

World Almanac and Book of Facts, 1993. New York: Pharos Books, 1993, 808, 811.

World Bank. *World Development Report 1988.* New York: Oxford University Press. 1988.

World Bank. *Adult Health in Brazil: Adjusting to New Challenges.* Brazil Development Report No. 7807–BR. 1989:1–133.

World Bank. *Road Safety, a Lethal Problem in the Third World.* The Urban Edge, 1990;14(5).

World Bank. *World Development Report 1993: Investing in Health.* New York, NY: Oxford University Press, 1993:1–32.

World Health Organization. Mercury. Geneva: WHO. *Environmental Health Criteria*, No. 1, 1976.

World Health Organization. *Lay Reporting of Health Information.* Geneva: WHO, 1978a.

World Health Organization. *Manual of the International Statistical Classification of Diseases, Injuries, and Causes of Death.* Ninth Revision. Vols I & II. Geneva: WHO, 1978b.

World Health Organization. *International Classification of Impairments, Disabilities, and Handicaps—a Manual of Classification Relating to the Consequences of Disease.* Geneva: WHO, 1980.

World Health Organization. Changing patterns in suicide behaviour: report on a WHO working group. Copenhagen. *EURO Reports and Studies*, 1982:74.

World Health Organization. Paraquat and diquat. Geneva: WHO. *Environmental Health Criteria* Series No. 39, 1984a.

World Health Organization. Aquatic (marine and freshwater) biotoxins. Geneva: WHO. *Environmental Health Criteria*, No. 37, 1984b: 39–41, 48–51.

World Health Organization, Walsh B, Grant M, eds. *Public Health Implication of Alcohol Production and Trade.* Geneva: WHO Offset Publication No. 88, 1985a:1–55.

World Health Organization, Grant M, ed. *Alcohol Policies.* Copenhagen: WHO Regional Office for Europe, WHO Regional Publications, European Series No. 18, 1985b:1–153.

World Health Organization, Mosner J, ed. *Alcohol Policies in National Health and Development Planning*. Geneva: WHO Offset Publication No. 89, 1985c:1–102.

World Health Organization. Ottawa charter for health promotion. *Can J Public Health* 1986;77:425–430 (see also 384–443).

World Health Organization. Carbamate pesticides: a general introduction. Geneva: WHO. *Environmental Health Criteria*, No. 64, 1986(a).

World Health Organization. Report of the second global liaison meeting on accident and injury prevention. Geneva: WHO, IRP/APR 218 m21A, September 1986(b).

World Health Organization. Accidents in children and young people. *World Health Statistics Quarterly* 1986(c);39(3):1–62.

World Health Organization. Organophosphorus insecticides: a general introduction. Geneva: WHO. *Environmental Health Criteria*, No. 63, 1986d.

World Health Organization. *Report of the Asian Seminar on Road Safety*. Geneva: WHO, IPR/APR 218 G, March 1987.

World Health Organization. *Global medium-term programme: accident prevention*. Geneva: WHO, APR/MTP/88.1, March, 1988a.

World Health Organization. Pyrrolizidine alkaloids: a general introduction. Geneva: WHO. *Environmental Health Criteria*, No. 80, 1988b: 183–217.

World Health Organization. *World Health Statistics Annual*. Geneva: WHO. 1988c.

World Health Organization. Manifesto for safe communities: safety—a universal concern and responsibility for all. 1st World Conference on Accident and Injury Prevention. Stockholm, Sweden, 1989.

World Health Organization. New approaches to improve road safety. Geneva: WHO, *WHO Technical Report Series* No. 781, 1989a:1–62.

World Health Organization. *Research Development for Accident and Injury Prevention*. Geneva: WHO, IPR/APR 216 m 8923E, 1989b.

World Health Organization. *World Health Statistics Annual*, 1990. Geneva: WHO, 1991.

World Health Organization. International statistics on causes of disability. *World Health Statistics Annual*, 1990. Geneva: WHO, 1991(a).

World Health Organization. *World Health Statistics Annual* 1992.

World Health Organization. *Toxic Oil Syndrome*.

Copenhagen: WHO, Regional Publications European Series No. 42, 1992(a):1–163.

Wotton K, Allen-Peters J, Fletcher D, McDowell M. Introducing participatory action research. In: Pickering JL, ed. *Health Research for Development: a Manual*. Ottawa, ON: Canadian University Consortium for Health in Development, 1997:18–47. (Available from; International Health Office, Dept. of Epidemiology, Biostatistics and Occupational Health, McGill University, 1020 Pine Avenue, West, Montreal, Quebec, Canada H3A 1A2.

Wright PH, Robertson LS. Priorities for roadside hazard modification: a study of 300 fatal roadside object crashes. *Traffic Engineering* 1976;46: 24–30.

Wright PH, Zador P. A study of fatal overturning crashes in Georgia. *Transport Res Rec* 1981;819: 8–17.

Wright R. The biology of violence. *New Yorker* 1995, Mar 13, 68–77.

Wu S, Malison MD. Motor vehicle injuries in Taiwan. *Asia Pacific J Public Health* 1990; 4:72–75.

Wyatt GB. The epidemiology of road accidents in Papua New Guinea. *Papua New Guinea Med J* 1980;23:60–65.

Xin LS. Problem of electrostatic hazard concerned in occupational injuries. In: Preprints: *Accident Prevention in Developing Countries*. International Conference on Strategies for Occupational Accident Prevention. Stockholm, Sweden: National Board of Occupational Safety and Health, 1989:1–6.

Xing-Yuan G, Mai-Ling C. Vital statistics. In: Health services in Shanghai County. *Am J Public Health* (suppl) 1982;72:44–77.

Yates DS, Heath DF, Mars E, Taylor RJ. A system for measuring the severity of temporary and permanent disability after injury. *Accid Anal Prev* 1991;23(4):323–329.

Yip W, Paul FM. Drowning in Singapore children. *J Singapore Pediatr Soc* 1975;17: 1103–1112.

Young TK. Mortality pattern of isolated Indians in Northwestern Ontario: A 10-year review. *Public Health Reports* 1983;98(5):467–475.

Young TK. Are Subarctic Indians undergoing the epidemiologic transition? *Soc Sci Med* 1988;26(6):659–671.

Young TK, Moffatt EK, O'Neill. An epidemiological perspective of injuries in the Northwest Territories. *Arct Med Res* 1992;51: Suppl. 7: 27–36.

Zador P. How effective are daytime motorcycle headlight use laws? *Am J Public Health* 1983; 73:808.

Ziedler F, Pletschen B, Scheunert D, Mattern B, Alt B, Miksch T, Eichendorf W, Reiss S. Development of a new injury cost scale. *Accid Anal Prev* 1993;6:675–687.

Zemach R. What the vital statistics system can and cannot do. *Am J Public Health* 1984;74: 756–758.

Zhang J, Feldblum PJ, Fortney JA. Moderate physical activity and bone density among perimenopausal women. *Am J Public Health* 1992; 82(5):736–738.

Zimicki S. Approaches to assessment of the cause structure of mortality: A case-study from Bangladesh. In: Vallin J, D'Souza S, Palloni A, eds. *Measurement and Analysis of Mortality: New Approaches*. International Studies in Demography, International Union for the Scientific Study of Population. Oxford: Clarendon Press, Oxford University Press, 1990:99–122.

Zimicki S. Old and new approaches to assessment of the cause structure of mortality: a case study from Bangladesh. *Seminar on Comparative Studies of Mortality and Morbidity*: Siena, Italy: International Union for the Scientific Study of Population and Institute of Statistics, University of Siena, 1986:1–33.

Zimicki S, Nahar L, Sander AM, D'Souza S. *Source Book of Cause-specific Mortality Rates 1975–1981*. Demographic Surveillance System—Matlab, Vol 13. Dhaka: International Centre for Diarrhoeal Disease Research 1985;63:26–61.

Zwi A, Ugalde A. Towards an epidemiology of political violence in the Third World. *Soc Sci Med* 1989;28(7):633–642.

Zwi A, Ugalde A. Political violence in the third world: a public health issue. *Health Policy and Planning* 1991;6:203–217.

Zwi A, Ugalde A. Victims of war. *World Health* 1993;1:26–27.

Bédard G. *Self-financing as a Peasant Process—the Amazing Strength of Warm Money in Micro-Credit—the Savings and Credit Clubs of Mayo-Kebbi in Chad*. Outremont, Quebec: The Partnership Publishing, 1997:1–83.

Centers for Disease Control. CDC recommendations for a community plan for the prevention and containment of suicide clusters. *MMWR* 1988;37 (suppl. no. 5–6):1–12.

Forjuoh S, Li G. A review of successful transport and home injury interventions to guide developing countries. *Soc Sci Med* 1996;43: 1551–1560.

Marsh D, Sheikh A, Khalil A, Kamil S, Jaffer-uz Zaman, Qureshi I, Siray Y, Luby S, Effendi S. Epidemiology of adults hospitalized with burns in Karachi, Pakistan. *Burns* 1996;22: 225–229.

Marzuk PM, Tardiff K, Leon AC., et al. Fatal injuries after cocaine use as a leading cause of death among young adults in New York City. *N Engl J Med* 1995;332:273–1757.

Masson I, Barss P. Personal flotation devices (PFDs) among recreational boaters: a pilot survey assessing the rate of wearing of PFDs and the reasons why the majority of users do not wear them. (Abstract) *Conference Proceedings, Working with a Net: Fostering Relationships and Collaborative Efforts in Injury Prevention*, Kingston, ON: Queens University, Centre for Injury Prevention and Research, 1996:32–33.

Michels R, Marzuk DM. Progress in psychiatry (second of two parts). *N Engl J Med* 1993; 329:628–638.

Pauls J. Stair-related falls: environmental documentation and regulatory controls (Abstract and text of poster). *Proceedings of the Third International Conference on Injury Prevention and Control, Melbourne, Australia*. Adelaide, SA: National Injury Surveillance Unit, Australian Institute of Health and Welfare, 1996, 65. (Full text available from: Jake Pauls Consulting Services in Building Use and Safety, 12507 Winexburg Manor Drive, Suite 206, Silver Spring, Maryland 20906–3442, USA.)

Zwi AB, Forjuoh S, Murgusampillay S, Odero W, Watts C. Injuries in developing countries: policy response needed now. *Trans R Soc Trop Med Hyg* 1996;90:593–595.

Acknowledgments

Dr. Richard G.A. Feachem, Director of the Population, Health, and Nutrition Division of the Population and Human Resources Department of the World Bank and former Dean of the London School of Hygiene and Tropical Medicine, first sponsored the initiation of this document as a background paper for the World Bank Project on Adult Health, and for his own book *The Health of Adults in the Developing World.* He later recommended it be expanded to a book, and provided vital encouragement during the process of research and writing, which took place over ten years. Dr. Anthony R. Measham, former Division Chief of the Population, Health, and Nutrition Division of the World Bank was also encouraging and helpful.

Dr. Peter Barss was a Medical Research Council of Canada Fellow at the Johns Hopkins University Injury Prevention Center during the initial phases of preparation of this publication, and earlier was assisted by a Canadian International Development Agency scholarship. Staff of the Papua New Guinea Institute of Medical Research at Tari and Goroka provided considerable assistance with rural dissertation research on injury mortality; Dr. Deborah Lehmann deserves special mention. While employed in the Department of Health of Papua New Guinea, the author acquired considerable knowledge from the rural people and health workers of Papua New Guinea about their injuries and environment. Québec colleagues in the Module de Prévention des Traumatismes and the Module du Nord Québécois of the Direction de la Santé Publique, Régie Régionale de la Santé et des Services Sociaux de Montréal-Centre and at McGill University provided insights into multisectoral injury coalitions and the prevention of injuries among indigenous peoples. Among others, these included Mme. Ginette Beaulne, Dr. Yvonne Robitaille, M. Jean-Guy Breton, Mme. Claudette Lavallée, and Dr. Elizabeth Robinson. Dr. Bruce Brown of the Charles LeMoyne Community Health Department provided materials and advice on traffic injuries. Ms. Cindy Lyon, Ms. Kim Richardson, Ms. Dawn Stegan, Ms. Paula Hadden-Jokiel, Mme. Caroline Gagnon, Mme. Isabelle Masson, and other members of the Water-Related Fatalities Research Group of the National Division of the Canadian Red Cross Society shared many ideas during collaboration on drowning surveillance and research. Dr. Marcel Sylvestre of the Public Health Unit of the Montreal General Hospital provided practical information on surveillance and prevention of occupational injuries. Dr. Joyce Pickering of the McGill University International Health Program reviewed the entire manuscript and made many helpful suggestions.

Dr. Jeffrey S. Hammer, senior economist in the Population, Health, and Nutrition Division of the World Bank, gave many helpful comments on an earlier version of the manuscript, as did Jo M. Martins in a constructive review. Dr. Carlos Doria of the World Bank provided suggestions during early development.

Dr. Raymond Zilinskas, of the Department of International Health of the Johns Hopkins School of Hygiene and Public Health, provided insights into public health and epidemiological aspects of war and violence. Dr. Charles Mock, of the Department of Surgery of the University of Washington, Seattle, reviewed the chapter on the role of the health sector. Dr. Garen Wintemute, of the University of California at Davis, gave background information on motor vehicle and other injuries.

The Johns Hopkins Center for Injury Research and Policy provided financial support for creating and revising the manuscript. At the Center, Ms. Laura Higgins worked on the book from its inception, preparing tables, revising text, and ensuring the excellence of the final product; Ms. Diane Reintzell worked intensively on checking and finalizing the references and on the reorganization and revision of the manuscript; and Ms. Li-Hui Chen prepared figures and updated the tables. Ms. Edie Stern of The Johns Hopkins University provided valuable editorial and technical advice.

The advice of Oxford University Press editor Jeffrey House and the outside reviewers were also essential during the revision. Susan Hannan's timely help throughout the final stages is greatly appreciated.

Index

About the authors

Peter Barss, MD ScD MPH FACPM FRCPC, is Head of Health Intelligence and Territorial Epidemiologist for the Canadian Arctic and based in Yellowknife and Iqaluit in the Northwest Territories and Nunavut. He is an Adjunct Professor in the Department of Epidemiology, Biostatistics, and Occupational Health at McGill University. He worked as a Consultant Physician in the Injury Prevention Module of the Montreal Public Health Department in Quebec, Canada, during which time he collaborated with injury surveillance and research for indigenous communities with the Northern Quebec Module of the Montreal General Hospital, Cree Health Board, Nunavik Inuit, and Health Canada. He is an epidemiological advisor to The Canadian Red Cross Society and The Lifesaving Society and helped to develop the Canadian Surveillance System for Water-Related Fatalities. He has served as a consultant on injuries for the Canadian government and in developing countries for the World Bank. As Medical Superintendent of a provincial hospital, he was responsible for surgical care and emergency evacuations of trauma patients in rural provinces of Papua New Guinea and Angola for ten years.

Gordon S. Smith, MB ChB MPH, is Associate Professor in the Johns Hopkins University Center for Injury Research and Policy. A New Zealander, he worked in Papua New Guinea for four years as a clinician and medical epidemiologist. He later served as an epidemiologist at the U.S. Centers for Disease Control. His current research interests include the epidemiology of drownings, injuries and alcohol, occupational injuries, and disasters. He has served as a consultant on injuries to a number of national and international organizations and participated in the Tenth Revision of the section on injuries of the World Health Organization's International Classification of Diseases.

Susan P. Baker, MPH, is Professor of Health Policy and Management, The Johns Hopkins School of Hygiene and Public Health, with joint appointments in Environmental Health Sciences, Pediatrics, and Emergency Medicine. She was the founding director of the Johns Hopkins Center for Injury Research and Policy. Her research, teaching, and articles address a variety of injury problems in the United States and other countries. She directed a World Health Organization Course on injuries in developing countries, is senior author of *The Injury Fact Book*, and has received national and international awards for her work in injury control.

Dinesh Mohan, PhD, is a Professor at the Indian Institute of Technology, Delhi, where he is the Coordinator of the Transportation Research and Injury Prevention Programme and Head of the WHO Collaborating Centre for Research and Training in Safety Technology. His research interests include biomechanics of human injury mechanisms, traffic crash, and rural injuries. He is an advisor to the WHO in injury prevention and control and on the editorial board of many national and international journals in the field. He received the 1991 Award of Merit from the Association for the Advancement of Automotive Medicine, and the Medal for outstanding achievement in the field of traffic medicine from the International Association for Accident and Traffic Medicine.